American Medical Association

Guide to
Preventing and
Treating Heart Disease

American Medical Association

Guide to
Preventing and
Treating Heart Disease

Essential Information You and Your Family Need to Know about Having a Healthy Heart

American Medical Association

Martin S. Lipsky, MD

Marla Mendelson, MD

Stephen Havas, MD, MPH

Michael Miller, MD

John Wiley & Sons, Inc.

This book is printed on acid-free paper. ∞

Copyright © 2008 by the American Medical Association. All rights reserved

Published by John Wiley & Sons, Inc., Hoboken, New Jersey
Published simultaneously in Canada

Wiley Bicentennial Logo: Richard J. Pacifico

Design and composition by Navta Associates, Inc.

Illustration Credits: Copyright © 2005 American Diabetes Association from www.diabetes.org, reprinted with permission from the American Diabetes Association, pp. 108 and 110; adapted by the American Medical Association from the American Heart Association Web site www .americanheart.org, pp. 81, 91, 121, and 276; © Comstock, p. 77 (bottom left); © Creatas Images, p. 244; National Cancer Institute, p. 85; photo courtesy of ON-X valves, p. 207; © PhotoDisc, pp. 53, 77 (top left, middle right, bottom right), and 174; Texas Heart Institute, www.tex-asheartinstitute.org, p. 78; © Thinkstock, p. 77 (middle left)

The information contained in this book is not intended to serve as a replacement for professional medical advice. Any use of the information in this book is at the reader's discretion. The author and the publisher specifically disclaim any and all liability arising directly or indirectly from the use or application of any information contained in this book. A health care professional should be consulted regarding your specific situation.

For general information about our other products and services, please contact our Customer Care Department within the United States at (800) 762-2974, outside the United States at (317) 572-3993 or fax (317) 572-4002.

Wiley also publishes its books in a variety of electronic formats. Some content that appears in print may not be available in electronic books. For more information about Wiley products, visit our web site at www.wiley.com.

Library of Congress Cataloging-in-Publication Data:

Lipsky, Martin S.
  American Medical Association guide to preventing and treating heart disease : essential information you and your family need to know about having a healthy heart / Martin S. Lipsky, Marla Mendelson, Stephen Havas, Michael Miller.
    p. cm.
  Includes index.
  ISBN 978-0-471-75024-6 (paper: alk. paper)
  1. Heart—Diseases—Popular works. 2. Cardiology—Popular works. I. Mendelson, Marla. II. American Medical Association. III. Title.
  RC672.L57 2007
  616.1'2—dc22

                                                          2006022016

Printed in the United States of America

10 9 8 7 6 5 4 3 2 1

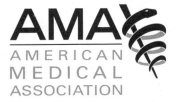

Contents

Introduction

For many years, the number one cause of death in the United States has been heart disease, which kills more than 650,000 people per year. In addition, almost 25 million people were living with a diagnosis of heart disease in 2004, according to the National Center for Health Statistics. The American Medical Association wants people to know and understand that aside from some inherited or congenital conditions, heart disease is largely preventable. It is important to remember, too, that preventive medicine is for every age group and should start in childhood; parents can guide their children to a healthy adulthood by helping them control their weight, make good food choices, enjoy regular physical activity, learn to control stress, and refrain from smoking.

In recent years, more and more children have become obese or overweight, and many cases of type 2 diabetes are reported earlier in life—that is, in teenagers or young adults—than was ever heard of in former years. Good lifestyle choices at an early age help set the course for a healthy life and specifically help minimize chances of heart disease and other chronic diseases.

In the *American Medical Association Guide to Preventing and Treating Heart Disease*, you will learn more about the importance of cholesterol, also called blood cholesterol, a substance that occurs in our body cells and also in some foods. If levels are high, cholesterol can be deposited in blood vessel walls as plaque (fatty deposits). One of the major risk factors for cardiovascular disease is a high total blood cholesterol level of 240 mg/dL or more. Adults of any age—whether young adults, middle-aged, or seniors—should know their cholesterol levels. A total cholesterol level of less than 200 mg/dL is desirable, a level of from 200 to 239 mg/dL is borderline high, and a level of 240 and above is considered dangerous. Control of LDL (low-density lipoprotein, or "bad" cholesterol) is essential for good heart health.

High blood pressure (hypertension) is another major risk factor for heart disease and stroke. One of three American adults has high blood pressure, and the numbers are increasing as our country ages and becomes more overweight. Having high blood pressure can affect your body in several ways. It can lead to atherosclerosis (hardening of the arteries), stroke, an aortic aneurysm, an enlarged heart, kidney damage, or eye damage. All adults, besides knowing their blood cholesterol numbers, should also know their blood pressure numbers. If you are black or have a family history of high blood pressure, you are at special risk and should therefore be especially aware of your blood pressure numbers. A healthy reading in an adult is 120/80 mm Hg or lower. Prehypertension is diagnosed after two or more readings between 120/80 mm Hg and 139/89 mm Hg, and changes in lifestyle are recommended to prevent the development of hypertension.

To help prevent cardiovascular disease, quitting smoking is another lifestyle change you can make to reduce your risk. Tobacco smoke endangers you by damaging the lining of your arteries, increasing the deposits of plaque, and causing your blood to clot more easily. Smoking also decreases your HDL (high-density lipoprotein, or "good") cholesterol. Furthermore, the nicotine and carbon monoxide in smoke reduce the amount of oxygen that your blood can carry and thereby make your heart beat faster and work harder.

Eating a sensible diet and exercising regularly, in tandem, are also vital to preventing heart disease. This volume explains the benefits of the DASH diet, a comprehensive eating plan developed by the National Heart, Lung, and Blood Institute. DASH stands for Dietary Approaches to Stop Hypertension, and it calls for foods low in saturated fat, cholesterol, total fat, and sodium, while emphasizing fruits, vegetables, and low-fat dairy products such as fat-free, or skim, milk. Together with regular exercise, using the DASH diet plan can lower your blood cholesterol levels and your blood pressure in as little as 2 to 4 weeks.

Another way you can take control of your cardiovascular health, as mentioned above in connection with diet, is to start a regular exercise program. A sedentary lifestyle is hard on your entire body. Thus, being inactive is a major risk factor for cardiovascular disease—right along with elevated blood cholesterol, high blood pressure, and smoking. Besides helping you to manage your blood pressure, exercising regularly, along with sensible eating, is necessary for controlling your weight. To stay heart healthy, doctors recommend that people take time to exercise at least 5 days a week, but preferably every day. If your current fitness level is low, talk to your doctor about appropriate exercise for you; he or she will probably recommend that you start by taking walks.

Besides the risk factors already mentioned, other contributing factors for cardiovascular disease are being overweight, having diabetes mellitus, and stress. Even if you are significantly overweight, taking off as little as 10 pounds can significantly lower your blood pressure and risk of heart attack or stroke. The ever-increasing incidence of diabetes and insulin resistance in the United States is due to weight gain and lack of exercise. Probably another contributing factor can be stress. Stressful situations cause our bodies to release hormones that raise blood pressure, injure the linings of the arteries, and also raise the heart rate.

To stay healthy or regain health, people are advised to see a physician promptly if worrisome symptoms appear and treat any disease that is diagnosed. Diabetes mellitus, whether type 1 or type 2, and obesity are major risk factors for heart disease, so people who have been diagnosed with diabetes or are overweight or obese should follow their doctors' recommendations on needed lifestyle changes and checkups or screening for heart disease.

The *AMA Guide to Preventing and Treating Heart Disease* includes not only the basics of prevention but also valuable, up-to-date information on treatment of heart attacks, strokes, arrhythmias, heart valve problems, congestive heart failure, and other problems. In these pages the reader will find information on symptoms, diagnosis, treatments (including surgery and medications), and self-care. A chapter on physical examinations and tests explains basic information about tests your doctor might prescribe, such as echocardiography; for each test, information is included on any needed preparation and whether the test is invasive. Finally, a special chapter deals with women and heart disease, including how pregnancy and menopause may affect heart conditions.

To help the reader understand and absorb the information in this book, all terms are clearly defined when first introduced, and a glossary at the end of the book recaps brief definitions of important terms for handy reference. A comprehensive index helps readers pinpoint where to find needed information on prevention and treatment of heart disease.

1

Your Heart and Circulatory System

Your heart is a vital organ, tirelessly pumping blood throughout your body whether you are resting, carrying out your daily activities, or exercising strenuously. It is the muscular powerhouse at the center of your circulatory system, and its healthy function keeps you alive, delivering nourishing blood to every cell of every tissue in your body.

The heart and the circulatory system together make up your cardiovascular system, which accomplishes the complex function of distributing oxygen and other nutrients to body cells, as well as carrying away carbon dioxide and other waste products of cellular function for elimination. Your heart provides the pumping action and force to push your blood first through the lungs to take on oxygen, and then out into the circulatory system. Your circulatory system ferries the blood out to body tissues via arteries, then back to the heart through veins. More than 60,000 miles of blood vessels are involved in this vast network.

The heart itself is about the size of a fist and weighs less than a pound. To "put your hand over your heart," you place it just to the left of your sternum, or breast bone, which is located in the center of your chest. You can usually feel your heart's regular beat, because the right side of the roughly cone-shaped organ tilts closest to your chest wall at this point. Behind the heart are the lungs. These organs are well protected within the bony structure of your chest cavity, with the spinal column and ribs behind them.

The Structure and Function of the Heart

In the heart, blood makes a figure-eight passage. It enters on the right side through two major veins, moves through the two right chambers, loops back through the lungs to pick up oxygen, then passes back into the left chambers and out through the aorta. The blood flow is propelled through the heart and body as the heart's muscles contract. Flow is directed by the opening and closing of one-way heart valves between the chambers of the heart and the great vessels, or veins and arteries.

The Heart Chambers

The heart is constructed of four chambers: the right atrium and the right ventricle, and the left atrium and the left ventricle. These four chambers function as two side-by-side pumps, each of which sends blood through a completely different system of circulation. The right side of the heart pumps blood through the less forceful pulmonary circulation of the lungs, where oxygen-depleted blood is replenished in lung tissue with oxygen from the air we breathe. The left side of the heart pumps blood into the rest of your blood vessels, allowing

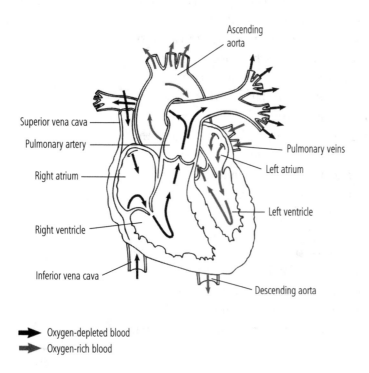

Ascending aorta

Superior vena cava

Pulmonary artery

Right atrium

Right ventricle

Inferior vena cava

Pulmonary veins

Left atrium

Left ventricle

Descending aorta

➡ Oxygen-depleted blood
➡ Oxygen-rich blood

How your heart pumps blood

The four chambers of your heart function as two side-by-side pumps. On the right side, oxygen-depleted blood that has circulated through the body passes into the right atrium through the superior vena cava and inferior vena cava. The right atrium pushes it into the right ventricle, which moves it into the pulmonary artery to flow into the lungs. In the lungs, the blood is enriched with fresh oxygen. Then the oxygen-rich blood flows through the pulmonary vein into the left side of the heart. The left atrium sends the blood into the left ventricle, which contracts forcefully enough to pump the blood into the aorta, the major artery at the top of the heart. From the aorta, the oxygen-rich blood is distributed throughout the body to nourish cells.

nourishing, oxygen-rich blood to leave the heart and travel throughout the rest of the body.

The atria receive blood from the body on the right side and from the lungs on the left side. The two ventricles are the pumping chambers that expel the blood. The two pumps operate in synchronized fashion, the two atria and then the two ventricles contracting and relaxing simultaneously. The two sides of the heart are separated by a thick muscular wall called the septum, which prevents blood from passing directly from one side of the heart to the other.

To understand the mechanics of pulmonary (lung) circulation, you can trace the path of about half a cup of blood— the amount pumped in a given heartbeat— through the right side of the heart. Blood enters the right atrium of the heart through two large veins: the superior vena cava, which collects blood from your head and upper body, and the inferior vena cava, which collects blood from your legs and abdomen. At this point, the red blood cells in the blood returning to the right atrium have delivered oxygen and nutrients to other body tissues. The depleted blood has a low oxygen content. The right atrium contracts and sends the blood through a one-way valve into the right ventricle, which in turn contracts and pushes the blood out through the pulmonary artery into the lungs. As the blood circulates through the lungs, it unloads carbon dioxide, a waste product of cellular function that it has carried from body tissues. The red blood cells then pick up fresh oxygen, and the blood is enriched, or oxygenated.

Similarly, on the upper left side of the heart, circulation to the rest of your body starts with the left atrium. Bright red, oxygen-rich blood enters the chamber via the pulmonary vein, from the lungs. The walls of the left atrium contract and push the blood through a one-way valve into the left

Heart Tissue

Your heart is composed of cardiac muscle: specialized, involuntary muscle tissue that is structured differently from the muscle tissue elsewhere in your body. The muscular wall of your heart chambers is called the myocardium. The fibers of cardiac muscle are uniquely networked to respond to the electrical impulses that initiate a heartbeat and coordinate the continuous, rapid, rhythmic contractions of the heart. At a cellular level, individual muscle cells shorten, causing the wall to tighten and the chamber to squeeze blood out. When the cells lengthen, the wall relaxes and the chamber becomes larger and allows blood to enter.

A layer of tissue called the endocardium lines the interior of the heart, including the surfaces of the valves. This membrane is smooth muscle tissue.

In addition, a layer of smooth, protective tissue covers the outer surface of the myocardium. This outer membrane, the pericardium, is actually a two-layer fibrous sac that encases the heart itself and the base of the major blood vessels. The outer sac holds the heart in place, while the inner sac is attached to the heart muscle. A lubricating fluid forms a film between these three layers to allow the heart to move freely within the pericardium.

ventricle. Then the left atrium relaxes while the powerful left ventricle contracts with the considerable force required to propel the blood into the aorta—the major artery at the top of the heart that directs the blood throughout the body. The left ventricle is the main pump and the strongest muscle tissue in the heart.

The Heart Valves

The blood flow through the heart needs to be one-way and carefully regulated. Four one-way valves between the chambers ensure that the blood moves through the heart and lungs in sequence and never dams up or back-flows. All the heart valves are constructed of overlapping flaps (leaflets or cusps) that open and close to control blood flow. The valves differ by structure and function.

The pulmonary and aortic valves between a ventricle and the great artery are called the semilunar valves because of their crescent-shaped leaflets. The tricuspid and mitral valves between the right and left atria and a ventricle are also called atrioventricular valves. The leaflets of the two atrioventricular valves are attached to the ventricular walls by fibrous cords. When the ventricle contracts and the valve closes, the cords secure the leaflets in place so they are not blown backward by the force of the contraction.

The tricuspid valve, on the right side of the heart, is named for its three leaflets, or cusps. Returning, oxygen-depleted blood flows through this valve into the right ventricle.

As the blood flows out of the right ventricle and into the pulmonary circulation, it passes through the pulmonary valve. The pulmonary valve's three leaflets open as the right ventricle contracts and close again as it relaxes.

As the oxygen-enriched blood passes back into the left atrium, it passes through the mitral valve (named for its shape, which resembles a type of bishop's hat called a miter). This valve has just two highly mobile cusps that can close rapidly when the powerful left ventricle contracts. This valve is attached by cords to muscles within the ventricle.

Finally, as the blood flows out of the left ventricle and into the aorta, the three-part aortic valve opens against the walls of the aorta. When the blood has passed into the aorta, the valve falls shut.

The Heartbeat

The continuous function of your heart is probably easiest to understand if you break it down into a single unit of pumping action, the heartbeat. A healthy heart beats between 50 and 75 times per minute, so a single heartbeat may occur in less than a second. It involves two distinct phases, the systole and the diastole. The systole is the pumping phase and the diastole is the resting phase.

The systole actually occurs in two sequential pumping actions: the atrial systole and the ventricular systole. The lub-dub that is heard through a stethoscope is the sound of the heart valves closing during the heartbeat's pumping cycle. The first heart sound, the "lub," coincides with the closing of the mitral and tricuspid valves. The second heart sound, the "dub," occurs with the closing of the aortic and pulmonary valves.

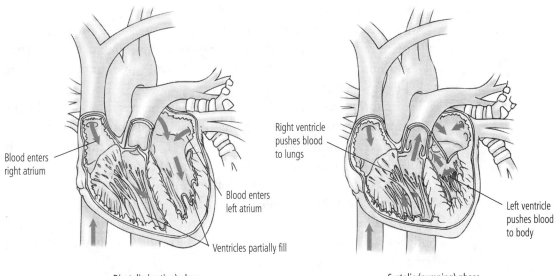

Blood enters right atrium

Blood enters left atrium

Ventricles partially fill

Diastolic (resting) phase

Right ventricle pushes blood to lungs

Left ventricle pushes blood to body

Systolic (pumping) phase

The heartbeat

A single heartbeat moves a quantity of blood through the heart in two phases: a resting, or dilating (diastolic), phase and a pumping, or squeezing (systolic), phase. During the diastolic phase, the heart relaxes and fills, as oxygen-depleted blood flows into the right atrium from the body, and oxygen-rich blood flows from the lungs into the left atrium. The ventricles fill partially. Then, during the systolic phase (right), an electrical impulse causes the heart to contract. First, the atria contract and completely fill the ventricles with blood. Then the ventricles contract, pumping blood out of the heart.

The diastole, the first and longer resting phase, occurs as blood collects in the two (right and left) atria. In the right atrium, depleted blood enters from the body, and in the left atrium, oxygen-rich blood flows in from the lungs.

Systole begins when an electrical signal from the heart's pacemaker cells stimulates the atria to contract and empty. The tricuspid and mitral valves open and blood flows into the two ventricles.

When the ventricles are full, the electrical impulse passes into an area just above the ventricles and triggers the ventricular systole, the third and final step. All four valves are in action: the tricuspid and mitral valves close to prevent backflow from the ventricles to the atria, and the pulmonary and aortic valves are pushed open as blood surges out. On the right side of the heart, oxygen-poor blood travels from the right ventricle into the pulmonary artery on its way to the lungs to acquire oxygen. On the left side of the heart, oxygen-enriched blood flows from the left ventricle through the aorta and into the general and coronary circulation.

After the blood has left the ventricles, they relax, and the pulmonary and aortic valves close. As the ventricles relax, the pressure in the ventricles lowers, allowing the tricuspid and mitral valves to open, and the cycle begins again.

Throughout this cycle, the two adjacent pumps move exactly the same amounts of blood; the volume of blood that enters and leaves the right chambers is the same as the volume that passes through the left chambers. Any change in the amount of blood entering the right side of your heart—in response to exertion, stress, or temperature changes, for example—causes a corresponding change in the amount of blood passing through the left side. Your brain is constantly monitoring the conditions that might require a change in blood supply and adjusting your heart's function accordingly.

The Heart's Electrical Conduction System

The electrical activity that stimulates and paces the heartbeat is critical. In order to deliver an appropriate blood supply to body tissues, the heart must beat at an adequate rate, and the timing and sequence of muscular contractions must be precisely coordinated.

Your heart's natural pacemaker is the sinoatrial (SA) node, a

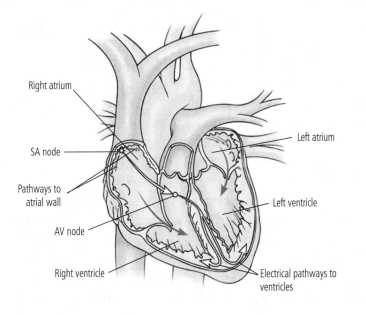

Right atrium

SA node

Pathways to
atrial wall

AV node

Right ventricle

Left atrium

Left ventricle

Electrical pathways to
ventricles

Your heart's electrical activity

Areas of specialized cells in heart tissue can initiate and conduct electrical impulses. The sinoatrial (SA) node, an area of electrical cells at the top of the right atrium, fires an impulse that initiates each heartbeat. The impulse first stimulates the walls of the atria to contract, allowing blood to fill the ventricles, and then travels to the atrioventricular (AV) node (over the ventricles). The AV node acts as a relay station for the signal before passing the impulse into the ventricles via branching electrical pathways.

microscopic group of specialized electrical cells located at the top of the right atrium. Each heartbeat originates in the SA node when it fires off an electrical impulse. This impulse travels via specialized pathways to the cells in the muscle tissues of the heart wall. The impulse first stimulates the upper chambers, the atria, to contract and squeeze blood out into the ventricles.

Then the impulse moves to another area of electrical cells called the atrioventricular (AV) node, located over the ventricles. This node acts as a relay station, allowing for a brief interval during which the atria empty completely before releasing the impulse along branching pathways that travel to the two ventricles to stimulate ventricular contraction. The ventricles similarly contract and empty, and blood is pumped into the pulmonary artery and the aorta.

The SA node speeds up when your body needs more blood. It also slows down during rest or in response to some medications. The message to increase or decrease the rate of impulses is controlled by the autonomic nervous system—the part of the nervous system that controls unconscious, automatic body functions including heart rate, blood pressure, and breathing. Autonomic nervous system activity regulates the release of the hormones epinephrine and norepinephrine, which act as accelerators for the heart's electrical impulses during times of stress or exercise.

Your heart's electrical activity can be followed and recorded on paper as an electrocardiogram (ECG, see pages 122–125). The initial impulse from the SA node is seen as a wave on the ECG, followed by a more static interval. The ECG recording shows spikes as the impulse travels from the AV node through the ventricular pathways and is again followed by a static interval that is a segment of recovery.

Coronary Circulation

Because your heart must operate continuously to supply the rest of your body with blood, it works harder and requires a richer blood supply of its own than any other muscle in your body. It cannot extract oxygen and nutrients from the blood that moves through it, so it maintains its own dedicated circulatory system of arteries and veins. This coronary circulation begins with two coronary arteries that branch off of the aorta just above the aortic valve (on the left side). These arteries extend over the surface of the heart and branch into smaller vessels that penetrate the heart muscles to provide oxygen. After the muscles of the heart have been nourished, the blood travels through coronary veins into the coronary sinus and then the right atrium. At this point, it flows in with the oxygen-depleted blood from the rest of the body.

The left coronary artery supplies blood to most of the powerful left ventricle. The circumflex coronary artery is really a branch of the left coronary artery. It wraps around the back of the heart and has several smaller branches. The right coronary artery supplies part of the left ventricle and most of the right ventricle. Interestingly, the configuration and even the sizes of the coronary arteries differ significantly from person to person.

The coronary arteries deliver oxygen-rich blood to the cardiac muscle cells according to the demand at the moment. If you are exerting yourself physically, your heart beats faster and more vigorously, and your coronary arteries expand to allow greater blood flow.

Your Heart's Performance

Both the rate at which your heart beats and the volume of blood your heart moves in a single beat determine how efficiently your heart pumps blood. Cardiologists calculate cardiac output to measure your heart's efficiency. Cardiac output is, quite simply, the amount of blood your heart pumps through your circulatory system in one minute. It is calculated by multiplying how much blood the left ventricle squeezes out in a single contraction (stroke volume) by the number of times the heart contracts in a minute (heart rate).

Most typically, when your body needs more blood (for instance, when you are running up stairs) the heart increases its output by beating faster. If your heart beats at a fast rate for very long, the muscle begins to tire and the resting phase of the heartbeat becomes too short for the chambers to fill adequately. If you are physically fit, your heart muscle is stronger and can pump more blood with each contraction. That is, your stroke volume is higher, so your heart can deliver adequate blood to your body without tiring as quickly. A physically fit person may actually have a low resting heart rate, because he or she has strengthened the heart muscle so that it can pump more blood, delivering adequate oxygen to the body with fewer strokes. When a fit person exercises, he or she may have the same heart rate as someone who is less fit, but the fit person is able to do more work, such as run longer without tiring.

A healthy resting heart rate is usually between 50 and 75 beats per minute. When you exercise, your heart rate may increase to as much as 165 beats or more. Age plays a role in determining your maximum heart rate; the maximum number of beats per minute can be very roughly predicted by the formula 220 minus your age. A number of other factors can cause your heart rate to increase, including stress, some medications, caffeine, alcohol, and tobacco. When a healthy person sleeps, his or her heart rate may dip to as low as 40 beats per minute. As you age, your heart rate may decrease somewhat.

Stroke volume in most people is about 3 ounces. That means that the ventricles pump out about half the blood they contain. A good athlete may be able to increase his or her stroke volume by 5 percent or more. A diminishing stroke volume is one of the first signs of a failing heart.

A pregnant woman's body demands more blood flow and oxygen for the developing placenta. Stroke volume increases early in pregnancy, and later the heart rate increases to maintain a cardiac output 40 to 50 percent above normal. These changes reverse after the baby is delivered.

The Circulatory System

Your systemic circulation is the vast highway system that carries blood from your heart to every part of your body, and then returns it to the heart. The vessels that carry blood away from the heart are the arteries; the vessels that carry blood back to the heart are veins. Like a system of roads, your circulatory system keeps branching off into successively smaller vessels that carry blood to and from the smallest structures and finally individual cells in body tissues. At a cellular level, single red blood cells exchange oxygen and nutrients with single body cells through the walls of microscopic capillaries.

The Arteries and the Capillaries

The aorta, the largest artery in your body, emerges from the left side of your heart. About 1 inch in diameter, it ascends from your left ventricle engorged with oxygen-rich blood, then arches down the chest into the abdomen. Major arteries branch off it to supply different areas of your body. The carotid and vertebral arteries travel to your head and neck. The subclavian arteries supply the arms. The abdominal (descending) aorta provides branches to your stomach, liver, kidneys, and intestinal tract. The aorta then divides into the iliac arteries and then the femoral arteries of the legs.

The pulmonary artery carries blood from your heart to your lungs. Exiting from your right ventricle, it transports oxygen-depleted blood into your lungs to replenish the oxygen. This pulmonary circulation functions similarly to your systemic circulation but is limited to the lungs, where oxygen exchange occurs at a cellular level.

The arteries subdivide into smaller vessels called arterioles. The arteries and arterioles have flexible muscular walls that can dilate (widen) and contract, with a critical impact on directing blood flow. Blood flows more easily to areas where there is less resistance, so arteries that widen increase the circulation to that area, while a constricted artery reduces blood flow. Branching off from the arterioles are the smallest vessels, the capillaries. Most capillary walls are only one cell thick. Specialized capillaries in different types of body tissue allow the passage of different types of molecules through their walls. In the lungs, for example, molecules of carbon dioxide (a waste product) pass into the tissue to be breathed out, while molecules of oxygen pass into the blood cells. In your intestinal system, nutrients from digested food pass through the capillary walls into the blood.

The Veins

At the level of individual cells throughout your body, the capillaries receive spent blood from body tissue that has a lower level of oxygen. The capillaries flow into larger vessels called venules, which converge and form still larger veins. The pressure in veins is significantly lower than the pressure in arteries, and the walls are thinner, which is why blood samples are typically taken from a vein. As with arteries, the walls of veins can expand or contract. Any tensing of your muscles squeezes the veins, helping to counteract gravity and keep blood flowing toward your heart. Larger veins also have a system of one-way valves that keep the returning blood flowing the right way.

Venous blood from the body enters the heart via two major vessels: the superior vena cava, bringing blood from the upper part of the body, and the inferior vena cava, returning blood from the lower part. These large veins enter the right atrium, where the blood is sent into the pulmonary circulation for oxygen pickup.

Blood

Blood is the fluid vehicle by which oxygen, enzymes (proteins that promote body processes), and other life-sustaining nutrients are brought to body cells in order to maintain an optimal environment for growth. Blood is composed of specialized blood cells—red blood cells, white blood cells, and platelets—and of plasma, the fluid in which the blood cells are suspended.

The vast majority of blood cells are red blood cells, also called erythrocytes or red corpuscles, which do the work of oxygen transport. An individual red blood cell is saucer-shaped to maximize its surface area for efficient oxygen exchange. Chemically, a red blood cell contains large quantities of hemoglobin, an iron-rich protein that is the body's oxygen transport carrier molecule. As red blood cells travel through the lungs, where oxygen levels are high, the hemoglobin readily combines with oxygen. When the blood cells reach body tissues where oxygen levels are relatively low, the hemoglobin just as effectively releases oxygen. The red blood cells also pick up the waste product carbon dioxide and carry it back to the lungs, where it is released and then exhaled out of the body. Red blood cells are formed in the bone marrow at the rate of about 8 million a second, or many billion in a single day. They live from 3 to 4 months.

White blood cells, or leukocytes, play a critical role in protecting the body against infection. One type of white blood cell, called a lymphocyte, identifies invading microorganisms or other harmful substances in the body and triggers the body's immune response. The number of white blood cells increases when your body is fighting infection. Also suspended in the plasma are cell fragments called platelets, which initiate a blood-clotting response when you are injured or a blood vessel is damaged. White blood cells and platelets make up about 1 to 2 percent of blood volume.

About 55 percent of the blood volume is plasma, a yellowish, watery substance that contains proteins, glucose (sugar), cholesterol, and other components. Proteins in the plasma perform varied roles such as carrying nutrients, contributing to the clotting factor, and acting as infection-fighting antibodies in an immune response.

The Lungs and the Respiratory System

The story of oxygen transport to body cells is not complete without a look at the respiratory system, which brings oxygen from the air into the body, transfers it to the blood, and then rids the body of the waste products of cellular energy. When you breathe, the organs of your respiratory system perform the physical job of bringing air into the body and expelling it. The same organs are the site of the more complex biochemical process of respiration, the oxygenation of blood at a cellular level.

When you inhale air, it passes down your trachea, into the tubular bronchi that branch into your lungs, and through a system of subdividing air passages that end deep in lung tissue as microscopic tubes called bronchioles. The bronchioles open into tiny, elastic air sacs called alveoli.

Parallel to these branching air passages, a network of blood vessels brings blood into lung tissue. Minute capillaries cover the surface of the alveoli, and through the walls of these capillaries oxygen passes from the air sacs into the blood. Carbon dioxide molecules, carried in the blood from body tissues, pass into the alveoli. The oxygen-laden blood flows

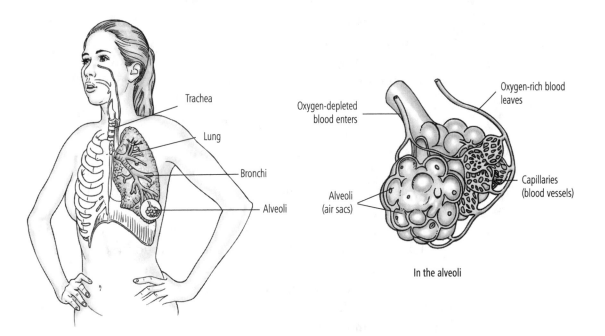

The respiratory system

When you inhale, you bring air into your lungs via the trachea, or windpipe. In the lungs, branching air passages (bronchi) end deep in lung tissue in microscopic clusters of air sacs called alveoli. In these clusters, networks of tiny blood vessels (capillaries) cover the air sacs. Oxygen exchange takes place through the walls of the alveoli and capillaries, as oxygen passes from lung tissue into the bloodstream and waste products (such as carbon dioxide) pass from the bloodstream into the lungs to be exhaled out of your body.

back into the heart, where it then can be circulated throughout the body, while the carbon dioxide moves back through the lungs to be exhaled.

The Heart and Other Body Systems

Your heart beats and your blood circulates with little or no conscious awareness on your part. Even though circulation is an involuntary function, it is a dynamic one. Your cardiovascular system is constantly adjusting to changes in the external environment or to demands you place on it. It adapts quickly, or directs other systems to adapt to changing conditions in order to maintain a constant flow of blood to body tissues. Even the simple act of standing up requires increased blood flow to the legs, because the heart must work harder to counteract the effects of gravity. This means that either blood flow to other parts of the body must be decreased or the heart must pump blood faster or in greater volume to accommodate the activity.

The two main systems that help regulate cardiac function are first, the brain and the nervous system, and second, the kidneys.

The Brain and the Nervous System

Nervous system receptors throughout your body constantly gather information about factors such as stretching of the arterial walls or the amount of oxygen in the blood. This information is relayed to the brain by chemicals called neurotransmitters. In the brain stem, at the base of the brain, regulatory centers involved with automatic body functions including heart rate, blood pressure, and respiration receive the messages and formulate a response. Neurotransmitters such as adrenaline carry messages back that direct a response in the target tissue, such as commands to constrict the blood vessels or increase the rate of respiration to deliver more oxygen to your lungs.

The Kidneys

The kidneys influence the volume of fluids in the body, so they can change the volume of circulating blood. In this way, they significantly affect blood pressure. They release enzymes that can raise blood pressure by constricting blood vessels, raising sodium levels, and increasing water retention. The kidneys can adapt to changing environmental conditions by, for instance, concentrating your urine if your body is dehydrated. If, on the other hand, you eat a lot of salty foods and start to retain water, your kidneys will produce less urine.

Preventing Heart Disease

Cardiovascular disease is the leading cause of death of men and women in the United States. Cancer, the second most common killer, accounts for the deaths of only half as many people. Heart and blood vessel disease takes many forms: high blood pressure, coronary artery disease, valvular heart disease, congestive heart failure, atherosclerosis, and stroke. Because of the enormous toll that the burden of these diseases has taken on the nation's health, extensive research has focused on preventing these problems. Over a period of decades, numerous studies involving hundreds of thousands of people have identified the major risk factors that indicate an individual's chances of developing cardiovascular disease. Understanding these risk factors and how you can control them gives you a good chance to prevent or modify heart disease in your own body. Even though cardiovascular disease is still a major threat, the death rates today are substantially lower than they were because so many people have been able to make effective changes in their lifestyle that prevent the development or the worsening of the disease.

These preventive changes—including how we eat, how physically active we are, and how we approach risky habits like smoking or drinking—make common sense in part because of the nature of heart disease and its treatment. Cardiovascular disease develops slowly and often without symptoms. Factors such as cholesterol buildup or rising blood pressure can start in childhood but may not become apparent as disease for decades, so prevention is the best answer.

About half the deaths from heart disease are sudden—an unexpected fatal occurrence that leaves little opportunity for intervention. Many treatments—for instance, the coronary artery bypass procedures that have become so common—can have side effects and are inappropriate to perform on every person at risk. Other technologies, such as balloon angioplasty or drugs, can treat a problem, but they cannot stop the underlying disease process.

Most positively, the picture that emerges from decades of research is that the healthy lifestyle choices that prevent heart disease also reduce the risk of other major diseases such as cancer and diabetes.

Risk Factors for Heart Disease

Some risk factors for heart disease are within your control, while others are not. The number of risk factors that affect you may change over the course of your lifetime. Having one or more of the major, proven risk factors doesn't mean that you will develop cardiovascular disease or die of it. But generally, the more of these factors that apply to you, the more likely you are to develop the disease at some point. By knowing your own constellation of risk factors, you can control as many as possible and reduce your risk. These are the factors you can't control:

- **Gender.** Men are more likely than women to have a heart attack at a younger age. Women are generally protected from heart disease by their sex hormones until menopause. Cardiovascular disease is still the leading cause of death for women, however. After menopause, a woman's risk of heart disease starts to rise. After the age of 65, a woman's chance of having coronary artery disease is about the same as a man's, and after 75, a woman is at even greater risk than a man is.

- **Increasing age.** Your risk of disease increases as you grow older. More than 80 percent of people who die from heart disease are over 65. As you age, your heart's function tends to weaken. The heart is less able to pump blood, the walls of the heart may thicken, and the walls of the arteries may stiffen and narrow. In addition to atherosclerosis, other conditions such as hypertension may compound the problem. Clearly this process is affected by lifestyle, including diet and exercise.

- **Heredity.** Cardiovascular disease runs in families, and you are more likely to develop it if your parents or siblings have coronary artery disease. Increased risk is linked to a family history of death from heart disease at a young age. Specifically, this is defined as coronary artery disease in men before age 55 and women before age 65. Your racial or ethnic background is another aspect of your heredity. In the United States, blacks are at higher risk than whites, in part because of higher rates of high blood pressure. The risk of heart disease is also somewhat higher in Mexican Americans and native Hawaiians. You can't change your heredity, but it gives you strong motivation to manage other factors that you can change.

The major proven risk factors for heart disease that you can modify, control, or treat are:

- **High blood cholesterol.** High blood cholesterol directly increases your risk of heart disease. Cholesterol is a fatlike substance that is carried in your blood, but excess cholesterol enters your body through foods derived from animals (meat, eggs, dairy products).

- **High blood pressure (hypertension).** High blood pressure increases your risk of several forms of cardiovascular disease: coronary artery disease, heart attack, kidney failure, congestive heart failure, and stroke. Other factors, such as obesity, alcohol abuse, unhealthy diet, or physical inactivity can contribute to high blood pressure, but you can also have it independent of those other influences. (See chapter 3.)

- **Obesity and overweight.** Excess body fat contributes to the risk of heart disease, independent of other risk factors, because it increases the heart's workload. It also raises blood pressure, adversely affects cholesterol levels, and contributes to the development of diabetes.
- **Physical inactivity.** An inactive lifestyle increases the risk of becoming overweight and developing high blood cholesterol levels, high blood pressure, and diabetes. Even moderate amounts of regular exercise will lower your risk of heart disease.
- **Type 2 diabetes.** Having diabetes puts you at serious risk; about 65 to 75 percent of people with diabetes die from some form of cardiovascular disease. Controlling your diabetes may help control your risk of heart problems.
- **Smoking.** If you smoke, you are more likely to develop cardiovascular disease than a nonsmoker is—in addition to the risk of lung cancer. Smoking increases your heart rate, constricts your arteries and contributes to their obstruction with plaque, and can cause irregular heartbeat. It also increases your risk of blood clots, which cause heart attack or stroke. Even exposure to other people's smoke increases a person's risk of heart disease.
- **Early menopause.** Women who have early menopause, whether naturally or as a result of surgery, have a higher risk of coronary artery disease.

Other influences, called contributing factors, are linked to heart disease, but their significance is not fully understood or measured yet. These factors are:

- **Stress.** Stress, particularly in some people, appears to increase the risk of heart problems, perhaps because it raises your heart rate and blood pressure, damaging your arteries over time. It may also

Heart Disease and Genetics

Because heart disease tends to run in families, having parents or siblings with the disease is a major risk factor. But there is no single gene for cardiovascular disease; in fact, geneticists think that more than a thousand separate genes may influence the overall cardiovascular system. There are separate genes for obesity, high blood pressure, and diabetes, all risk factors for heart disease. Scientists are still identifying these genes and studying how they interact with one another—and with other influences such as diet—in an individual or a family. Many geneticists believe that one of the most effective approaches for a person at high genetic risk of heart disease is to ensure that the person follows a healthy lifestyle.

Other avenues of research include developing drugs that target a specific genetic predisposition, along with developing genetic tests that can screen for high-risk patients. The ultimate implications of genetic research for testing and treatment of heart disease are still far in the future.

contribute to other harmful behaviors such as overeating, smoking, or drinking too much.

- **Alcohol.** Drinking more than a moderate amount of alcohol can raise blood pressure, negatively affect cholesterol and triglyceride (blood fats) levels, and cause irregular heartbeats. However, modest amounts of alcohol may actually reduce the risk of heart disease. Since so many Americans drink to excess, doctors are reluctant to recommend moderate drinking to improve heart health, for fear that "moderate" usage will change to "excessive" use. Alcohol, whether wine, beer, or liquor, but only in moderate amounts, may be helpful to your health.

- **Birth control pills.** If you smoke or have high blood pressure, and especially if you are over 35, birth control pills may increase your risk of heart disease. Today's birth control pills contain much lower levels of hormones than early ones and are generally considered safe, independent of other risk factors. You should not smoke and take birth control pills, especially over age 35, due to the increased risk of heart attack and blood clots.

2

Managing Your Cholesterol Level

Cholesterol, also called blood cholesterol, is a natural waxy substance that occurs in all your body cells. It is one of several types of fats (lipids) that circulate in your bloodstream. Your body uses it to form cell membranes and to make certain hormones, and therefore at healthy levels it is an essential component of cells and blood. Your liver makes as much cholesterol as your body needs—about 1,000 milligrams (mg) per day.

You consume cholesterol (dietary cholesterol) in the foods you eat, especially animal products such as meats, eggs, and dairy foods. If cholesterol levels are high, cholesterol can be deposited in the blood vessel walls as a major component of plaque (a fatty deposit). A buildup of plaque restricts the blood flow, a process called atherosclerosis, and puts you at greatly increased risk of heart disease.

Triglycerides are the true blood fat that exists in the body as well as in food. Triglycerides circulate in your blood along with cholesterol and are fuel for your body's energy production. Together, cholesterol and triglycerides in the blood are called plasma lipids. Excess calories that you consume in foods are converted to triglycerides and are carried to fat cells for storage. In between meals, hormones control the release of triglycerides to meet your body's need for energy. Like cholesterol, triglycerides can build up in the blood and contribute to atherosclerosis.

Because neither cholesterol nor triglycerides can dissolve in the blood, they have to be moved to and from cells by carriers called lipoproteins. The two most common types, the ones you hear the most about, are low-density lipoproteins (LDL), the "bad cholesterol," and high-density lipoproteins (HDL), the "good cholesterol." LDLs have a lower density of protein (about 25 percent) and more cholesterol. HDLs have a higher density of protein (about 50 percent) and less cholesterol.

If too much LDL accumulates in your blood, it causes fatty plaque to collect on your arterial walls, and the process of atherosclerosis begins. If the buildup reduces blood flow in the arteries that supply your heart, you may experience the chest pains known as angina. If a blood clot forms near the plaque and stops the blood flow, you have a heart attack. If a clot blocks blood flow to your brain, you have a stroke. Your LDL levels increase when you consume foods that contain lots of fat, cholesterol, or both. Foods rich in saturated fats and trans fats, such as butter fat, cheese, red meat, processed meats, and bakery goods, are the most harmful, along with tropical oils found in some products like crackers (see also pages 27–29).

High-density lipoproteins carry cholesterol back from your cells to your liver, where it can be passed out of the body. Most doctors think that HDL can actually slow down the development of plaque by removing cholesterol from it. A high level of HDL seems to protect against heart attack, and a low level places you at greater risk of heart attack and stroke.

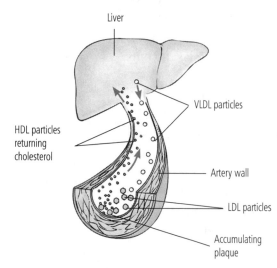

Liver

HDL particles returning cholesterol

VLDL particles

Artery wall

LDL particles

Accumulating plaque

Cholesterol transport

Your liver produces blood cholesterol, a waxy substance that your body uses to build cells and make hormones, and you consume additional cholesterol in foods. Cholesterol is transported to cells through the bloodstream on carrier particles called lipoproteins. Low-density lipoprotein (LDL) consists of less protein and more cholesterol, and it can be harmful at high levels when it builds up on the walls of your arteries as plaque. Very low-density lipoprotein (VLDL) is another form of cholesterol that can convert to LDL and cause problems. High-density lipoprotein (HDL; shown as smaller units), which consists of more protein and less cholesterol, can absorb some of the cholesterol in plaque and return it to the liver to be excreted. So you need to try to reach a high enough level for HDL in your bloodstream to help protect against heart attack and stroke.

Testing Cholesterol Levels

High cholesterol does not cause any symptoms, so people can have excessively high levels without knowing it. High blood cholesterol (defined as a level of 240 mg/dL or higher) is among the most important risk factors for developing heart disease. In countries such as Japan, which until recently had cholesterol levels averaging only 150 mg/dL, heart disease has been very rare.

All adults over the age of 20 should have their cholesterol measured at least once every 5 years with a blood test called a full lipoprotein profile. Children in families with premature heart disease may be screened starting at age 2. A full lipid profile measures not only the total cholesterol but also HDL and triglycerides. Your doctor looks at all of these numbers, as well as your other risk factors for heart disease, and then can use a risk assessment tool to estimate your chances of having a heart attack in the next 10 years. Knowing your risk enables you to take steps to improve your cardiovascular health and lower your chances of heart disease and stroke.

To have your cholesterol tested, you need to go to your doctor or a medical laboratory. The results from tests performed at shopping centers or health fairs are not as reliable as having your blood sample analyzed at an approved laboratory. Reliable testing requires a fasting blood sample. A nonfasting sample does not allow an accurate determination of LDL, which is the most important indicator of your heart attack risk. You should do the following to prepare for the blood test:

- For 10 to 12 hours before testing (often overnight), you may not eat or drink anything except water.

- You can eat as you usually do until 10 to 12 hours before the test.

- You might be asked not to drink any alcohol for several days before testing, because alcohol can affect triglyceride levels.

Home Cholesterol Testing

You may see home cholesterol testing kits for sale in some drugstores. Some measure only total cholesterol, or only total cholesterol and HDL. At least one is designed to test HDL, LDL, triglycerides, and total cholesterol. There is no harm in trying one of these devices, or having your cholesterol checked at a health fair, but these tests do not take the place of a laboratory-analyzed lipoprotein profile (which requires you to fast before the test).

If you try one of these methods and the results indicate that your total cholesterol is 200 mg/dL or more, follow up with a full profile done by trained professionals.

Most laboratories do not measure your LDL directly but calculate it by subtracting your HDL from your total cholesterol level, then subtracting one-fifth of your triglyceride level. This figure is your LDL. In cases of markedly elevated triglycerides, direct testing of LDL is needed.

- If you are sick on the appointed day, the test should be rescheduled.
- Before the day of the test, check with your doctor as to which of your regular medications, if any, you should take at home in the morning.

Interpreting Test Results

Cholesterol readings are expressed in milligrams per deciliter of blood (mg/dL), and the numbers are classified by level of health risk. Your reading can change somewhat from day to day, and the classifications are based on ranges. Of course, being in a high range doesn't guarantee that you will develop heart disease, nor does being in a low range assure that you will not. The impact of your cholesterol readings on your overall risk for heart disease or stroke depends on other factors, including your family history, conditions such as diabetes or high blood pressure, and other health habits such as smoking or physical inactivity.

Total Cholesterol Level

The total cholesterol level is the most common screening measurement. About half the adults in the United States have a reading in the desirable range of 200 mg/dL or less, indicating a lower risk of developing heart disease. Even if you are at this level, it's still a good idea to eat foods that are relatively low in saturated fats and trans fats, and to exercise regularly. Continue to get a full lipoprotein profile every 5 years.

The total needs to be interpreted, along with how the cholesterol is packaged in the bloodstream. A total level of 200 to 239 mg/dL is called borderline high and places you at up to two times the risk of heart attack as someone with a reading below 200 mg/dL. Your doctor will discuss this reading and the rest of your profile with you, as well as other factors that contribute to your risk. Some people, such as menstruating women before menopause or young, active men, may have an elevated total cholesterol reading but may not be at high risk for heart disease. The reason is that although the total cholesterol is elevated, it is the HDL, or good cholesterol, that is elevated, and LDL, the bad cholesterol, is within target range. Talk to your doctor to interpret your results.

Total Cholesterol Guidelines

Level (mg/dL)	Category
Less than 200	Desirable
200–239	Borderline high
240 and above	High

Source: All cholesterol levels adapted from the National Institutes of Health's National Health Education Program Adult Treatment Panel III.

If your total cholesterol is above 240 mg/dL, you are more than twice as likely to have a heart attack as someone with a borderline high reading. You are also at a higher risk of stroke. Again, you need to discuss your overall profile with your doctor and get started trying to bring your level down to a healthy target.

HDL Level

HDL is the good cholesterol that, at higher levels, appears to reduce your risk of heart disease. People with a low level of HDL are at increased risk for heart disease. In the average man, HDL levels range from 40 to 50 mg/dL. In an average woman, they are higher, 50 to 60 mg/dL, because the female hormone estrogen raises HDL. After menopause, a woman's HDL levels may fall, increasing her risk of heart disease. For a man or a woman, a reading below 40 mg/dL is considered too low. People who are overweight or physically inactive are more likely to have a low HDL reading.

If your reading is low, your doctor may recommend that you get more exercise, lose weight if you are overweight or obese, and quit smoking if you are a smoker. Although treatment for high cholesterol usually focuses on lowering LDL cholesterol, doctors are placing increasing emphasis on the importance of raising HDL as well. A key strategy for raising your HDL cholesterol levels is eating more fish and less red meat. Further, consuming omega-3 fish oil reduces triglycerides and raises HDL.

The ratio of total cholesterol to HDL is a more meaningful indicator of risk than is total cholesterol alone. This is especially true because a normal total cholesterol number (less than 200 mg/dL) may pose increased risk if it is associated with a low HDL level. To calculate that ratio, divide your total cholesterol by your HDL value. A number greater than 5 shows a higher risk level. The lower your ratio is, the lower your risk of heart disease is. Try to keep your ratio lower than 4 to 1.

HDL Guidelines

HDL Level (mg/dL)	Category
Less than 40	Low
40 to 59	Desirable; the higher the better
60 and above	High

LDL Levels

LDL is the harmful cholesterol that can slowly build up plaque in the arteries. Of your lipid readings, it is the single most important indicator of your risk of cardiovascular disease. A reading of less than

LDL Guidelines

LDL Level (mg/dL)	Category
Less than 100	Optimal
100–129	Near or above optimal
130–159	Borderline high
160–189	High
190 and above	Very high

100 mg/dL is considered optimal, but not everyone needs to be that low if their other risk factors are under control.

You and your doctor will talk about your target LDL reading level in the context of other aspects of your cardiovascular health and other risk factors. Medical conditions that increase your risk include high blood pressure (120/80 mm Hg or higher) or being on medication for high blood pressure, other vascular disease, type 2 diabetes (fasting blood glucose of 126 mg/dL or higher), or having had a heart attack. Other risk factors are:

- Smoking cigarettes or long-term exposure to second-hand smoke
- An HDL reading of less than 40 mg/dL
- A family history of early heart disease (heart disease in your father or brother before age 55 or in your mother or sister before age 65)
- Age (45 years or older if you are a man; 55 years or older or menopausal if you are a woman)
- Menopause, at any age
- A sedentary lifestyle

Target LDL Readings

Risk Status	Target LDL (mg/dL)
Low risk (no other high-risk medical conditions and one or no risk factors)	Less than 160
Moderate risk (no other high-risk medical condition and two or more risk factors)	Less than 130 or less than 100, depending on overall risk assessment
High risk (a high-risk medical condition is present)	Less than 100
Very high risk (diabetes, known coronary artery disease, or other high-risk medical condition is present)	Less than 70

Source: National Cholesterol Education Program.

To lower your LDL reading, a diet low in saturated fat, trans fat, and cholesterol and high in fiber is your first step (see below and pages 30–32). You also need to lose weight if you are overweight, and get more exercise. If your level of LDL is high, however, drug therapy may be started while you work on lifestyle changes. Lifestyle measures will go a long way to improve your LDL level and condition your heart and blood vessels. But if they do not bring your reading down to your target, your doctor may prescribe medication (see box page 244). A combination of cholesterol-lowering drugs and lifestyle changes will bring LDL levels down in most people.

Triglycerides

A high triglyceride level may contribute to your risk of developing heart disease, but it is not clear to what degree high triglycerides alone are a risk factor. Doctors do know, however, that a combination of high LDL level and high triglyceride level raises the risk of a heart attack to a greater extent than either one does on its own. People with high triglycerides are often obese or have low levels of HDL, high blood pressure, or diabetes. Extremely high triglycerides (more than 500 mg/dL) can lead to a life-threatening inflammation of the pancreas called pancreatitis.

If you have an elevated triglyceride reading, you will benefit from staying at a healthful weight, eating a diet low in saturated fat and trans fat, limiting intake of sugar and other carbohydrates, drinking in moderation if at all (see page 97), and exercising regularly. You should also have a fasting blood sugar test to monitor for early signs of diabetes. Elevated triglycerides can be a sign of metabolic syndrome, also called insulin resistance syndrome.

Triglyceride Guidelines

Triglyceride Level (mg/dL)	Category
Less than 150	Desirable
150–199	Borderline high
200–499	High
500 and above	Very high

Eating to Control Your Cholesterol

Choosing foods that are low in saturated fats, trans fats, and cholesterol can lower your cholesterol. You might think that cholesterol in food is the major contributor to elevated blood cholesterol, but that is not the case. The biggest culprits are saturated fats and trans fats. The first step toward lowering your cholesterol through diet is to understand the different types of fats in foods and their impact on blood cholesterol.

Fats That Raise Cholesterol

Two types of fats are known to raise your cholesterol: saturated fats and trans fats. If you have high cholesterol, current guidelines recommend that you limit your intake of saturated and trans fats to total no more than 7 percent of the total calories you consume in one day. Saturated fats, which your body uses to make bad LDL cholesterol, mostly come from animal products. Beef, veal, lamb, pork, and whole-milk dairy products including butter, cream, milk, and cheeses are all high in saturated fat. Plant sources of saturated fats include tropical oils (coconut, palm, and palm kernel oils) and cocoa butter. These foods are also high in dietary cholesterol. However, the fat in cocoa butter appears to be more neutral and less likely to raise LDL levels.

Trans fat or trans fatty acid is an unsaturated fat, but it can also raise your LDL levels and lower your HDL levels. Trans fats are made when hydrogen is added to vegetable oils to make them solid and longer lasting. Trans fats are widely used in commercial baking (crackers, cookies, and cakes) and in restaurants, particularly for frying. They also occur naturally in some foods such as meat and whole milk. Recently the Food and Drug Administration mandated that the amount of trans fatty acids in any prepared food product be spelled out on the food label (see sample label on page 94). Also recently, the American Heart Association recommended that people limit their consumption of trans fatty acids to no more than 1 percent of their total calories each day. However, a label may state "0 g trans fat" but still contain up to 0.5 g of trans fats per serving, so to be confident you are controlling the amount of trans fats, make sure the label says the product contains no hydrogenated oil or "partially hydrogenated oil." The New York City Department of Health recently banned the use of trans fats in restaurants in the city.

Fats That Lower Cholesterol

Some fats may actually lower your cholesterol. Both polyunsaturated and monounsaturated fats alike have qualities that help lower your cholesterol. They are both good substitutes for saturated or trans fats, but you still need to moderate your intake of fats in order to keep down your total calorie intake. To lower your cholesterol, your intake of all fats combined should be 25 to 35 percent of your total calorie intake per day.

Monounsaturated fats are found in oils and fruits, such as olive oil and avocadoes. In your body, these fats help your body's cells resist absorption of fat and cholesterol and slow the buildup of plaque in your arteries. Polyunsaturated fats are found in many nuts and seeds, corn, and soybeans and their oils. It is important to recognize that canola oil has the lowest content of saturated fat among the various pressed oils that are available.

Foods rich in omega-3 polyunsaturated fats may be especially health-ful, reducing your risk of coronary artery disease, high triglycerides, blood clotting, abnormal heart rhythms, and sudden death. The American Heart Association recommends that you eat at least two servings of baked or grilled fish, preferably fatty fish, each week. Omega-3 fats or fatty acids are found in fish, especially fatty fish such as sardines, mackerel, lake trout, salmon, and albacore tuna. However, concerns about the high levels of mercury in mackerel, swordfish, and tuna have led experts to recommend that adults limit themselves to eating no more than one serving of these fish per week. A fetus may be especially vulnerable to mercury, so doctors often recommend that pregnant women limit their consumption of mercury-containing fish even more. As an alternative to fish, several plant sources are rich in omega-3 fats, including flaxseed and flaxseed oil, soy-bean oil, and walnuts. Soy, though high in total fat, is very low in saturated fat and might have a beneficial effect on lipids. Soy may be consumed in various forms including tofu, soy milk, and edamame beans.

Dietary Cholesterol

Cholesterol is found exclusively in animal-based products. Red meat, whole-milk dairy products, egg yolks, and organ meats are especially high in cholesterol. To lower cholesterol, current guidelines recom-mend that you limit your cholesterol intake to less than 300 milligrams per day, on average. Keep in mind that plant-based foods—fruits, vegetables, grains, nuts, and seeds—don't raise your cholesterol level, so you can eat more of them.

Fiber

Eaten as part of a diet low in fat and saturated fats, fiber can help lower your cholesterol. A high-fiber diet is linked to lower death rates from coronary artery disease and heart attack.

Soluble fiber (a type of fiber that is partially broken down in your intestine) effectively lowers cholesterol about 5 percent by chemically binding to cholesterol-based substances to remove them from the bloodstream. Adding more fiber to your diet is one means of enhancing the effects of your overall cholesterol-lowering diet. Soluble fiber is found in oatmeal and oat bran, beans, peas, barley, citrus fruits, strawberries, and apples. By contrast, the insoluble fiber found in wheat products has no cholesterol-lowering effects.

Plant Stanols and Sterols

Your doctor may recommend that you start using soft margarines containing plant stanols and sterols. These substances are the plant equivalent of cholesterol, and they may significantly reduce your body's absorption of dietary cholesterol from other sources. Margarines containing these substances are available at most grocery stores. Liquid margarine, spray margarine, or soft margarine in tubs are recommended over hardened margarines in sticks, because those contain hydrogenated fat or trans fat.

TLC Diet Recommendations

The Therapeutic Lifestyle Change (TLC) diet is a set of concise dietary guidelines for people who need to lower their cholesterol levels. If your blood cholesterol is not lowered enough by the TLC diet, your doctor may increase your intake of soluble fiber and plant sterols. See also information on the DASH diet, pages 47–50.

Dietary Intake	Recommended Daily Allowance
Total fat	25–35 percent
Saturated fat	Less than 7 percent
Monounsaturated fat	Up to 20 percent
Polyunsaturated fat	Up to 10 percent
Cholesterol	Less than 200 milligrams
Fiber	20–30 grams
Protein	About 15 percent
Total calories	As needed to maintain desired weight

Source: Adapted with permission from R. S. Lang and D. D. Hensrud. *Clinical Preventive Medicine*, 2nd ed. Chicago: AMA Press, 2004.

Alcohol and Cholesterol

You may have read about some studies suggesting that moderate use of alcohol may actually raise your good HDL cholesterol. However, the benefits are not clear enough to recommend that you start drinking alcohol if you don't drink now. People who drink in moderation—one drink a day for women, two drinks a day for men, on average—have a lower risk of heart disease than nondrinkers. But drinking in higher amounts is dangerous to your cardiovascular health in many ways, contributing to your risk of developing high blood pressure, obesity, and stroke. Also, for women, more than one alcoholic drink per day increases the chances of breast cancer.

Medications to Lower Your Cholesterol

If a healthful diet, regular exercise, and weight loss do not bring your total cholesterol or LDL levels down to your target, your doctor may prescribe a cholesterol-lowering medication, or a combination of more than one. You also may need to take these drugs if you have even moderately high cholesterol and also have a medical condition such as heart disease, thyroid disease (hypothyroidism), diabetes, or kidney disease. Your doctor will consider your age and family history as well as your risk status (see box, page 21) to determine what target cholesterol level is appropriate for you, and whether drugs are needed.

If you are at high risk or very high risk, your doctor may recommend drugs to lower your LDL cholesterol aggressively, to less than 70 mg/dL. If you are at moderate risk, drugs will probably be recommended if your LDL is higher than 130. On the other hand, drug therapy is not necessarily appropriate for everyone—for example, for frail elderly people who have high cholesterol levels but who do not have heart disease or diabetes.

It is important to discuss your medical history and lifestyle with your doctor before you begin taking cholesterol-lowering medications. Tell him or her about any other medications, vitamins, or herbal supplements you are taking. (Some drugs can interact with one another in a harmful way.) You and your doctor will also need to talk about what other illnesses you have, particularly if you have had liver problems, diabetes, gout, ulcers, or kidney or gallbladder disease, because some cholesterol-lowering medications can make these problems worse.

There are five main types of cholesterol-lowering drugs, each with a different method of action in your body.

- **Statins (or HMG CoA reductase inhibitors).** The most commonly prescribed cholesterol-lowering drugs are statins, which block the activity of an enzyme (HMG CoA reductase) in your body that helps you make cholesterol. As your cholesterol production slows down, your liver makes more LDL receptors. These receptors attract LDL particles in your blood and further lower your LDL levels. In addition to lowering cholesterol levels, statins may have other positive effects such as reducing inflammation and improving the working of the cells that line the blood vessels. Many people can take statins without difficulty, but the drugs can cause side effects in some people such as constipation, abdominal pain, or cramps. These side effects are likely to lessen or disappear the longer you take the drug. Statins are usually taken at bedtime, because the body produces more cholesterol in the evening. If you develop any muscle cramps or muscle weakness, alert your physician because this might represent a more serious side effect. Muscle aches affect both sides of the body and commonly occur in large muscle groups such as those in the shoulders and the thighs. While taking statins, you need to have a blood test periodically to make sure your liver is not being affected by the drugs. Examples of statins include lovastatin, pravastatin, simvastatin, atorvastatin, and rosuvastatin.

A Cholesterol-Lowering Lifestyle

You can lower your cholesterol, and keep it lower, by developing several simple habits:

- Get a fasting lipoprotein profile as often as your doctor recommends. Know your numbers for total cholesterol, LDL, HDL, and triglycerides.

- Talk to your doctor about your risk for heart disease, considering your cardiovascular health and your lifestyle, and determine your target cholesterol level.

- Calculate or look up your body mass index (page 101) and determine a healthful weight for you. If you need to take off some pounds, work with your doctor or nutritionist to make a plan to help you lose weight and reduce your intake of fats and dietary cholesterol.

- Try to work in at least 30 minutes of moderate exercise every day (or at least four or five times a week); one hour per day is ideal.

- **Bile acid sequestrants (or resins).** Your liver uses cholesterol to produce bile, an acid involved in the digestive process. These drugs bind chemically to bile in the intestine, preventing the bile from being reabsorbed; the bile is subsequently eliminated from the body in the stool. Your liver responds by using more cholesterol, which is a building block of bile, to make more bile. As a result, less cholesterol is left to enter your bloodstream. Bile acid sequestrants may have side effects such as constipation, stomach bloating, upset stomach, or heartburn. Examples of bile acid sequestrants are cholestyramine, colestipol, and colesevelam.

- **Nicotinic acid (niacin).** This product is a form of vitamin B that slows the liver's production of certain components of LDL. It also can lower triglycerides and raise HDL. Possible side effects of nicotinic acid include flushing, upset stomach, a gout attack, or abnormal heart rhythms. The flushing can be reduced by taking an aspirin 30 minutes before taking the nicotinic acid. If niacin is prescribed, it should be started at low doses and increased gradually. Alcohol should not be consumed for two hours after taking niacin because of a possible increase in flushing. Episodes of flushing may be curbed with a chewable adult-dose aspirin or liquid ibuprofen (like aspirin, a nonsteroidal inflammatory product).

- **Fibric acid derivatives (or fibrates).** These drugs inhibit the production of the particles that may contain triglycerides and also stimulate enzymes that break down fats. Fibric acid derivatives may be prescribed to lower your triglycerides. They can cause side effects such as upset stomach, vomiting, gas, or headache, and they may increase the risk of gallstones. Examples of fibrates include gemfibrozil and fenofibrate.

- **Cholesterol absorption inhibitors.** This is a newer class of drugs that inhibits the uptake of cholesterol by the small intestine. Ezetimibe is the first drug developed in this category, and it can be given with any statin. Currently, the statin drug simvastatin is manufactured with ezetimibe in a combination pill. Ezetimibe is often prescribed for people with high cholesterol levels who cannot take a statin. Side effects may include stomach pain, feeling tired, or allergic reactions such as swelling in your throat. Inform your doctor promptly if these side effects occur.

You may not have any side effects at all from your medications, or you may experience some that are not mentioned here. Be sure to tell your doctor immediately if you think you might be experiencing side effects from the drugs you are taking. But don't stop taking them without checking with your doctor first; going off medication abruptly can make your condition worse. These drugs should not be used during pregnancy (with the exception of bile acid sequestrants) because the effects on developing fetuses are not yet known.

3

High Blood Pressure

Today, high blood pressure (hypertension) is probably the most modifiable common major risk factor for heart disease and stroke in the United States. About one out of every three American adults has high blood pressure, and the numbers are increasing as our country ages and becomes more overweight. High blood pressure can cause damage to the heart, blood vessels, and, over time, the kidneys.

Current findings suggest that high blood pressure is an even more widespread health problem than previously understood. Today, at age 55, even a person who does not yet have high blood pressure has about a 90 percent chance of developing it at some point in his or her life. Furthermore, recent evidence shows that the damage to arteries that leads to heart disease, stroke, and other major problems begins at blood pressure levels that doctors once considered normal. Independent of other risk factors such as high blood cholesterol level or being overweight, the higher your blood pressure, the higher your chance of heart disease or stroke.

About one third of Americans who have high blood pressure don't know it. Hypertension is often called the silent killer because by itself it does not cause symptoms, but over time it can cause stroke, heart attack, and kidney failure, any of which can be fatal. Most people who know they have the condition still do not have it under control; that is, their blood pressure levels are higher than is considered healthy.

These numbers make clear how important it is to get your blood pressure checked, and to start as early as possible to prevent or treat the development of high blood pressure. The very good news is that it's easy to be tested and treated. Even better, high blood pressure is largely preventable.

Just What Is Blood Pressure?

As your heart pumps blood through your arteries, the moving blood exerts pressure against the arterial walls. This force is measured as blood pressure. Your blood pressure rises normally in response to many everyday influences, such as exercise, caffeine, medications, or stressful situations, and then returns to a normal level. But if the pressure in your arteries is consistently higher than is healthy, your heart needs to work harder and your blood vessels and heart can become damaged.

Blood pressure is determined by the force of the heart as it contracts (systole) and the resistance of the main arteries and smaller arteries (called arterioles) to blood flow. The other force is diastole or relaxation. Healthy arterioles are muscular and highly elastic and stretch easily as blood is pumped into them. Their ready squeezing action keeps blood moving. When the heart is pumping more blood, as during exercise, many of the arterioles expand to accommodate greater blood flow. Healthy arteries are also wide open, clear of any buildup or obstruction so that blood can flow freely. Diseased arteries lose their elasticity, and pressure rises.

Measuring Blood Pressure

Because your heart pumps in pulses, your blood pressure naturally rises and falls with each surge, even when you are at rest. Blood pressure peaks when the heart's ventricles contract (the pumping or systolic phase) and falls to its lowest level after the contractions (the resting or diastolic phase). To accurately assess blood pressure, you need a reading for both phases, systolic and diastolic.

You have probably had your blood pressure measured many times—just about every time you have any kind of a physical checkup. The familiar instrument your doctor uses, the blood pressure cuff and pressure gauge, has an unfamiliar name: sphygmomanometer.

This instrument works by measuring how high the pressure in an artery in your arm can raise a column of mercury, so the measurement is expressed in millimeters of mercury (mm Hg). The reading is always expressed with the systolic (pumping) pressure on the top and the diastolic (resting) pressure on the bottom. A healthy reading in an adult is less than 120/80 mm Hg.

Healthy adults should have their blood pressure checked at least every two years. If you have not had it checked recently, make an appointment to do so soon. It is an easy, painless, and inexpensive test. You can have a reliable blood pressure check in many different settings—a hospital clinic, a nurse's office, a company clinic. You may be tempted to consult the free blood pressure testing units that you see at some drugstores or shopping malls, but you should not rely on them alone. They may not be checked regularly for accuracy, and they may suffer from wear and tear. If you try out one of these machines, record the reading and then compare it with a reading from your doctor's office.

When you know you are going to have your blood pressure checked, you can do several things to help ensure an accurate reading:

- Do not drink coffee or smoke 30 minutes before the check; both caffeine and nicotine raise your blood pressure temporarily.

- Try to arrive at your doctor's office at least 5 minutes before the check and sit comfortably, so you are not feeling hurried.

- Wear short sleeves.

Some people have a response called "white-coat hypertension," which means that their blood pressure actually rises when they are undergoing a checkup. This phenomenon is quite common. If you or your doctor thinks you may be responding this way, you can try having your blood pressure checked in another setting, or you can buy a blood pressure device to do your own reading at home (see page 55). Your doctor can compare your home and office readings to get a clearer idea of your average blood pressure.

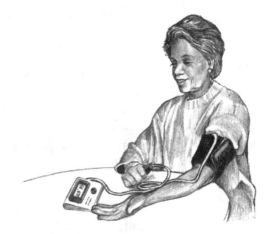

Checking your blood pressure

If you have been diagnosed with high blood pressure, your doctor will encourage you to acquire and use a device for monitoring your own blood pressure at home. This is especially important if you are taking new medications or if your drug dose has been changed.

If your doctor is concerned about your blood pressure, he or she will initially take measurements on several different days, because there are so many normal variations. It is not unusual to have a high measurement on a single day and then have it return to normal when you are tested again. Your doctor will probably not diagnose you as having high blood pressure unless your measurement is high on two or more readings taken at separate visits.

If your readings are 120/80 mm Hg or greater over several different days, your doctor will evaluate your condition in other ways. He or she will take a detailed medical history to determine if you have other risk factors for heart disease or stroke. He or she may use an instrument called an ophthalmoscope to look at the blood vessels in your eyes. This is the only place in your body where a doctor can directly look at your blood vessels to see if they are damaged. Thickened, narrowed, or burst vessels in the eyes can be another indication of high blood pressure.

If your doctor diagnoses high blood pressure, he or she may order several tests. These tests are used to determine if there is an underlying cause of high blood pressure, to detect any organ damage, to assess other risk factors for heart disease, and to identify other conditions that might affect the course of treatment.

In addition to conducting blood tests, your doctor also might order a chest X-ray (see page 128) to check the size and condition of your heart and lungs. An electrocardiogram (ECG; see page 122) may provide evidence about whether your heart is enlarged and if there is any damage to the heart muscle. It is not uncommon to have a routine ECG in the doctor's office that reveals signs of an enlarged heart or a previously unknown heart attack.

You may have blood and urine tests to determine if your kidneys are working properly or if there are any underlying problems causing the blood pressure to rise. In rare cases, people may have an intravenous pyelography, a procedure that examines kidney function by injecting a

How Blood Pressure Testing Works

The instrument used to test your blood pressure has four parts: an inflatable cuff, a pump, a pressure gauge, and a stethoscope. When you have a checkup, the tester wraps the cuff around your arm and inflates it so that the pressure in the cuff is higher than the pressure in your artery. The flow of blood is momentarily stopped and your heartbeat is inaudible through the stethoscope. As the cuff deflates, the tester checks the pressure gauge as soon as he or she hears your heartbeat again. At this moment, the pressure in the cuff is the same as the pressure in your artery, and the reading is your systolic pressure. As the cuff deflates further, the tester listens for the moment the sound of the heartbeat disappears again— when the cuff pressure goes below the resting pressure in your artery. This reading is your diastolic pressure.

harmless dye into an artery and watching its passage on an X-ray screen. A few people may need more advanced tests to evaluate blood flow, such as an MRI (magnetic resonance imaging; see page 141), a nuclear scan stress test (see page 135), or a coronary angiogram echocardiogram (see page 146).

Factors That Increase Your Risk for High Blood Pressure

The vast majority of people—90 to 95 percent—with high blood pressure have a type called essential or primary hypertension, which means that the exact cause or causes are unknown. In other people, high blood pressure may occur because of an underlying problem such as a blood vessel abnormality, kidney disease, or thyroid disease.

However, there are well-known factors that increase your risk of developing high blood pressure or tend to worsen an existing condition. If one or more of these risk factors applies to you, you are at greater risk.

You may have these factors contributing to hypertension, some of which are not within your control:

- **Gender** Men are somewhat more likely to develop high blood pressure until age 70 than women, but after age 70 women are at greater risk.
- **Race** Blacks develop high blood pressure more often than whites, and it tends to develop earlier and be more severe.
- **Family history** If your parents or siblings have high blood pressure, you are more likely to develop it.
- **Age** Generally, the likelihood that you have high blood pressure increases as you age. However, it is not a normal part of aging, and some people never develop it. Men tend to develop it after age 35. Women are more likely to have it after menopause.

Other factors are within your control:

- **Weight** As your body weight increases, your blood pressure rises.
- **Lack of exercise** An inactive lifestyle increases your likelihood of being overweight and of having high blood pressure.
- **Salt** Many people with high blood pressure are sensitive to salt; eating too much salt raises blood pressure in most people.

- **Unhealthy diet** A diet low in fruits and vegetables or high in fat increases your risk of developing high blood pressure.
- **Drinking too much alcohol** Heavy regular intake of alcohol can increase blood pressure significantly.
- **Medication** Over-the-counter decongestants and nutritional supplements may increase blood pressure. Birth control pills may also increase blood pressure in some women.

A Diagnosis of High Blood Pressure

If your doctor diagnoses you as having hypertension, your first reaction may be surprise, because you feel fine. That is not unusual. High blood pressure usually has no symptoms, and many people go for years without knowing they have it. Your heart, brain, and kidneys can handle increased pressure for a long time, and you can live for many years without any symptoms or discomfort. But getting treatment to lower your blood pressure is extremely important, because hypertension is a major risk factor for serious disease.

High blood pressure can affect your body in six main ways:

- **Atherosclerosis** Uncontrolled high blood pressure can cause the walls of the arteries to thicken and become less flexible. Fatty deposits are more likely to form on the rigid walls, and the channel in the artery narrows.
- **Stroke** If a blood clot forms and lodges in a stiffened artery traveling toward your brain, it can cause a stroke. If the clot is in an artery that supplies blood to your heart, it can cause a heart attack. High blood pressure may also cause a stroke if a weakened blood vessel ruptures.
- **Aortic aneurysm** High blood pressure contributes to the widening of a weakened aorta, and an aortic aneurysm can be fatal if untreated.
- **Enlarged heart** High blood pressure forces your heart to work harder. Over time, the muscle thickens and stiffens, or the heart muscle may enlarge and weaken. As it weakens, it pumps less efficiently, and you will feel weak and tired more often. Fluid may back up and congest the lung tissue.
- **Kidney damage** The kidneys filter waste products from the blood. If the vessels of the kidneys are thickened and damaged,

your kidneys will begin to fail, causing waste to build up in the bloodstream. Treatment for kidney failure requires dialysis, a mechanical means of filtering the blood.

- **Eye damage** If you have diabetes, high blood pressure can cause the capillaries in your eyes to bleed. This condition, called retinopathy, can eventually lead to blindness.

These potential complications of blood pressure are genuinely alarming, but remember, blood pressure can be significantly lowered with treatment. The great decreases in death from heart disease and stroke in this country in recent years are partly the result of successful treatment of high blood pressure, specifically:

- The incidence of stroke can be reduced by 35 to 50 percent.
- The incidence of heart attack can be decreased by 20 to 25 percent.
- The incidence of heart failure can be decreased by more than 50 percent.

What Your Blood Pressure Reading Means

National guidelines place your blood pressure into one of three categories: normal, prehypertensive, or hypertensive (see box on page 44). Normal blood pressure is considered to be less than 120/80 mm Hg. If your blood pressure is equal to or higher than this for two or more readings on different days, you are classified as either prehypertensive or hypertensive. The guidelines, based on the impact of high blood pressure, are aimed at getting you and your doctor started as soon as possible to bring your blood pressure down to healthy levels.

Prehypertension

If you have prehypertension (with readings consistently 120/80 or higher but below 140/90), you are in a group that used to be called high normal. Almost one-third of the U.S. adult population now falls

The Silent Disease

Some people think that high blood pressure causes symptoms such as nervousness, sweating, or difficulty sleeping. None of these is a symptom of hypertension, and these are not necessarily related. Many people who look and feel perfectly fit have high blood pressure, while some people who are overweight, smoke, or show other risk factors for heart disease have normal blood pressure. That's why the only way to know for sure if you have high blood pressure is to be tested.

A person with severe, untreated high blood pressure may have headaches, dizziness, or nosebleeds, but probably not until the condition has reached an advanced, life-threatening stage. Again, even many people with uncontrolled high blood pressure still do not have any of these symptoms. Getting tested and getting treatment are the only answers.

into the prehypertensive category. The most recent guidelines identify this range as a warning zone, because people in it are considerably more likely to develop true hypertension later in life. The designation of "prehypertension" reflects evidence showing that the risk of heart disease actually begins to climb at readings above 115/75 mm Hg. From that level, every increase of 20/10 mm Hg doubles the risk of death from heart disease. Changing to a healthy lifestyle is the only way to prevent this progression into high blood pressure.

If you are in the prehypertensive category, you have a good reason to get motivated to start managing your blood pressure immediately through nondrug treatment. Even though you do not have high blood pressure, you can start making changes in your lifestyle that will bring your readings down to a lower, healthier level without medication; see pages 46–47. Lifestyle changes alone are likely to help you at this early stage. You and your doctor can start talking about setting priorities and taking definite steps to form some new habits.

Start with your eating habits. Eat 8 or more servings of fruits and vegetables each day and less fat and saturated fat. Limit salt intake to less than 1,500 mg per day, or about ⅗ of a teaspoon of salt. If you are overweight, losing weight can be important. The benefits of weight reduction start early, with a loss of as little as 10 to 15 pounds, because with every 3 pounds you lose, there is an average corresponding drop of about 2 mm Hg in your systolic pressure. Build just 30 minutes of exercise into your schedule, at least five days a week. Limit your alcohol intake to no more than one drink per day for women and two drinks for men (whether hard liquor, wine, or beer). These changes may not seem easy at first, but they will pay big dividends if they mean you will not have to take medications.

Systolic Hypertension

The guidelines also say that systolic pressure (the top number) of more than 140 mm Hg should be treated regardless of the diastolic level (bottom number). Either your systolic or your diastolic number—or both—may be elevated. As you get older, your diastolic pressure usually decreases and the systolic pressure begins to rise.

If only your systolic reading is high and your diastolic reading is normal, you have the most common form of high blood pressure. It is called isolated systolic hypertension, and new guidelines emphasize its importance. Treating isolated systolic hypertension early, with lifestyle changes and medications if necessary, reduces the future risk of developing heart disease and stroke. For example, with each reduction of 5 mm Hg in your systolic blood pressure, death from stroke is reduced about 14 percent and from heart disease by 9 percent. The potential impact on your quality of life is enormous.

Treatment Strategies

Lifestyle changes or medication, or a combination of both, can lower your blood pressure. Lifestyle changes are recommended for everyone with elevated readings of any kind. For many people, the results of losing weight, exercising, limiting salt, and generally adopting a healthy eating plan can be as significant as the use of any single medication. Many different types of medications are available, and different drugs or drug combinations work better for some people. You and your doctor have lots of options, and your treatment will be most successful if you work together to find the treatments that work best for you.

Your doctor will help you set a target reading and determine how to reach it. Do not hesitate to tell your doctor as much as you can about your eating, smoking, and drinking habits; whether you exercise regularly; or what other medications or supplements you take. The more you understand about the factors that contribute to your high blood pressure reading, the more likely you are to bring it down.

Your doctor will approach your treatment by considering three factors: the blood pressure reading itself; whether there is already some damage to your arteries or other organs; and whether you have other conditions, such as diabetes, that might affect your treatment. If you are still in the prehypertensive category and have no other complications, you may be able to bring your blood pressure down to less than 120/80 mm Hg in a year just by changing your lifestyle (see below).

If you have stage 1 or stage 2 hypertension without organ damage or complicating conditions, the goal will be to bring your reading down to a prehypertensive level. Doctors have found that many people will need to take more than one medication to reach their target blood pressure. If you are at stage 1, lifestyle changes are an essential first step. If lifestyle changes fail to achieve your target blood pressure, your doctor may subsequently prescribe a diuretic and maybe other drugs as well (see page 59). If you are in stage 2 hypertension (a reading of 160/100 mm Hg or higher) without complications, you will almost certainly need to take more than one drug, one of which will probably be a diuretic, to achieve good blood pressure control. But continue making lifestyle modifications—improvements in your diet and exercise habits—while taking the medications.

If you have high blood pressure (stage 1 or stage 2), and you have another condition—for instance, you have already had a heart attack, you are at high risk for developing coronary artery disease (see page 211), or you have kidney disease or diabetes—your doctor will prescribe medications that have proven to be beneficial for your conditions. Of course, a healthier lifestyle is a must as well. With these conditions, achieving a blood pressure goal as low as 130/80 mm Hg may be the wisest course.

Warning: Be alert for any signs of stroke. These include headache, confusion, weakness, numbness, difficulty speaking, slurred speech, or weakness on one side of the body. If you have any of these signs, seek emergency treatment at a hospital promptly.

No matter what your blood pressure reading, personal medical situation, history, or treatment plan, sticking to the treatment is the only way to reach your goal. That goal starts with a number, but it is much more than that.

Prevention: A Healthier Lifestyle

By now you've gotten the picture: preventing your blood pressure from creeping up, or bringing it down to a desirable level, always begins with healthy choices in many areas of your life. The benefits are by no means limited to your blood pressure alone; they also improve your heart health, reduce your chances of stroke and kidney disease, and give you an overall sense of well-being. No matter how many predisposing factors for high blood pressure apply to you—being male, being black, having hypertension in your family, being older—you can reduce your blood pressure somewhat with changes in lifestyle. These are the areas to work on:

- Start eating a low-fat, low-salt diet such as the DASH diet (see below).
- Lose weight if you are overweight.
- Exercise regularly.
- Drink alcohol in moderation.
- If you smoke, quit.
- Learn to manage stress.
- Do not take over-the-counter medications that can raise blood pressure, including decongestants or "energy products."

The DASH Diet

The National Heart, Lung, and Blood Institute (part of the National Institutes of Health) has developed a comprehensive eating plan called the DASH (Dietary Approaches to Stop Hypertension) diet. The DASH diet is low in saturated fat, cholesterol, total fat, and sodium. It emphasizes fruits, vegetables, and low-fat dairy foods; it includes whole grain products, fish, poultry, and nuts; and it recommends less red meat and fewer sweets. Major studies have demonstrated that the DASH plan works better than other heart-healthy eating plans to help most people reduce their blood pressure. Most people who stick to the plan for a month can significantly lower their blood pressure, and the effect lasts as long as you stay on the plan. The DASH plan also works for people with normal blood pressure who are trying to prevent an increase. In any case, along with following the DASH diet you should make or continue modifications to your lifestyle, including exercising and stopping smoking.

Following the DASH diet may enable some people to go without medication, or to use fewer medications than they otherwise would. However, do not discontinue any medication or lower the dose without talking to your doctor first.

The DASH plan is two-pronged, involving the eating plan itself and lowering sodium intake as a means of treating hypertension. The diet can be adapted to different levels of sodium intake, depending on a person's individual sensitivity to salt. The reduction of blood pressure is greatest at the lowest level (1,500 mg or less of dietary sodium per day).

In many instances, diets or eating plans are based on the ideas or theories of one or two people, sometimes doctors but not always. In the case of the DASH diet, you can be assured the benefits of the DASH eating plan were proven in two research studies funded by the federal government and conducted in several cities.

The DASH diet coupled with sodium reduction is a remarkable approach for treatment of high blood pressure for many reasons:

- It works for a wide variety of people—those with or without high blood pressure, old and young, men and women, blacks and other races, obese or slender, active or inactive.

Following the DASH Plan

The abbreviated DASH eating plan shown here gives you an idea of what types of foods are recommended and in what amounts. This plan is based on 2,000 calories per day. Servings can be adjusted depending on your calorie needs and your desired level of sodium intake. You and your doctor can tailor a plan to suit you.

Food Group	Daily Servings	Serving Sizes
Grains and grain products	7–8	1 slice bread; 1 ounce dry cereal; ½ cup cooked rice, pasta, or cereal
Vegetables	4–5	1 cup raw or ½ cup cooked; 6 ounces vegetable juice
Fruits	4–5	1 medium fruit; 6 ounces juice; ¼ cup dried
Low-fat or fat-free dairy	2–3	8 ounces milk; 1 cup yogurt; 1½ ounces cheese
Meats, poultry, fish	2 or fewer	3 ounces cooked
Dry beans and nuts	4–5/week	⅓ cup nuts; ½ cup cooked dry beans or peas
Fats and oils	2–3	1 teaspoon soft margarine; 2 tablespoons light salad dressing; 1 teaspoon vegetable oil
Sweets	5/week	1 tablespoon sugar; 1 tablespoon jelly; 8 ounces lemonade

Adapted from the National Heart, Lung, and Blood Institute.

Cutting Back on Salt and Sodium

Small amounts of sodium occur naturally in fresh foods, but most processed foods are high in sodium content. Most is added in manufacturing and processing. Most restaurants add a lot of salt to foods they prepare. The only way to know for sure is to check the nutrition label carefully. You can cut back on sodium substantially by remembering a few general tips:

- Start by eliminating your use of table salt; an herbal salt substitute—available in a variety of flavors—is often helpful.

- Learn to use spices instead of salt. Flavor your food with herbs, spices, lemon or lime juice, vinegar, or salt-free seasoning blends.

- When you buy vegetables, choose fresh or frozen without sauce instead of sauced or canned.

- Rinse canned foods, such as beans or tuna, to remove some of the sodium.

- Always choose low-salt or no-salt products when you can.

- Buy fresh poultry, fish, and lean meat rather than canned, smoked, or processed forms.

- Limit cured foods (such as bacon or ham), foods in brine (such as pickles, olives, and sauerkraut), and condiments (such as MSG, mustard, ketchup, and barbecue sauce). Limit even low-sodium versions of soy sauce or teriyaki sauce (which contain lots of MSG); measure them as you would table salt.

- Cook rice, pasta, and hot cereals without salt. Cut back on flavored rice, grain, or pasta mixes; they are loaded with salt.

- Rely less on frozen dinners; canned soups, broths, and sauces; and bottled salad dressings. You can make a large quantity of something like tomato sauce using a low-salt recipe, and freeze it in smaller amounts for later use. You can make simple vinegar-and-oil salad dressings in small quantities to use for a few days.

- Most restaurants add a lot of salt to the foods they prepare. When you eat in a restaurant, ask which items can be prepared without adding salt. Ask if other spices can be used.

- The diet is more effective in lowering blood pressure than other heart-healthy diets, and the low-sodium version is even more effective than other low-sodium diets.

- The plan works quickly, lowering blood pressure readings in as little as 2 to 4 weeks.

- In addition to its effectiveness at lowering blood pressure, it also lowers blood cholesterol levels, another important factor in prevention of heart disease (see page 23).

The DASH eating plan is especially rich in fresh fruits and vegetables (eight or more ½-cup servings per day) in part because these foods are low in salt. They are also rich in potassium, calcium, and magnesium. Grains and grain products are another major component of the diet (seven to eight servings per day) because they supply energy and fiber. The plan limits the amount of meat, sweets, and sugary drinks in order to reduce intake of fats and sugars, as well as sodium. The plan teaches you to sharply reduce your salt intake by avoiding processed foods, which are the source of most of the salt that Americans eat.

If you are on the DASH plan, as with any other diet, the foods that you eat at one meal or over the course of a day may add up to more than the recommended servings. You also might consume more sodium on one day than on another. The important point is that your average for several days or a week should be close to the recommended amounts in order to derive the health benefit.

You also need to keep in mind that if your doctor has prescribed medication for your high blood pressure, you should not stop taking it. If you feel that following the DASH diet (or another diet plan) may have lowered your blood pressure, have your blood pressure checked at your doctor's office and discuss the numbers with him or her.

Managing Your Weight

One of the most important things you can do to control your blood pressure—and prevent heart disease—is to keep your weight at a healthy level. If you are overweight, you are more than twice as likely to develop high blood pressure than if you maintain a healthy weight. Even if you are only 10 pounds more than you should be, taking off that little bit of extra weight can significantly lower your blood pressure. Your weight interacts with other factors, such as cholesterol levels and risk of diabetes, to affect your overall cardiovascular health in more complicated ways (see pages 99–104). But the relationship between your weight and high blood pressure is relatively easy to understand.

As you gain weight, you put on mostly fatty tissue. Like any other tissue in your body, fat requires oxygen and nutrients to live. As your fatty tissue increases, the amount of blood circulating through your body also must increase. You retain more sodium and water, which increase your blood volume, and a larger volume of blood causes greater pressure against your arterial walls. When you take off weight, those negative effects are reversed, and your blood pressure comes down to a healthier level. (For more about heart-healthy weight control, see pages 83–98.)

Healthful Eating Habits

Limiting sodium and following a healthful diet that is low in fat helps prevent or control hypertension, even in people of normal weight. Potassium helps protect against high blood pressure, in part by enhancing the excretion of salt. This nutrient occurs in certain foods, especially fruits and vegetables. If you take potassium in supplements, you will not derive the same benefit that you get from consuming it in your diet. Most people get enough potassium through eating foods that contain it; the exception is those on diuretic drugs, who may need to take supplements.

Your intake of sodium (salt) in foods is a critical factor in controlling blood pressure. Too much salt causes you to retain water, thereby increasing blood volume and blood pressure. Although sodium is an essential mineral, health experts recommend that a person consume less than 2,400 milligrams (mg, or 2.4 g) per day, which is only about 1 teaspoon of table salt. That includes all salt contained in foods, as well as the salt you add while you are cooking or at the table. A typical American diet often includes about 4,000 mg (4 g) of salt—far more than a person needs. To control high blood pressure, or if you are over 50 or black, limit daily sodium intake to 1,500 mg or less.

All animal products, such as meat and dairy products, contain sodium. Processed and restaurant foods are notoriously high in sodium; to see a clear example of that, check the nutrition label on a can of soup or a bottle of ketchup. You can consume significant quantities of salt without ever picking up a salt shaker. Three-fourths of the salt that people in the United States consume comes from processed or restaurant food. By contrast, fresh fruits, vegetables, and grains have little or no sodium unless you add it.

What Is Salt Sensitivity?

In most people, the body regulates salt concentration carefully, and any excess salt will be eliminated in the urine or in perspiration. But for many people, eating too much salt causes their blood pressure to rise, a condition known as salt sensitivity.

For reasons that are not clear, some groups of people are more likely to be salt-sensitive than others. For example, as many as 70 percent of black people are salt-sensitive. Older people are also more likely to react this way. Almost half the people with high blood pressure are salt-sensitive, which is why salt reduction is such a prominent part of treatment. There is no way to test for salt sensitivity except to eat less salt for a while to see if your blood pressure goes down. The cumulative effects of a high-salt diet eventually raise blood pressure in most people.

Exercise Regularly

Being physically active is a great way to help manage your blood pressure and benefit your overall health in many other ways at the same time. During aerobic exercise, the heart works harder and pumps more blood to supply oxygen to the hard-working muscles. You might think that this action would increase blood pressure over time. But the increase in heart output is accompanied by widening of the blood vessels that supply the muscles, substantially reducing the resistance to blood flow. Regular exercise actually increases the number of capillaries that supply muscle tissue, further reducing resistance. Your heart, arteries, and lungs become more fit, helping to protect you against heart disease.

Also, exercise is the essential calorie-burning partner to sensible dieting as a means of controlling your weight. A moderate exercise program combined with a healthful diet will make it much easier to lose that extra ten pounds (or more), which can significantly lower your blood pressure. The benefits of exercise do not stop there: physical activity helps protect against not only high blood pressure, but also against heart disease, diabetes, stroke, and cancer. Plus, exercise lifts your mood, protects against osteoporosis, and helps you manage stress, so it enables you to work toward several of your goals at once.

You do not need to become an athlete. Aerobic exercise (which means exercise that causes the body to use oxygen to fuel the muscles) includes a broad range of activities such as walking, bicycling, climbing stairs, social dancing, and gardening. In order to get the cardiovascular benefits, you should aim for exercising 20 to 30 minutes at a time at least 5 days a week; recent government recommendations advise 1 hour a day if you are overweight. Most people can start a moderate exercise plan without consulting their doctors. If you are already moderately active, you will get greater benefit from exercising longer or more often, or choosing a more vigorous form of activity. If you are not sure how to get started, try a simple walking program. Set aside time 5 days a week or more to walk around your neighborhood, take a lunchtime break from work, or go to a gym or a shopping mall.

- **Week 1.** Walk slowly for 5 minutes to warm up your muscles, walk briskly for 5 minutes to get your heart working, then walk slowly for 5 minutes to cool down.
- **Week 2.** Do 5 minutes of warm-up walking, increase your brisk walking to 7 minutes, then cool down for 5 minutes.

- **Week 3 and beyond.** Walk slowly for 5 minutes, then increase your brisk walking by 2 minutes each week until you are up to 30 minutes or more, followed by 5 minutes of slower walking.

Many people can start their exercise program more intensively, walking 20 minutes briskly, rather than 5 minutes, in week 1, then increasing that baseline of 20 for weeks 2 and 3. However, if you are over 50 and have not been physically active, if you have already had a heart attack, or if you have a family history of heart disease, talk to your doctor before increasing your level of activity. If you have heart disease already, your doctor might use a stress test to assess your capacity to exercise and to individualize your exercise program.

Even if you do not engage in formal exercise or set aside a special time for walking, you can increase your fitness by becoming more active in your daily life. Examples include walking rather than driving short distances, parking far away from a store or mall entrance, and walking up one flight or down two flights of stairs. Purchase and use a pedometer to measure how many steps you walk every day, and gradually increase your activity until you walk at least 10,000 steps per day.

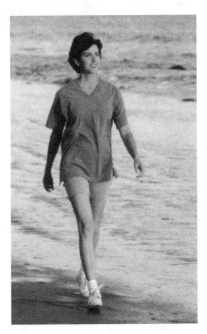

Exercise to control blood pressure
Exercise helps control blood pressure in several ways: it actually helps widen blood vessels, it helps control your weight by burning calories, and it helps you deal with stress.

Quitting Smoking

Tobacco smoke contains literally thousands of substances that, alone or in combination, damage your health in many ways. In addition to damaging your lungs, smoking does harm throughout your cardiovascular system. It does not directly cause persistent high blood pressure, but it temporarily raises your blood pressure by constricting the diameter of the arteries to your heart, depriving your heart muscle of blood and oxygen. Every time you smoke a cigarette, your blood pressure goes up for about 30 minutes. A pack-a-day habit keeps your blood pressure up for 10 hours.

Exposure to tobacco smoke over time damages the protective lining of your artery walls, making them more susceptible to the formation of plaque. Plaque narrows the arteries and interferes with blood flow to your heart, your brain, and the rest of your body. Smoking also causes

Aids to Help You Stop Smoking

Stopping smoking is very hard work, but there are many aids to help you quit and improve your health and life expectancy. Nicotine replacement products are very popular; these include the nicotine patch, gum, lozenges, and nasal spray. These products are effective for many, but if you already have high blood pressure, nicotine products can raise your blood pressure and so should be used only with the advice of your doctor. Bupropion is a prescription medication that increases the likelihood a smoker will successfully quit.

Many people have quit successfully with the help of antismoking group therapy or classes, often available at a local hospital or community college. Antismoking telephone hotlines can also be helpful. Others find that regular exercise helps relieve stress and reduce the temptation to light up a cigarette. Meditation techniques may help alleviate feelings of nervousness; hypnosis and biofeedback have also been effective with some people. For those—usually women—who say they smoke for weight control (that is, to avoid consuming candy or other fattening treats), keep a supply of carrot sticks and celery sticks on hand for snacking.

your blood to clot more easily, for reasons that are not fully understood. The clots more easily adhere to the inner surfaces of arteries roughened by plaque. Smoking also decreases the good cholesterol in your blood; see "Managing Your Cholesterol Level," page 23.

Smokeless tobacco products are not the way out. Although it is difficult to give up any tobacco habit, the enormous health benefits make it worth it. So if you smoke, quit. (For tips on aids to help you stop smoking, see the box above.) If you do not smoke now, do not even think about starting.

Managing Stress

Though stress does not cause high blood pressure, it can keep your blood pressure up when you are upset. The body normally responds to stress with the so-called fight-or-flight response, which prepares the body either to meet challenges or to avoid them. A temporary increase in heart rate and blood pressure is a part of this physiological response, and it is stronger in some individuals than in others. Although stress is somewhat difficult to measure, research demonstrates some general findings:

- In some individuals, blood pressure spikes in response to stressful situations, and these people are at greater risk of developing high blood pressure.
- Some people cope with stress in unhealthy ways, such as overeating, smoking, or drinking alcohol, which become contributing factors to high blood pressure.

You may not be able to alter your body's unconscious response to stress, and you cannot always avoid stressful situations, but you can learn relaxation techniques or coping activities like physical exercise that will help modify the harm to your health. You can also talk to your doctor about the level of stress in your life as one of the factors involved in your high blood pressure (see pages 113–115).

Limiting Alcohol Consumption

Over time, heavy drinking increases your chances of developing high blood pressure. It also contributes to the development of heart disease in other ways. If you are taking hypertension medications such as beta-blockers, alcohol may interfere with their action. If you have high blood pressure, talk to your doctor specifically about how alcohol in large quantities affects your blood pressure. In moderation, drinking has beneficial effects and is associated with lower risk of developing heart disease. Moderation generally means up to two drinks a day for men or one drink a day for women (see pages 97–98), whether each drink is a glass of wine, a beer, or a mixed drink.

Home Monitoring

Your doctor may ask you to start taking your blood pressure at home and recording it. Doing so will give both you and your doctor a more complete understanding of how much your blood pressure varies during the day, and how well your medication is working to control your condition. It also eliminates the "white-coat hypertension" factor (see page 39), which can complicate the process of diagnosis. Self-measurement is never a substitute for having your blood pressure checked by a health-care professional; it complements and confirms the measurements taken at your doctor's office. If there is a large discrepancy between readings at home and in the doctor's office, bring in your home blood pressure monitor for your doctor or nurse to check for you.

You will need to purchase a blood pressure monitor (see below) that you feel comfortable using at home. You can find a selection of these devices at any pharmacy or medical supply store. You may wish to learn more about them by reading a consumer review magazine, and your doctor can help you decide which one will work best for you. You can choose between two basic types: a digital monitor or an aneroid monitor.

Digital Monitors

A digital, or automatic, monitor is the most popular blood pressure measuring device because it is easy to use. The gauge and the stethoscope are in one unit, the digital screen is easy to read, and the deflation is automatic. You can choose between an automatic or a manual inflation device. The chance of human error is much less than it is when using an aneroid monitor. To use a digital monitor, follow these steps:

1. Place the cuff around your upper arm. Turn on the machine.
2. Push the button to activate the inflation device, or squeeze the hand bulb on a semiautomatic model. After the cuff is inflated, the instrument will automatically start to deflate.
3. Look at the digital screen to see your reading. Both your systolic and diastolic measurements will appear. Write the numbers down, with the systolic reading over the diastolic reading.
4. Press the exhaust button to fully deflate the cuff.
5. If you want to repeat the measurement, wait 2 or 3 minutes.

A drawback of the digital monitor is that it is highly sensitive, and body movements or an irregular heartbeat can affect its accuracy. Be careful about the placement of your arm and application of the cuff. The device requires batteries and needs factory repair or readjustment when problems arise. Digital monitors are somewhat more expensive than aneroid devices, depending on what model you choose. A fully automatic model may be twice the cost of an aneroid device, and the most expensive ones can be several hundred dollars.

Aneroid Monitors

An aneroid, sometimes called a spring gauge, monitor is relatively inexpensive, lightweight, and portable. (Aneroid means "containing no liquid.") Some cuffs have a built-in stethoscope, which is easy to work with. The gauge has a round dial that indicates the amount of pressure in the cuff, and you can read it easily in just about any position, as long as you are looking directly at it. Some models have a large, easy-to-read gauge, a cuff with a ring closure for one-handed use, and a deflation valve that works automatically. To use an aneroid monitor, follow these steps:

1. Put the earpieces for the stethoscope into your ears, with the earpieces facing forward.

2. Extend your arm at about the level of your heart on a table or a chair arm, and wrap the cuff snugly around your upper arm, with the lower edge of the cuff about an inch above your elbow. Place the dial where you can see it clearly.

3. Place the stethoscope disk on the inner side of your elbow crease (over the pulse).

4. Rapidly inflate the cuff by squeezing the rubber hand bulb to a reading 20 or 30 points above your last systolic (top) measurement. (Inflating the cuff a little at a time gives an inaccurate reading.) When you stop pumping, you will not hear any pulse sound because the cuff is temporarily stopping the flow of blood through your artery.

5. Deflate the cuff slowly (about 2 or 3 mm Hg per second on the dial). Keep your eye on the dial and listen carefully for the first sound of the blood flow returning. Write down the number the pointer is on; that is your systolic blood pressure.

6. Continue deflating the cuff. Listen until you no longer hear your heartbeat, and note the reading. This number is your diastolic blood pressure.

7. Record the numbers with the systolic reading over the diastolic reading (for example, 140/80).

8. If you want to repeat the procedure to confirm your reading, wait 2 or 3 minutes before you reinflate the cuff.

There are some disadvantages to using an aneroid monitor. It is a fairly delicate, complex device that can be easily damaged. You will need to have it checked for accuracy at your doctor's office or pharmacy at least once a year, or if you drop it or bump it. If it is damaged, it will need factory repair. It may be difficult to use if your hearing or sight is impaired, or if you have difficulty squeezing the hand bulb.

Other Types of Monitors

You may see mercury monitors, which are considered the standard for blood pressure measurement. The mechanism is simple and works by gravity, giving consistent, accurate readings. However, a mercury monitor is generally not recommended for home use because of the danger of mercury spills. The device has a long glass or plastic mercury tube that must be carefully protected against breakage. The device is bulky and must be kept upright, and the gauge must be read at eye level. It is difficult to use if you have a hearing or vision impairment.

You may see finger or wrist monitors that look convenient. These devices are not very accurate, however. They are highly sensitive to position and body temperature and are usually significantly more expensive than other types of monitors.

You can also buy portable devices that continuously monitor and record your blood pressure day and night. For some people, this method is the most effective way to get a clear picture of blood pressure variances and the effect of medications. Your doctor will tell you whether you require this type of monitoring.

Home Monitoring Tips

You may need some practice, but before long, taking your own blood pressure will be easy. Here are a few suggestions to get started on your monitoring at home:

- Wait half an hour after drinking a cup of coffee or smoking a cigarette. Either of these can temporarily raise your blood pressure.

- Sit comfortably with your feet flat on the floor and your back supported. Relax quietly for approximately 5 minutes before taking a reading.

- Rest your arm on a table or the arm of a chair. Let your arm muscles relax.

- Wrap the cuff smoothly around your bare arm. It should fit snugly, but you should be able to slip one finger under it. The bottom edge of the cuff should be about 1 inch above the crease in your elbow.

- Record the date, time of day, and your measurements, with the systolic reading over the diastolic reading. Use a small notebook to keep your readings orderly and easy to refer to.

- Do not be alarmed at a single high reading. Your blood pressure normally varies throughout the day. It may be higher if you are worried about something. If you have a high reading, take several more readings the next day to see if your blood pressure is persistently elevated, before calling your doctor.

- Store your monitor in a place where you can easily find it.

Take your time making your choice about what kind of home monitor to buy. Talk to your doctor about which kind is most suitable for you. As you shop, consider these features:

- **Cuff size.** Cuffs come in different sizes—including children's models—and the right size is very important for accurate measurement. Your doctor's office or pharmacy can tell you what size you will need. If you need a size that is not standard, it can be ordered for you.
- **Readable numbers.** Be sure that the numbers on the gauge are easy for you to read.
- **Cost.** Do not assume that the most expensive is the best. You have many models to choose from and a wide price range. The most important consideration is accuracy.
- **Care and storage.** Some models may require storage in a certain position, protection from bumps, or protection from heat.

After you have bought a device, take it to your doctor's office and have it tested for accuracy. Ask a health-care professional to show you exactly how to use it and what to do if you get an elevated reading. Find out how to get your device checked and recalibrated periodically.

Medications for High Blood Pressure

In addition to lifestyle changes, many people with high blood pressure must take at least one medication or a combination of drugs to keep their blood pressure at a healthy level. These drugs, called antihypertensives, are highly effective and are an extremely important factor in reducing your risk of stroke, heart disease, and other major diseases related to high blood pressure. Many different types of drugs and combinations of drugs have been developed, so you and your doctor can work together to find the ones that will successfully control your blood pressure with the fewest possible side effects. Although antihypertensives are powerful drugs, they have fewer unpleasant side effects today than ever before.

If you have not been taking medications until now, and especially if you feel fine, you may not look forward to the idea of taking drugs that may have side effects and may be expensive. It could take some time to tailor your drug regimen to your needs, but do not get discouraged. Tell your doctor as much as you can about how the drugs make you feel. If you experience side effects, your doctor will probably substitute another medication that does not have the same effect on your body. Some people are able to reduce their need for medication if they can bring their blood pressure down and maintain it for a year or more, particularly if they lose weight as needed and adopt a healthier lifestyle generally. But you usually cannot stop treatment altogether. If the cost of your drugs is a problem, talk to your doctor about that, too. There may be lower-priced alternatives.

Once you start taking prescription medications, do not stop or change your regimen without talking to your doctor first. Even if the medicine is working and your blood pressure goes down, you need to continue taking the drug in order to get the benefit. If you hear about a new drug or you talk to someone who is taking something different from what you are taking, talk it over with your doctor. Everyone responds differently to these medications and has a different medical history, so not every drug will be right for you. The most important goal is to get your blood pressure to a healthy level and keep it there for the rest of your life. Make sure to take your medication every day, even if you feel fine; if you have forgotten a dose, look at the patient information sheet that comes with your prescription to determine if you should take a "catch-up" dose or if it is preferable to wait till the next dose is due.

There are eight major categories of antihypertensive medications, each with a different mechanism of action in your body. Within these eight categories, individual drugs have generic names and a brand name registered to a particular pharmaceutical company. Whatever the category of medication, taking medication may lead to a decrease of up to 10 percent in your systolic blood pressure and 5 percent in your diastolic blood pressure. Many of these drugs are also prescribed for heart disease, so you can find more information about them on pages 165–173 and 241–246. Here is a summary of the broad categories and their method of action:

- **Diuretics** rid your body of excess fluids and sodium through urination, lessening the volume of blood that your heart has to pump. Your treatment will almost certainly begin with a diuretic, alone or in combination with another medication. Diuretics are sometimes also used to enhance the blood-pressure-lowering effects of other drugs. Common examples include amiloride, bumetanide, chlorothiazide, chlorthalidone, hydrochlorothiazide, indapamide, metalozone, and spironolactone. The adverse effects of diuretics may include urinary frequency and low potassium levels.

- **Angiotensin-converting enzyme (ACE) inhibitors** lower the levels of angiotensin, a chemical in your body that constricts your blood vessels, so your vessels expand, reducing resistance to blood flow, and allowing your heart to pump more efficiently. Examples include benazepril, captopril, enalapril maleate, and lisinopril. ACE inhibitors should not be used in pregnancy. They have a low incidence of side effects compared to other medications for high blood pressure. The most common side effect is a cough, which develops in 5 to 15 percent of cases. Rarely, people will have swelling in the face, a potentially dangerous side effect that means you should discontinue the drug immediately. However, talk to your doctor promptly to report your reaction and get another prescription.

- **Angiotensin-2 receptor blockers** inhibit the effect of angiotensin (rather than lowering the level), so they too prevent angiotensin's effects on your heart and vessels. They are often prescribed for people who cannot take ACE inhibitors. Examples include losartan, candesartan, and valsartan. Side effects may include nausea or a headache.

- **Alpha-blockers** prevent your arteries from constricting and block the effects of the stress hormone epinephrine, which elevates blood pressure. These drugs are no longer highly recommended but are prescribed occasionally. Examples include doxazosin, prazosin, and terazosin. The major side effect is dizziness.

- **Beta-blockers** (see illustration on page 62) decrease your heart rate and cardiac output, which lowers your blood pressure. Examples include atenolol, metoprolol, and propranolol. Beta-blockers are commonly used to treat angina and are good choices for people with coronary artery disease and hypertension. Fatigue is a common side effect.

- **Calcium channel blockers** inhibit the movement of calcium into your heart and blood vessels, which relaxes the muscles in the arterial wall that constrict the artery, preventing the narrowing of the artery. Examples include diltiazem, amlodipine, and verapamil. Side effects include leg swelling and constipation.

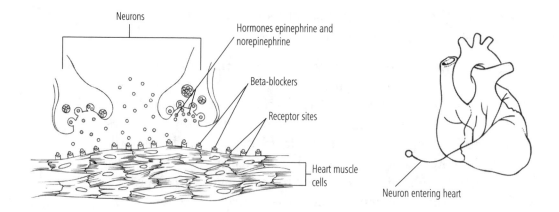

Neurons

Hormones epinephrine and norepinephrine

Beta-blockers

Receptor sites

Heart muscle cells

Neuron entering heart

Beta-blocker action

Beta-blocker drugs, often prescribed for hypertension, work by blocking the effects of epinephrine and norepinephrine—hormones that stimulate heart muscle cells and cause a more rapid heart rate. The drugs occupy receptor sites on the muscle cells to interfere with the hormones, preventing the increase in heart rate and lowering the force of heart contractions. Both the heart rate and the strength of the contractions are controlled by neurons that carry nerve signals from the brain to the heart (see figure at right).

- **Centrally acting drugs (or central alpha agonists)** act on the brain and the nervous system to lower your heart rate and prevent the arteries from narrowing but are rarely used now. Examples include clonidine, guanfacine, and methyldopa. Clonidine is unique in that in addition to being available in oral form, it is available in a skin patch, which is applied once a week. Side effects of centrally acting drugs include sedation, dizziness, dry mouth, and fatigue.

- **Vasodilators** cause the muscular walls of the blood vessels to relax so that the vessels can dilate (widen). These drugs are used only in emergencies or for people whose blood pressure cannot be controlled with other drugs. Examples are hydralazine and minoxidil. Minoxidil may cause you to retain fluids, so it should be used in combination with diuretics, which will help remove fluid from your system.

The more familiar you are with your drug program, the easier it will be to talk to your doctor about it and take the medications correctly so that they work as they should. Here are some important points to know about your high blood pressure medication or that of a family member whom you are assisting:

- The name of the medication
- What it does in your body
- How often to take it and how much to take
- What time of day to take it
- What food, drink, or other medications you should avoid while taking it
- How to store it (is it sensitive to heat or dampness?)
- What reactions or side effects might occur and what to do if you get them
- What to do if you miss a dose
- Specific side effects if you are a woman and you become pregnant
- When you need to refill your prescription so you do not run out.

High Blood Pressure in Special Groups

Although high blood pressure is a common disease among all Americans, some groups are at higher risk, for reasons that are not fully understood. People in some racial or ethnic groups are more likely to develop high blood pressure. Some people are at higher risk because of other diseases, such as diabetes. Often these factors are interrelated; for instance, diabetes occurs frequently in people who are overweight, people with diabetes often have high blood pressure, and overweight is a contributing factor in high blood pressure. Metabolic syndrome—also called insulin resistance syndrome—is a constellation of related factors such as obesity, high cholesterol levels, diabetes, and high blood pressure. The point is to know the factors that put you at risk for high blood pressure and then to take steps to bring your blood pressure under control.

Black Americans

No one knows why, but black men and women are more likely to develop high blood pressure than white Americans. It often develops at a younger age, and it tends to be more severe. As a result, blacks are also more likely than whites to develop hypertension-related health problems such as an enlarged heart, retinopathy (damage to the blood vessels in the eye), heart disease, kidney disease, and stroke. The solution to these disproportionate common health problems is awareness and treatment:

- If you are black, it is especially important to have your blood pressure checked regularly. If it is elevated, you and your doctor can begin treatment immediately.

- A healthy lifestyle will go a long way to prevent and control your high blood pressure and reduce your risk of serious problems. Understanding that you are in a high-risk group is good motivation to, for instance, start building eight or nine ½-cup servings of fruits or vegetables per day into your diet.

Women

Almost half the 65 million Americans with high blood pressure are women. The disease is more common among black and Hispanic women than in any other group. As a woman grows older, her chance of having high blood pressure becomes greater than a man's. A woman may have had normal blood pressure throughout her life, but after menopause, she is considerably more likely to develop hypertension.

A woman's reproductive life may also affect her blood pressure. In some women, using birth control pills or becoming pregnant can raise blood pressure. Here are some considerations to keep in mind:

- If you have high blood pressure and you are pregnant or considering pregnancy, work with your doctor to control your blood pressure before and during the pregnancy. Many women with high blood pressure have healthy babies, but prenatal health care is especially important. If you are on medications for high blood pressure, talk to your doctor about whether you should be taking them while you are pregnant. Some blood pressure medications such as ACE inhibitors should not be used during pregnancy. However, do not stop taking the medications without consulting your doctor first.

- High blood pressure during pregnancy (called gestational hypertension) occurs in about 6 to 8 percent of pregnancies. It is more common among women with chronic hypertension or diabetes. Gestational hypertension can lead to a condition called preeclampsia, which can be life-threatening to both the mother and the fetus.

- If you have had gestational hypertension or preeclampsia during a pregnancy at some time in your life, you may be at higher risk for developing high blood pressure or other cardiovascular problems later in life. Your doctor should know about this part of your medical history.

- Blood pressure usually does not increase significantly as a result of hormone therapy for menopause in most women, with or without high blood pressure. However, hormone therapy can increase blood pressure in some women, so if you need to take hormone therapy for menopausal symptoms, your doctor will want to check your blood pressure initially and then monitor your blood pressure regularly. Also, using oral contraceptives may cause blood pressure to rise.

- Even if high blood pressure has never been a problem for you, take extra care to monitor yourself after menopause. Get your blood pressure checked regularly.

- Every woman can reduce her risk of developing high blood pressure, or help control high blood pressure, by eating more healthfully, being physically active, and drinking in moderation. High blood pressure is a highly preventable condition.

People with Diabetes

Diabetes, a condition in which your body cannot make or respond properly to the hormone insulin, is occurring at an ever-increasing rate among Americans. Research suggests that, for reasons that are not completely understood, as many as 60 million Americans may have a condition called insulin resistance—an inadequate response to their own insulin—that greatly increases their chances of developing diabetes and heart disease at some time in their lives. Many authorities attribute the increase in the number of individuals with insulin resistance to lifestyle changes in the population, particularly weight gain and lack of exercise. The most common cause of diabetes-related death is cardiovascular disease, but many people are unaware of this link.

Secondary High Blood Pressure

About 5 to 10 percent of people diagnosed with high blood pressure have secondary hypertension, meaning that their condition is a secondary result of another problem. These underlying problems may include a kidney abnormality, a structural abnormality of the aorta, a narrowing of certain arteries, or certain types of hormone abnormalities. These secondary causes of high blood pressure are more common in children and young adults.

These problems can usually be corrected, causing blood pressure levels to drop to healthy levels. For example, a surgeon can repair a narrowed or defective artery.

When your doctor examines you, he or she can usually rule out these problems as causes of high blood pressure by taking a careful medical history, giving a thorough physical examination, taking blood tests, performing urinalysis, and taking some further tests. These tests generally do not require a hospital stay.

Diabetes has a hereditary component, and people who have family members with diabetes are at greater risk for developing the disease. More women are affected than men, and black, Hispanic, and Native American people are especially susceptible. People with diabetes often have high blood pressure, high cholesterol, or both, which increases their likelihood of developing heart disease still further.

People with diabetes are classified by whether they produce sufficient amounts of insulin. A person with type 1 diabetes does not produce any and must take insulin as a medication. Most people with diabetes (more than 90 percent) have type 2, meaning that they produce insulin (a hormone that changes glucose, or "blood sugar," into energy), but their bodies are resistant to insulin's action, and they do not utilize it properly. As a result the body cannot transfer sufficient amounts of energy from food to body cells. Because the cells are not taking in glucose, it builds up in the blood, leading to "high blood sugar" (hyperglycemia), or diabetes.

If you have type 2 diabetes, the changes in your body's chemistry brought on by high glucose levels can increase the buildup of fatty deposits inside the arteries (atherosclerosis; see page 152), which can impede blood flow. These changes can also make the blood clot more easily, which can lead to a heart attack or a stroke. High blood pressure and high blood cholesterol combined with diabetes make the risk for heart attack or stroke greater than the risk from either one. The bottom line is that if you have diabetes you can greatly reduce your chances of cardiovascular disease by bringing down your blood pressure or cholesterol as needed.

Awareness of these links is the place to start to improve your health. By working with your doctor to control your high blood pressure, you can help reduce the risk of complications from diabetes. Controlling your blood pressure and cholesterol levels is likely to prolong your life and greatly improve its quality.

Children

Even babies and children can have high blood pressure. Doctors used to think that high blood pressure in children was secondary (caused by some other condition). But now they know that children can have primary hypertension—that is, high blood pressure—for unknown reasons. The condition may be hereditary. It is more frequent and severe in black families, although scientists do not know why.

Living with High Blood Pressure

If you are being treated for prehypertension or hypertension, you can monitor your own health in several important ways:

- Be your own best advocate. Stay with your treatment plan—healthy lifestyle habits and medication—to get the best results.

- Know your blood pressure and have it checked regularly. Those already being treated for high blood pressure should have theirs checked more frequently; ask your doctor how often. Make sure that your family members (parents, brothers and sisters, children) have theirs checked regularly, too.

- Keep appointments with your doctor so that he or she can monitor your treatment and make adjustments if necessary. Ask your doctor or other health-care provider any questions that interest or concern you about your treatment.

- Follow a healthful diet, cutting down on fatty foods such as red meat and increasing your intake of fruits and vegetables and whole grains; also, exercise 5 times a week (or, more ideally, every day).

- Keep track of your blood pressure. Remember, you cannot tell from the way you feel how high your blood pressure might be.

- Keep a diary of your blood pressure reading every time you measure it at home, or have it checked by a health-care professional. Record the date and the reading. Find a handy place to keep the diary. Bring your diary to your doctor's appointment.

- Talk to your doctor about the names and dosages of your blood pressure medications and how to take them. Don't hesitate to ask questions. Again, keep a written record that you can refer to and show to family members. Keep a written list of your medications, including dosages, in your purse or wallet.

- If you notice any problems (side effects) that you think could be related to your medications, talk to your doctor about them. The problems may not be related to your medicine. Or you may need a change in dose, or perhaps another medicine might work for you without side effects.

- Refill your blood pressure medications before they run out, even though you feel fine.

- Tell your family members that you have high blood pressure and get their support for your treatment plan. If possible, have your partner or a family member go with you to your doctor's office to hear firsthand about your medications and how to make lifestyle changes.

- If you have a severe headache, changes in your vision, numbness on one side, or dizziness, seek emergency medical treatment immediately. You could be having a stroke.

- Have your eyes checked periodically by a qualified physician such as an ophthalmologist.

The average blood pressure level for children and teenagers has risen considerably over the past 25 years, mainly because of the increase in overweight and obesity. Today, guidelines for blood pressure in children include a prehypertension category, just as adult guidelines do. Like adults, children can have a syndrome of risk factors—including overweight, high blood pressure, and insulin resistance—that increases their risk of diabetes and heart disease.

Treatment for children with high blood pressure usually involves the same types of lifestyle changes that benefit adults: weight control, a healthful diet, and regular exercise. Doctors will prescribe medications if necessary. Ensuring that a child has a healthy weight and blood pressure early in life gives him or her a head start on preventing serious disease later on.

4

Quitting Smoking

The reasons to quit smoking are legion. In terms of your cardiovascular health, quitting smoking is a major way you can take control of your risk of coronary artery disease and other heart and blood vessel diseases. Briefly, these are the ways in which tobacco smoke endangers your cardiovascular system:

- **Atherosclerosis.** Smoking damages the lining of the arteries that supply your heart, brain, and the rest of your body with blood. The roughened, damaged walls are more susceptible to the formation of plaque. As the plaque forms, it restricts the flow of blood, a process called atherosclerosis. If your coronary arteries are affected, it dramatically increases your chances of a heart attack. If the arteries to your brain are blocked, you may have a stroke. Atherosclerosis is also a risk factor for developing peripheral artery disease, which affects the arteries to your arms and legs. In combination with other factors (high blood pressure, high cholesterol), it is even more dangerous (see page 71). Smoking even one cigarette a day can harm the endothelium, or inner lining of your blood vessels.

- **Blood clots.** Smoking causes your blood to clot more easily. Smoking encourages the formation of blood clots by causing platelets to stick together, which is often part of the cascade of events leading to a heart attack and stroke. A blood clot can block an artery and lead to heart attack, stroke, or peripheral artery disease. Some scientists think the blood-clotting effect of smoking is even more important than its role in inducing atherosclerosis.

- **High cholesterol.** Tobacco smoke decreases HDL cholesterol, or good cholesterol.
- **High blood pressure.** Although smoking does not directly cause high blood pressure, it temporarily constricts the diameter of the blood vessels to your heart.
- **Constriction of arteries.** Apart from the blockages within arteries caused by atherosclerosis, smoking causes your arteries to constrict, reducing blood flow.
- **Less oxygen in your blood.** The nicotine and carbon monoxide in smoke get into your blood and reduce the amount of oxygen it can carry. This effect causes your heart to beat faster in order to try to keep the oxygen supply adequate.
- **Family health.** A recent report by the Surgeon General confirmed that secondhand smoke in any amount carries health risks to those who live with smokers. The report summarized major research on how secondhand smoke can cause cancer, respiratory problems, and cardiovascular disease. To maintain or improve the health of your partner, children, or other people you live with, stop smoking now.

These harmful effects all interact to harm your heart and blood vessels. In addition, of course, smoking damages your lungs and increases your risk of developing cancers of the lung, throat, stomach, and bladder, and several other cancers.

How to Kick the Smoking Habit

Making a decision to quit smoking may be the smartest thing you ever do, but it is the beginning of a difficult process. You will find reams of materials to help you quit, backed by extensive scientific knowledge about how nicotine works in your body, why it's so hard to stop smoking, and what it takes to improve your chances of kicking the habit for good. But it's still up to you to do the work. Keeping at it even after several relapses is part of the challenge. The effects of nicotine addiction in your brain positively reinforce smoking (making you feel relaxed, less stressed, and more alert), and negatively reinforce not quitting smoking (by reversing all those positive sensations).

Making the decision to quit is the first step, and your doctor can help. Take some time at your next appointment to specifically discuss your smoking habits and what you may need to make quitting easier. Your doctor can counsel you as an individual, provide you with nicotine replacement therapy or other medication if you wish (see the warning on page 73), and offer effective ways to deal with nicotine cravings and relapses.

Preparing to quit is the second phase. You will need the support of family and friends. Identify the situations that tempt you to smoke (like drinking alcohol), and figure out ways to avoid them or handle them. Make plans to incorporate exercise as a means of helping you quit; you will have to address concerns like possible weight gain. You may wish to enroll in a structured smoking cessation program or consider working with a trained smoking cessation counselor. Ask your doctor to recommend one in your area. Also ask about smoking hotlines that provide telephone counseling to help you quit and resist the urge to relapse. Many states and large health-care plans offer these services, which are an effective way to give you the ongoing support you need to make this major change.

Stop Smoking: It's Worth It!

If you are a smoker, you've heard plenty about the damage you are doing to your body. If you have already had a heart attack or you have several other risk factors for heart disease, you are under even more pressure to quit. Among all the negative messages, here are a few encouraging words about the rewards of quitting smoking:

- One year after quitting, your risk of developing heart disease as a result of your smoking is cut in half.

- This reduction also applies to your risk of stroke: in 5 to 15 years, your stroke risk will be that of a nonsmoker.

- You'll live longer. Quitting before age 40 will add an average of 3 to 5 years to your life expectancy. Quitting at age 65 or more adds a year.

- If you're trying to quit, you're in good company. Four out of five smokers say they want to quit, and many thousands of people succeed every year and stay off tobacco for a year or more.

- When you stop smoking, your family—especially your partner and/or your children—and your friends will be healthier as well as you, because they won't be exposed to secondhand smoke.

- You will save money if you quit. Assume you smoke a pack a day at an average cost of $4. That totals up to about $1,500 a year or about $60,000 over a period of 40 years. Certainly you could use that extra money for your children's education, your retirement, health care, or other major expenses.

Once you have resolved to quit, you and your doctor can probably agree on a "quit date." Although some people try to taper off gradually, it's best to stop smoking altogether by going cold turkey on your quit date. If you are using nicotine replacement products or another drug, that treatment will begin on or maybe before your quit date.

Nicotine Replacement Products

Nicotine replacement products, including patches, gum, nasal sprays, and inhalers, can be a valuable part of your overall strategy to stop smoking. They do not work perfectly, but they are a valuable aid in reducing the symptoms of nicotine withdrawal while you learn to adjust to living without cigarettes. These products are closely regulated by the U.S. Food and Drug Administration, and they are safe and effective for most people when used as directed (see the warning on page 73). They work by delivering a safer form of nicotine (the addictive component of cigarette smoke) without any of the cancer-causing and otherwise harmful substances. They may also desensitize nicotine receptors in your brain to reduce the satisfaction from smoking.

Used properly, nicotine replacement products at least double your chances of success, and they are especially successful when used with other smoking cessation support methods, like telephone counseling or a formalized program. You still have to change your behavior in order to kick your dependence on nicotine, but the drugs substitute for a cigarette in the meantime. They are available in several forms and can be used individually or in combination. Always talk to your doctor or other health-care provider about how to use these products safely and for maximum effect. If you experience unpleasant side effects, report them to your doctor.

Patches

If you choose to use nicotine patches, you wear a patch every day for 6 to 8 weeks. The patches are easy to use; you can put one on under your clothes and leave it there all day without any other effort on your part. The patch delivers a low dose of nicotine for 16 to 24 hours, starting 4 to 6 hours after you put the patch on. The patches are available in different doses so that you can taper off gradually. The most annoying side effect is a rash on the patch application site in some people. Other side effects include dizziness, nausea, and increased blood pressure. If you use a patch and are scheduled for an MRI (magnetic resonance imaging) procedure, tell your doctor or technician about the patch. Remove the patch at home the morning of the test, unless instructed otherwise, to prevent burns (the radiofrequency waves used in MRIs heat the patch to a dangerous degree). Do not smoke while wearing a patch; this is dangerous.

Gum

Nicotine gum delivers nicotine through the mucous membranes in your mouth. It acts on your system in 20 to 30 minutes. Starting on your quit date, you will chew 10 or 15 pieces of the gum each day for about 3 months. You will have to learn the "chew-and-park" system in order for it to be effective: you chew the gum slowly until you get a distinctive taste or tingle in your mouth, and then "park" it between your gum and your cheek for a full 30 to 60 seconds. You repeat this chew-and-park cycle, without drinking any beverages, for about half an hour for each piece of gum. Some people get a sore jaw, hiccups, or nausea. These effects are usually mild.

Nasal Sprays

A nasal spray is a fast-acting nicotine delivery system. Starting on your quit date, you use the spray one or two times an hour, and if you get an urge to smoke, up to no more than five times an hour. You generally continue using the spray for about 3 months, tapering off gradually. Some people experience nose and throat irritations, which usually disappear after the first week or so of use.

Inhalers

A nicotine inhaler, available by prescription, is a plastic cylinder with a nicotine capsule inside. You place the device in your mouth and suck in nicotine vapor that is absorbed into the mucous membranes in your mouth. Some people like the inhaler because using it mimics some aspects of puffing on a cigarette. You need to puff on the device four or five times a minute for as long as 20 minutes to deliver an effective dose of nicotine. You will use the device 6 to 16 times a day for about 3 months, and then taper off for about another 3 months. Some people get slight mouth or throat irritations.

> **WARNING!**
>
> **Nicotine Replacement and Heart Disease**
>
> If you have certain types of heart problems such as irregular heartbeat or chest pain, nicotine replacement drugs may not be right for you. Although these products are safe for most people with heart disease, your doctor will evaluate your risk. Most of the products are over-the-counter drugs; don't start using them without checking with your doctor first.

Lozenges

The lozenge is a promising form of nicotine replacement. It is quick-acting and easy to use, because you just let it dissolve in your mouth without biting or chewing. You can use it similarly to nicotine gum.

You may use a combination of a slow-release product like the patch and one of the quick-release products like the gum, sprays, or inhalers to help you through the nicotine withdrawal process. There is no one product or combination of products that has proven to be more effective for long-term success. Talk to your doctor about how to manage your smoking cessation medications and how to bolster their effectiveness with counseling and support.

Drugs

A drug called bupropion hydrochloride, which contains no nicotine, is approved by the Food and Drug Administration for smoking cessation. It is a form of antidepressant that increases the level of a substance called dopamine in your brain, just as nicotine does. Bupropion may be appropriate for any smoker trying to quit, but it may be especially attractive to people who have tried nicotine replacement without success or who do not wish to use nicotine in any form. It may also help lessen weight gain after smoking cessation. If you use bupropion, you start about a week before your official quit date and continue for 2 to 3 months. Side effects in some people include dry mouth, sleep difficulties, and nausea, which tend to disappear over time. The drug may not be safe for people who have or have had a seizure disorder, brain injury, or eating disorders. You will need to thoroughly discuss your medical history before taking this drug (or any other); for safety's sake do not take bupropion prescribed for someone else.

Varenicline, a relatively new drug, works to block the action of nicotine in the body by blocking receptor sites on cell membranes. In a major research study, people who took varenicline were much more likely to give up smoking in a 12-week period than those who took a placebo (sugar pill) or bupropion. People who took varenicline in the study reported a reduced craving for nicotine and fewer other withdrawal symptoms than those taking a placebo. However, side effects of varenicline include nausea, headache, and insomnia.

5

Exercise and Physical Activity

Americans know exercise is good for them. A proliferation of health clubs and fitness centers, joggers in every park and walkers in every shopping mall, and constantly changing fashion trends in exercise gear are all evidence that we've gotten the message. Ironically, at the same time, advances in technology and labor-saving devices (along with other factors) have made us more sedentary and more overweight.

A sedentary lifestyle is hard on your entire body—muscles, bones, heart, lungs, arteries—because your body is a physical system that is built to move. In terms of cardiovascular benefit, exercise first strengthens your heart muscle and makes it pump blood more efficiently. In your bloodstream, it reduces harmful triglycerides, increases good HDL cholesterol, and improves the proportion of HDL to the bad LDL cholesterol. This effect is so important that being physically inactive is a major risk factor—just like smoking, high blood pressure, or high cholesterol levels—for developing coronary artery disease. It doubles your chances of having a heart attack.

At the same time, exercise tends to lower your blood pressure and reduce elevated blood sugar levels if you have diabetes, both of which in turn reduce your risk of heart disease. Of course, exercise also helps you control your weight and reduce obesity. So when you exercise, you are working on your high blood cholesterol, high blood pressure, or diabetes. You are less likely to develop these problems if you are active. Even a moderate increase in physical activity—30 minutes or more of brisk walking most days of the week—is enough to have a significant positive effect on your heart and blood vessels. Exercise can benefit you, no matter how old you are or what your current fitness level is.

Exercise also helps you modify the effects of some other factors that are harmful to heart health. It reduces stress, anxiety, and depression and their toll on your body. If you smoke, being active can make it easier to cut down or quit. Exercise never takes the place of other lifestyle changes you need to make to control as many of your risk factors as you can (quitting smoking, eating more healthfully, and so on). However, a major research study in *JAMA*, the *Journal of the American Medical Association*, showed that overweight women who exercised had a longer life expectancy than overweight women who were not physically active.

Types of Exercise

There are three categories of exercise: cardiovascular, strength-building, and flexibility. All three types condition your body and improve its performance in different ways. A well-balanced pattern of exercise that includes all three types will make you feel the best. Cardiovascular exercise is aerobic, which means that it makes your heart and lungs work harder because your muscles demand more oxygen. Strength and flexibility exercises do not have the cardiovascular effect of increasing your heart rate, but they make your muscles and bones stronger. Strength exercise, such as using weights or doing some floor exercises, requires short, intense effort that builds muscles. Flexibility exercise tones your muscles by stretching them and can prevent muscle and joint problems later in life.

Cardiovascular, or aerobic, activity usually involves continuous exercise of the large muscles in your arms and legs, such as brisk walking, jogging, or dancing. This form of exercise increases your heart's ability to pump blood and opens the blood vessels in your muscles. As your body responds to this conditioning by becoming more efficient, your heart rate actually goes down, both at rest and during moderate exercise. Your endurance improves; you are able to exercise more before becoming tired.

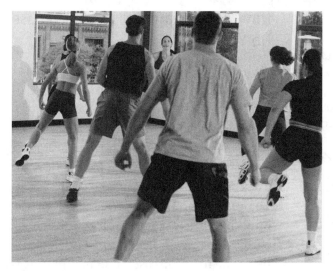

Exercise classes

Formal exercise classes are a good option for people who need help scheduling exercise time and enjoy a supportive group atmosphere. Be sure to select a class geared toward your particular fitness level. If you're not sure how vigorously you can exercise, check with your doctor before signing up for class.

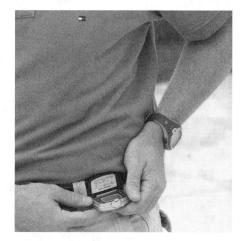

Using a pedometer

A pedometer is a small device that you wear on your belt or waistband that senses body motion and counts your footsteps. Doctors suggest setting a goal of from 2,000 to 10,000 steps per day depending on your physical condition. (Walking 2,000 steps is the equivalent of walking one mile so 10,000 steps is about five miles.)

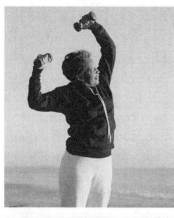

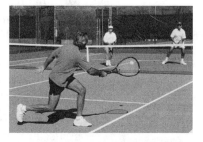

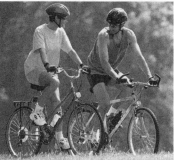

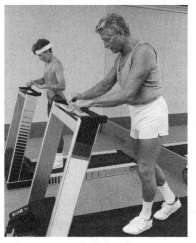

Varying types of exercise

Cardiovascular, strength-building, and flexibility are three forms of exercise that condition the body in different ways. Cardiovascular, also known as aerobic, exercises include tennis (top, right), walking or running on a treadmill (bottom, right), and riding a bicycle (bottom, left). All of these activities have the cardiovascular effect of increasing your heart rate and making your lungs work harder. Tennis is not only a cardiovascular exercise, but also a particularly good exercise to maintain flexibility. The woman stretching with small weights (top, left) is engaging in two kinds of exercise: strengthening exercise for her arm muscles and flexibility exercises for her torso and limbs.

How Much Cardiovascular Exercise Do You Need?

To promote cardiovascular benefit for most people, about 30 minutes a day of moderate to vigorous aerobic activity most days of the week is a good start; the latest recommendations, however, suggest that you work your way up to 1 hour of exercise per day if you are overweight. You can accumulate the total in 10- or 15-minute sessions if you want to, but check with your doctor if you are under treatment for heart disease. The main point is to make exercise a regular part of your lifestyle. Try to burn about 1,000 to 2,000 calories per week (see page 81). To get a sense of an effective exercise pattern, you can think in terms of the so-called FIT formula: frequency (days per week); intensity (how hard—moderate or vigorous) or percentage of heart rate; and time (amount of time in each session or day). You can adjust these elements to suit your schedule, just as long as you expend enough energy to accomplish your fitness goals. For instance, you can make a point of taking a longer walk three times a week and a shorter jog two times a week.

Frequency of exercise sessions and time spent in each session are easy to understand, even if it seems hard to find the time to exercise.

If you cannot exercise every day, try to plan your sessions on nonconsecutive days of the week. If you are breaking up your time into shorter sessions, don't forget to warm up and cool down briefly for each session. If your activity is more vigorous, the cool-downs and warm-ups are especially important.

Intensity can be as simple as identifying moderate-level activities that fit most naturally into your lifestyle, and then consciously sticking with them. A moderate activity raises your heart rate to at least 50 percent of its maximum (see box on page 78). A more practical definition of cardiovascular exercise might be any activity that raises your heartbeat to a level where you can still talk, but you start to sweat a little and breathe more heavily. If you have heart disease and your exercise is being planned with medical supervision, your peak heart rate achieved during exercise stress testing is a safe goal. But ask your doctor about this.

Examples of moderately active pastimes are:

- Brisk walking (3 to 4 mph)
- Gardening or yard work
- Active housework, such as vacuuming
- Swimming
- Tennis
- Golf, if you don't use a cart
- Dancing

More physically demanding forms of exercise, done regularly, raise your heart rate to 50 to 85 percent of the maximum and are especially beneficial:

- Aerobics classes
- Jogging or running
- Bicycling
- Games such as racquetball or basketball
- Cross-country skiing
- Handball

Exercise and Weight Loss

If you need to lose weight, you and your doctor or registered nutritionist can design a healthy diet plan, which will involve determining a level of calorie intake that is appropriate for you—but one that contains at least 1,200 calories per day. Your exercise plan should ensure that you burn more calories than you consume. The healthiest and most effective way to lose weight is to limit the energy consumed in food, and then increase the amount of energy burned off by exercise, to achieve a slow but steady weight loss. Most experts recommend losing 1 to 2 pounds per week.

To lose 1 pound in 1 week, you need to burn about 3,500 excess calories; that is, you need to burn about 500 calories more per day than you consume. Dieters are plagued by the plateau phenomenon. When you achieve about a 10 percent weight loss, your body compensates by slowing your metabolism. It is important to keep exercising and not get discouraged during this time.

Exercise as a Part of Every Day

Your plans to exercise more are much more likely to succeed if you think of exercise as a pleasure rather than an obligation. It is important to choose activities that you enjoy and then find ways to make them easier to do often. Here are some tips to keep you going:

- Develop a variety of physical activities that you can choose from so that you don't get bored. In addition to a walking routine, alternate sessions of some goal-oriented activity like gardening or a more intensive activity like bicycling to keep you interested.
- Find a friend or family member to exercise with you. You'll both enjoy the sociability and both get the physical benefits. Wear comfortable, appropriate clothing when you work out, including shoes that fit properly and suit your activity.
- Listen to music or watch television to keep yourself entertained.
- Avoid overdoing it. You don't need to be an athlete, and you don't need to exhaust yourself. Start with low-level or moderate

Where Do I Start?

If you are inactive, any level of activity is a start in the right direction. A basic walking plan that increases your level of exercise gradually is an excellent beginning (see page 81). The key is to start slowly and build up; the goal is not to start a program quickly that you will need to stop; it is to develop a lifetime habit of regular exercise. The benefits of being more active far outweigh any risks for most people. Talk to your doctor before starting to exercise more if:

- You have ever had any kind of a heart problem, especially a heart attack.
- You have a family history of premature coronary artery disease.

- You have diabetes.
- You have problems with your bones or joints, such as osteoporosis or arthritis.
- You have high blood pressure and are not on medication.
- You are very overweight.
- You have high levels of cholesterol in your blood.
- You smoke.
- You are over 60 and you are not accustomed to any regular exercise.

Physical Activity and Calorie Use

The following chart shows the approximate calories spent per hour by a 100-, 150-, and a 200-pound person doing a particular activity.

Sample Body Weights

Activity	100 Pounds	150 Pounds	200 Pounds
Bicycling, 6 mph	160	240	320
Jogging, 7 mph	610	915	1,220
Jumping rope	500	750	1,000
Running			
5.5 mph	440	660	962
10 mph	850	1,275	1,700
Swimming			
25 yds/min	185	277	370
50 yds/min	325	500	650
Tennis, singles	265	400	535
Walking			
2 mph	160	240	320
3 mph	210	315	416
4.5 mph	295	442	590

Adapted by the American Medical Association from the American Heart Association Web site www.americanheart.org.

exercise, then gradually increase the intensity and the time you spend, until you are up to a half hour or a full hour per day, most days.

- Look for ways to make your daily activities more physical. Do your own housework or yard work instead of hiring someone. Walk to the store instead of driving. Choose the long, hilly route instead of the shortcut.

You can also get more active in small ways that may not increase your heart rate but will burn up energy throughout the day. Instead of looking for ways to save effort, be imaginative about making yourself more active, whether you are at home, at the office, or on vacation. Here are a few tips to get you started, but you can think of dozens more:

- Stop using the TV remote. And if you want a drink while you're watching TV, don't ask someone else to get it for you—get up and walk to the kitchen.

- Stand up and walk around while you talk on the phone. If you are waiting at a train station or airport, walk around instead of sitting.

- In a parking lot, choose a space farther away from the store instead of the one closest. Or park several blocks from your destination and make a round trip to and from your errand.

- Take every opportunity to climb stairs, at home or in public. Take the stairs instead of an elevator or an escalator.

- Participate in charity events that require you to walk or play a sport.

- When you're traveling, take advantage of a hotel swimming pool or exercise room. Also, schedule a walking tour of a new city, rather than driving around.

- Consider buying exercise equipment like a stationary bicycle and use it while you listen to music or books on tape or watch TV.

- Make sure you are getting exercise during recreational time— walk instead of using a golf cart, rent a rowboat or a canoe instead of a motorboat, or play singles tennis instead of doubles.

- Purchase a pedometer, and walk with a goal of 10,000 steps a day. Every 2,000 steps equal about a mile.

Exercising if You Are Older or Disabled

If vigorous activities are not an option for you because of advanced age or physical disabilities, some daily exercise will still bring health benefits. If you can walk, garden, or swim, gradually increase to longer sessions to get more benefit without overdoing it. Some sports like table tennis, croquet, or shuffleboard are excellent ways to get moving. If you are in a wheelchair, you can spend 30 to 40 minutes a day doing arm exercises or actively using the chair to get some good exercise. If possible, join a class that offers a modified exercise plan that suits your ability. Such classes may be available through a senior citizen center, a retirement community, a hospital, or a YMCA.

6

Eating Healthfully for a Lifetime

Of all the advancements made in our understanding of heart disease and how to prevent it, perhaps the greatest is the clear, consistent link between healthful eating habits, coupled with regular exercise, and the prevention of heart problems. By following some fairly simple guidelines about how to eat healthfully, you can substantially improve your overall heart health and reduce your risk of developing high blood pressure, high blood cholesterol, and overweight or obesity, three of the major contributors to cardiovascular disease. The benefits don't stop there; very similar dietary habits also help you prevent breast, prostate, and other cancers; control type 2 diabetes; avoid osteoporosis (bone loss); and perhaps lengthen your life. For an excellent diet plan to improve your health, see the information on the DASH diet, pages 47–50.

As you start eating more healthfully, you will probably get the most satisfaction from the immediate benefits: you'll have more energy and you'll shed excess pounds. Today, eating better is also easier and more enjoyable because a delicious variety of fresh, good-for-you foods are more widely available for more seasons of the year than ever before.

Of course, there is also no shortage of diet advice, nutritional claims for specific food products, and conflicting headlines about the value—or the hazards—of certain foods. Don't let fads or eye-catching news stories distract you from a commonsense approach to your diet.

Eating Plan for Healthy Americans

The American Heart Association has designed these guidelines to help you reduce your risk of cardiovascular disease. Following this plan will improve your overall condition if you already show signs of heart and blood vessel problems, or even if you are currently enjoying good health. These are general guidelines; see also the DASH diet, pages 47–50.

- Eat a variety of fruits and vegetables (nine or more servings per day).
- Eat a variety of grain products, including whole grains (six or more servings per day).
- Include fat-free and low-fat milk products, fish, legumes (dried peas or beans), skinless poultry, and lean meats.
- Choose fats and oils with 2 grams or less of saturated fat per tablespoon and no trans fats, such as liquid and tub margarines, olive oil, and canola oil.
- Balance the number of calories you eat with the number you use each day. To arrive at that number, multiply the number of pounds you weigh now by 15 calories. This represents the number of calories you burn in one day if you are moderately active. If you exercise very little, multiply your weight by 13 instead of 15.
- Exercise to stay fit and to burn the number of calories you eat. Walk or exercise actively in some other way at least 30 minutes on most days of the week; one hour a day or more is considered optimal.
- Limit your intake of snacks, soft drinks, or candy that are high in calories.
- Eliminate foods high in saturated fat or trans fat, such as full-fat milk products, fatty meats, tropical oils, and partially hydrogenated vegetable oils. Instead, substitute more foods from the first four categories listed in the first column of this box.
- Trim your salt consumption.
- Drink alcohol in moderation, if at all. That's one drink a day if you are a woman or two drinks a day if you are a man. One drink is 12 ounces of beer, 4 ounces of wine, 1½ ounces of 80-proof spirits, or 1 ounce of 100-proof spirits.

You'll do better if you don't think about *dieting*, but about developing new ways of eating for the long term.

If you are trying to accomplish a specific goal, like lowering your blood pressure or your cholesterol levels, your doctor may work with you to develop an eating plan designed to help you achieve your target. But for those of you working on an overall heart-healthy eating pattern, the American Heart Association has developed a set of general guidelines to help you change your current habits for the better and maintain a healthy pattern throughout your life; see the box above.

Fruits and Vegetables

The good news just keeps pouring in about the healthy benefits of fruits and vegetables in your diet, especially for your heart. Fruits and vegetables are the best source of vitamins, minerals, and fiber. They have few calories and no cholesterol, and are low in fat and sodium. You can fill up on them at meals and snack on them in between. Generally, the most colorful fruits and vegetables are the most loaded with vitamins, including antioxidant vitamins.

Antioxidant vitamins are so called because they may slow down the process of oxidation in your arteries—a chemical process that enables cells in your artery walls to more easily absorb fatty acids and LDL cholesterol. As a result, antioxidant vitamins may reduce the accumulation of plaque in the arteries that can lead to atherosclerosis and stroke. The major antioxidant vitamins are vitamin E (found in vegetable oils, wheat germ, and nuts), vitamin C (found in green and red peppers, broccoli, spinach, tomatoes, potatoes, and citrus fruits), and carotenoids (found in yellow, dark green, and red vegetables and fruits). It is important to know that taking vitamin supplements does not have the beneficial effects of a balanced diet.

Any fruits and vegetables you choose are a healthy addition to your diet. Some major research shows that

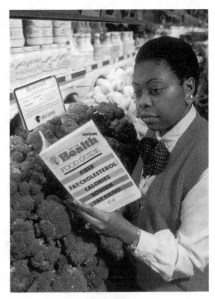

Eat your vegetables!
The produce department of your grocery store is loaded with vegetables and fruits that are naturally low in fat and cholesterol and packed with healthful nutrients and vegetable proteins. Eating a wide variety of produce is the best way to get adequate amounts of fiber and of vitamins A, C, and E, which help protect your heart.

Daily Servings of Fruits and Vegetables

Eat at least eight servings a day of fruits and vegetables—more is even better. Choose from all fruits and vegetables except coconut, which contains harmful tropical oils. Consider olives and avocados as fats (see page 90). Starchy vegetables such as potatoes are included in the category of grains and grain products (see page 86).

Examples of serving sizes:

- One medium piece of fruit
- ½ cup chopped, cooked, or canned fruit
- ¾ cup (6 ounces) fruit juice
- ¼ cup dried fruit
- ½ cup cooked or raw vegetables
- 1 cup raw leafy greens
- ¾ cup (6 ounces) vegetable juice

fruits and green, leafy vegetables (spinach, kale, collards) are especially associated with a reduced risk of developing heart disease.

Grains and Grain Products

Grains, grain products such as breads, and starchy vegetables are rich in complex carbohydrates, which provide you with energy. They also contain vitamins, minerals, and fiber. Contrary to what many people believe, they are also usually relatively low in fat and calories. If you are eating less fat and sugars (also a type of carbohydrate), you can healthfully fill up on grains. There are two important points to remember: choose whole grain products, and watch out for added fat, calories, and sodium in the preparation or processing of these foods.

Whole grains are healthier than refined grains because they retain the germ (the nutrient-rich core of the grain) and the bran (the outer layer of the grain, containing nutrients and most of the fiber). If you are unsure about whether a product is whole grain, check the label for the term "whole wheat" or "whole grain" as the first item in the ingredients list. Choose whole grain breads, English muffins, bagels, and breadsticks; whole grain pastas; and brown rice. Limit white rice, white bread, and egg noodles.

It's easy to consume hidden or not-so-hidden calories in the way you prepare foods or the way they are processed. Of course, limit high-fat and sweetened products such as croissants, sweetened cereal, crackers, and potato chips. (Unsalted pretzels and plain popcorn are better snack substitutes.) When you are cooking at home, cut back on butter and cheese and use seasonings liberally to boost flavor. Check sodium levels carefully if you use boxed grain mixes.

The fiber in foods comes in two forms: soluble (meaning that the fiber is partially broken down in your intestine) or insoluble (the fiber passes through your system without being broken down). Both types of fiber are part of a healthy diet. Soluble fiber is found in oat bran, oatmeal, beans, peas, citrus fruits, and apple pulp; it helps lower cholesterol. Insoluble fiber, found in whole wheat breads and cereals, cabbage, beets, carrots, cauliflower, and apple skin, encourages good bowel function but does not lower cholesterol.

Daily Servings of Grains and Grain Products

Eat six or more servings per day, preferably whole grain breads, cereals, pasta, and rice.
Examples of serving sizes:

- 1 slice bread
- 1 cup cereal flakes
- ¼ cup nugget or bud cereal
- ½ cup hot cereal
- ½ cup cooked rice or pasta
- ¼–½ cup starchy vegetables (potatoes, beets, corn)

Fat-free and Low-fat Milk Products

Dairy products provide you with protein, calcium, and nutrients including phosphorus, niacin, riboflavin, and vitamins A and D. Right now, the impact of calcium on the risk of heart disease is not entirely clear, but people who do not consume much calcium tend to have higher blood pressure, so dietitians recommend getting plenty of calcium from foods (1,000 milligrams per day for adults below the age of 50; 1,200 milligrams per day over 50). Fat-free or low-fat (½ percent or 1 percent) dairy products contain slightly more nutrients than whole or 2 percent milk but are much lower in fat, saturated fat, cholesterol, sodium, and calories. If you have difficulty giving up whole milk (3½ or 4 percent fat), try decreasing gradually to get accustomed to the difference.

> ### Daily Servings of Dairy Products
>
> Eat three or more servings a day if you are 19 to 50 years old, four servings if you are 51 or older, and three or four servings if you are a woman who is pregnant or breast-feeding.
>
> Examples of serving sizes:
>
> - 1 cup fat-free or low-fat (½–1 percent) milk
> - 1 cup fat-free or low-fat yogurt
> - 1½ ounces low-fat fresh cheese (such as cheddar or Swiss)
> - 2 ounces processed cheese (such as American)
> - ½ cup low-fat cottage cheese

For those who eat cheese, choose natural or processed cheeses with no more than 3 grams of fat per ounce and no more than 2 grams of saturated fats per ounce. Part-skim cheeses such as mozzarella are popular with those watching calories and fat content. If you like ice cream as a dessert, choose instead sherbet or sorbet, low-fat yogurt, low-fat ice cream, or low-fat pudding.

Meat, Poultry, and Fish

Eating relatively small portions of meat, poultry, or fish will still provide you with adequate amounts of protein, B vitamins, and iron. The trick is to limit your portion sizes and think of meats as a side dish or garnish rather than as the centerpiece of your meal. Try mixing small amounts of meats with pasta, rice, or vegetables for a filling entrée.

When you shop for meats, look for cuts with little or no visible fat. Choose "choice" or "select" rather than "prime" cuts of beef. Lean veal, lamb (leg or loin), and pork (tenderloin or loin chop) are good choices. Lean ham is a good choice, although cured ham and Canadian bacon are higher in sodium than other meats. Most ground meats today are clearly labeled with the percentage of fat; look for lean or

Eat no more than two servings (6 ounces total) of cooked lean meat, poultry, or fish per day. Choose fish two or more times a week.

Examples of serving sizes (3 ounces):

- A piece of beef the size of a deck of cards
- A hamburger 3 inches across and ½ inch thick
- Half a chicken breast
- A chicken leg and thigh without skin
- ¾ cup flaked fish

extra lean, with no more than 15 percent fat. Organ meats such as liver are high in cholesterol but are iron-rich. You can enjoy small portions of these meats once or twice a month. When you prepare meat, make sure that you trim off visible fat before cooking, and cook without adding fat: broil, roast, grill, or stir-fry with a little olive oil.

Poultry meats (chicken, turkey, Cornish hens) are low in fat if you take off the skin before you cook them. Ground turkey is low in fat; check the label for the percentage of fat in ground chicken. Low-fat processed sandwich meats (low-fat chicken or turkey, turkey ham, lean boiled ham) are available now, but check sodium levels on the label.

Fish, particularly oily fish, is an excellent source of protein but does not contain the saturated fats found in other meats. The recommended two servings a week are a minimum—eating fish and shellfish more frequently helps you lower your dietary fat and cholesterol. Choosing fish and seafood may be confusing at first because of some precautions about the health benefits of certain types. Here are a few key points:

- Oily or fatty fish are particularly good for you because they have high levels of omega-3 fatty acids (see box on page 89). Oily fish include mackerel, lake trout, herring, sardines, albacore tuna, and salmon.

- Swordfish, king mackerel, shark, and tilefish may contain undesirable levels of mercury, while farm-raised fish contain environmental contaminants. Exposure to mercury is a concern especially for children and for pregnant and nursing women. For the general population, however, the benefits of eating fish far outweigh the hazards. Eating a variety of fish reduces your risk of adverse effects caused by levels of mercury or other contaminants.

- Although some shellfish (such as shrimp and crayfish) are higher in cholesterol than most fish, they are lower in saturated fat and total fat than meats and poultry, so they are still a heart-healthy choice.

Q. I know that omega-3 fatty acids are supposed to be good for my heart, but why?

A. The exact effects of omega-3s on the heart are still being studied, but evidence clearly shows that they slow the growth of plaque in your arteries, decrease triglyceride levels, slightly lower blood pressure, and decrease the risk of arrhythmias, which can cause sudden death.

Q. What types of fish or seafood contain the most omega-3s?

A. All types of marine animals contain some, but some of the highest levels are found in salmon, sardines, albacore tuna, herring, halibut, and trout.

Q. Is fish the only food source?

A. No, you can also eat tofu and other forms of soybeans; and canola, walnut, and flaxseed and their oils. These foods contain alpha-linolenic acid (LNA), which is a type of acid that converts to omega-3 fatty acid in your body.

Q. How much omega-3 oils should I consume to get the benefit?

A. The ideal amount is not clear. For omega-3s, a range of 0.5 to 1.8 grams per day may have a preventive effect; for LNA, 1.5 to 3 grams per day may be beneficial. Two servings of fish per week puts you in the beneficial range.

Q. Can I take supplements to be sure I'm getting enough?

A. Omega-3 fatty acid supplements may reduce cardiovascular disease, as shown in a recent study. However, it may be better to try to get your omega-3s in foods. But if you are at high risk of coronary artery disease or you have very high triglycerides, you might want to talk to your doctor about supplements.

Other Protein Sources: Dried Beans and Eggs

Plant sources of protein and other nutrients, such as dried beans, peas, lentils, or soybean curd (tofu), can supplement your diet and substitute for meat, poultry, and fish. These foods are high in complex carbohydrates and are lower in saturated fats and calories than animal products such as meat.

Eggs are a good source of protein, B vitamins, and iron, and they are low in saturated fat and total fat. But they are also a source of confusion for many people because they are high in cholesterol. One whole egg contains almost three quarters of the daily limit for cholesterol, so if you eat a whole egg, try to avoid or limit other sources of cholesterol (meat, poultry, and whole-milk dairy products) that day. Limit your intake of egg yolks when possible

Daily Servings of Other Protein Sources

Eat a serving of legumes (dried beans) as an equivalent of a 2-ounce serving of meat, poultry, or fish. Eat eggs and nuts in moderate amounts as part of your overall diet.

Examples of serving sizes (equivalent to 2 ounces of meat):

- 1 cup cooked beans, peas, lentils, or tofu
- 4 ounces peanut butter

because that is where the cholesterol is. If you have heart disease or are at high risk, limit yourself to no more than three egg yolks per week; use egg-substitute products or egg whites instead. Baked goods such as doughnuts and coffee cake contain eggs, so be sure to include any eggs eaten this way in your total of three eggs per week.

Fats and Oils

Apart from the saturated fat and total fat you may consume in meat or dairy products, fats and oils from other sources increase your total fat intake per day. Nutrition labels measure fats in grams. How much total fat and saturated fat (in grams) you can consume depends on the number of calories you burn off each day. To arrive at that number, see the table on page 91.

Use fats and oils sparingly and shop for foods lowest in saturated fat and cholesterol. Use more poly- or monounsaturated oils (see pages 30–32). Check the labels on vegetable oils and margarines and choose products with liquid vegetable oil as the first listed ingredient and no more than 2 grams of saturated fat per tablespoon (canola, olive, corn, safflower, sesame, soybean, and sunflower oils). Use margarine as a substitute for butter and choose tub or liquid forms that are low in saturated fat and trans fat. When possible, use soft margarines that contain plant stanols and sterols. Switch to low-calorie salad dressings and mayonnaise.

Adjust your cooking style to use more low-fat cooking methods such as baking or roasting, grilling, poaching, and braising. Also, use a nonstick cooking spray instead of butter or oil for cooking or baking.

Several types of fat substitutes in foods have been developed to help people lower their fat intake. Any fat-modified product on the market has been approved by the U.S. Food and Drug Administration and is considered safe. But they have not been available long enough to fully assess the long-term benefits or risks. In the context of an overall healthful diet, you may find that using some fat substitutes gives you some extra options.

Daily Servings of Fats and Oils

Adjust your consumption of fats and oils to your desired calorie level (see the box on page 91). If you are trying to lose weight, limit yourself to 5 teaspoons or the equivalent per day.

Examples of serving sizes:

- 1 teaspoon vegetable oil or margarine
- 1 tablespoon salad dressing
- 2 teaspoons mayonnaise or peanut butter
- 1 tablespoon seeds or nuts
- ⅛ of an avocado
- 5 large olives

How Much Fat Should You Consume per Day?

Use this table to determine the recommended maximum amounts of total fat and saturated fat you can consume each day.

Daily Calorie Level	Total Fat 30% or Less (grams)	Saturated Fat Less than 10% (grams)	Saturated Fat Less than 7% (grams)
1,200	40 or less	Less than 13	Less than 9
1,800	60 or less	Less than 20	Less than 14
2,200	73 or less	Less than 24	Less than 17
2,500	83 or less	Less than 28	Less than 19

Adapted from the American Heart Association.

Desserts, Snacks, and Beverages

Traditional desserts are generally high in calories, saturated fat, cholesterol, and perhaps trans fat. You can save these treats for special occasions only and cut down your portion size. Your best choices for every day are fruits, fat-free yogurt with fruit, frozen no-fat yogurt or low-fat yogurt, low-fat ice cream (3 grams of fat per ½ cup or less), or flavored gelatin, ices, sherbets, or sorbets. Angel food cake is a healthier choice than denser cakes, and you can choose cookies in small quantities.

Choose snacks from healthful food groups: fruits; raw vegetables with or without low-fat dip; low-fat crackers; plain, unsalted, unbuttered popcorn; and unsalted pretzels are good choices. In the store, read labels carefully and avoid high sodium and trans fats.

Choose beverages such as water, vegetable juice, low-calorie soft drinks, coffee, or tea. All three of these areas—desserts, snacks, and beverages—offer an opportunity to get extra servings of fruits or vegetables as substitutes for junk food or sugary treats.

Sodium

The typical American diet is salty: most Americans consume about 4,000 to 5,000 milligrams (almost two teaspoons of salt) per day. That may not sound like much, but the recommended level of salt consumption is no more than 2,400 milligrams per day. And for those who have high blood pressure, are over age 50, or are black, less than 1,500 milligrams per day

What about Caffeine?

Headlines about the effects of caffeine on your body come and go, but no clear link between caffeine consumption and heart disease has been found. It appears that moderate coffee drinking (1 to 2 cups per day) is not harmful to your heart. Caffeine is also found in tea, many soft drinks, and chocolate. Caffeine does have the effect of temporarily raising your blood pressure slightly; stimulating your central nervous system; raising your heart rate; and affecting your kidneys to increase urination, which can dehydrate you slightly. Some people are especially sensitive to caffeine, and their doctors may recommend that they avoid it.

is recommended. Although the body's response to salt varies widely from person to person, people who reduce their sodium (salt) intake to the recommended level or below have lower blood pressure and are less likely to die from heart attack or stroke than those who don't. A lower salt intake is especially helpful as you grow older, when high blood pressure is more common and sensitivity to salt (see page 51) often increases.

If you already have high blood pressure and you are sensitive to salt, reducing sodium intake can lower your blood pressure. If you are on blood pressure medication, less sodium in your diet can improve the effectiveness of the drugs. If you are at risk for developing high blood pressure, you may be able to avoid it by eating less salt and changing your diet in other ways (see pages 83–91).

The salt that you shake onto your meal at the table is only a small part of the sodium you consume. Processed foods and restaurant foods are by far the biggest culprits in adding excessive salt to your diet. But even natural foods such as dairy products, meat, and vegetables have some sodium. To cut back on salt, try these tips:

- Read labels on packaged foods carefully. Look for the words *sodium*, *soda* (which is baking soda, a sodium compound), or the chemical symbol *Na*. All of these indicate sodium content.

- Choose fresh or frozen vegetables instead of canned as often as possible. If you do use canned products, drain and rinse them before adding them to other dishes.

- Select salt-free or low-sodium versions of products such as broths, nuts, crackers, and soups.

- If you buy frozen meals, purchase those with the lowest sodium levels.

- Limit your intake of salty snacks like potato chips. Avoid highly processed and high-salt products like most canned soups, frozen entrées, and sandwich meats.

- Use low-fat dairy products, which are also lower in salt content.

- Season your foods with herbs and natural flavorings like lemon or lime juice instead of salt. Try salt-free lemon pepper or other seasoning blends to boost flavor.

- At restaurants, ask to have your meal prepared without salt.
- Check the labels (ingredients list and warnings) on over-the-counter medicines such as antacids; many of these products contain significant amounts of sodium.
- Ask your doctor about the use of "lite" salt. Some people use so much of these products to get the flavor they want that they end up getting more sodium than they would from regular table salt.

Reading Nutrition Labels

Food labels tell you a great deal about the contents of foods, and they are a big help in making reasonable choices to limit the fat, sodium, and cholesterol in the foods you eat. Both the ingredients list and the nutrition facts panel are useful. By law, the ingredients list is in descending order of weight to give you an idea of the proportions of the ingredients in the package. The nutrition facts label tells you the number of servings in the package, as well as the amount and percentage of recommended daily values, such as total fat, saturated fat, cholesterol, sodium, fiber, and carbohydrates (including sugar). As the label tells you, these percentages are based on a diet of 2,000 calories a day. The label also tells you the fiber and sugar content of the food. At the bottom of the panel, the percentages for vitamins A and C, calcium, and iron are listed (see the following section, "Nutrients").

If you are concerned about heart disease, you will probably be paying closest attention to the percentages of fat, saturated fat, and sodium. As a general rule, choose foods that are low in saturated fat; avoid foods containing trans fats and sodium. A daily value of 5 percent or less saturated fat is low; 20 percent or more is high. If you consume a food high in fat at one meal, it is wise to try to balance that with low-fat items at the next meal.

Another item to look for is trans fat, which is formed when vegetable oil is hardened (hydrogenated) in the manufacturing process (see page 30). Like saturated fat and cholesterol, trans fat raises harmful LDL cholesterol levels in the blood. Check the ingredients list for trans fat, shortening, or hydrogenated or partially hydrogenated vegetable oil and limit your use of products containing them. Recently, the FDA began requiring that the amount of trans fat be listed on the nutrition panel under total fat and saturated fat. However, the labeling

Reading the Food Label

- *Serving size*   Check serving sizes carefully, and calculate the nutrient and calorie values for how much you actually plan to eat, not how much the label describes as one portion (often a small amount and only a small portion of the can, box, or other package).

- *Calories*   Know how many calories you can consume per day to lose weight or maintain your weight. Look for foods that have fewer than 30 percent of calories from fat.

- *Total fat*   Saturated fat and trans fat are the fats to limit. Add the amounts of these two fats for a combined total (for example, 3 g of saturated fat and 1.5 g of trans fat is a total of 4.5 g). Compare products and choose the one with a lower combined total. The percentage of trans fats should not exceed 2 percent.

- *Cholesterol*   Choose products with a low cholesterol count. Try to consume less than 300 mg of cholesterol each day, or follow your doctor's recommendations.

- *Sodium*   Try to keep your sodium intake less than 2,400 mg per day. Less than 1,500 mg is even better. Most Americans eat far more salt than they need.

- *Carbohydrates*   Many carbohydrates (bread, potatoes, fruits, and vegetables) are relatively low in fat and provide nutrients and energy. Cut down on fat and you can have more carbohydrates.

- *Fiber*   Dietary fiber helps reduce the risk of heart disease. Both soluble fiber and insoluble fiber are healthful.

- *Protein*   Most people get more than enough protein. Limit the fat content of your protein sources. Beans, grains, and cereals are low in fat and high in protein. Meat products, full-fat dairy products, and fish and poultry are higher in fat.

- *Vitamins and minerals*   Shoot for 100 percent of your daily values every day.

- *Daily values*   These percentages are based on a diet of 2,000 to 2,500 calories per day. As a quick guide, a daily value (DV) of 5 percent or less is low; 20 percent or more is high. Try to maximize your DVs for vitamins and minerals, while limiting your DVs for fats and cholesterol.

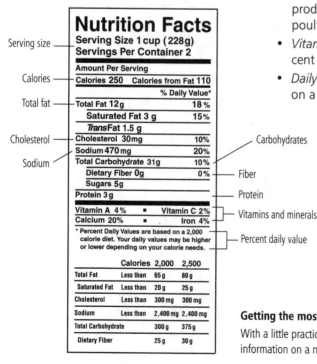

Getting the most from nutrition labels

With a little practice, you can learn to quickly analyze the wealth of information on a nutrition label.

regulations allow as much as 0.5 g of trans fat per serving to be listed as "0 g," so make sure the label does not mention hydrogenated oil or partially hydrogenated oil, both trans fats.

Nutrients

Whether you are at risk of cardiovascular disease or not, a healthy, balanced diet is one of the best ways to take care of your body. Eating a variety of fresh foods is beneficial in part because these are the best sources of nutrients that your body needs. A great deal of research has focused on specific vitamins and minerals in an effort to isolate those that are of particular benefit to your heart and blood vessels. At this time, many of these findings are inconclusive. Some physicians recommend taking a multivitamin and mineral supplements each day, but there is no evidence this is beneficial. (See page 89 for recommendations about omega-3 oil supplements.)

Antioxidants

Antioxidants are believed to slow oxidation of harmful LDL cholesterol, a process that may cause the development of fatty buildups in the arteries (see page 152). Antioxidant vitamins (E, C, and beta carotene, a form of vitamin A) are found in fruits, vegetables, whole grains, and nuts. These foods are all part of a heart-protecting diet. Experts recommend a diet rich in the food sources of antioxidants, but studies show no benefit to taking antioxidant supplements to prevent atherosclerosis or any other cardiovascular disease. In fact, one study showed negative effects from taking large doses of supplement vitamin E. This is probably because supplement forms of vitamin E are processed substances that differ from the natural vitamin E that occurs in the foods mentioned above.

Calcium

Doctors recommend getting plenty of calcium in your diet by eating low-fat dairy products and vegetable greens such as kale, broccoli, and soybean products. Daily calcium requirements vary by age and gender. The DASH diet, which is rich in calcium because it recommends eight servings or more a day of fruits and vegetables, as well as low-fat dairy, is proven to lower blood pressure (page 47). Use of calcium supplements to prevent high blood pressure has not been proven.

Iron

Some research has indicated that a high level of iron stored in the body may be linked to a greater incidence of heart attacks. But many other studies have failed to demonstrate this effect, and research continues. There is no evidence today to support reducing your iron intake or to justify screening of patients with cardiovascular disease to check their iron levels.

Minerals

Magnesium, a mineral found in leafy vegetables, dried peas and beans, nuts, and seeds, may have a positive effect on blood pressure. But the link is not clear enough to recommend the use of magnesium supplements. Magnesium-rich foods are good for you in any case.

The effects of other minerals on heart health are the subject of research, but there are no clear-cut conclusions. Fluoridation of public water supplies is not harmful to your cardiovascular system. A relationship between water hardness and heart health has not been demonstrated. Some sources of water are high in sodium, and a person with a tendency toward high blood pressure should avoid such drinking water. A number of trace elements including zinc, copper, cadmium, and lead have been studied without any demonstrable impact on cardiovascular disease.

Potassium

Potassium is an essential element that plays a role in balancing the fluid content between body cells and body fluids. Eating foods rich in potassium may protect some people from developing high blood pressure. Some people who take diuretics to control high blood pressure may be potassium-deficient because potassium is lost in increased urination. Doctors may recommend that these people take potassium supplements or eat foods rich in potassium. Bananas, cantaloupe and honeydew melons, oranges and grapefruit, prunes, raisins, tomatoes, and low-fat dairy products are all rich in potassium and are part of a healthy diet. On the other hand, some blood pressure medications such as ACE inhibitors cause the body to retain potassium, so your doctor may advise you to limit intake of potassium-rich foods (including salt substitutes containing potassium).

Moderating Your Alcohol Consumption

Drinking too much alcohol can be harmful to your cardiovascular system in numerous ways: it can contribute to high blood pressure, raise your level of harmful triglycerides, and add empty calories that contribute to overweight or obesity. Excessive drinking or binge drinking can lead to stroke, diseases of the heart muscle (cardiomyopathy), and disturbances of the rate or rhythm of the heartbeat (arrhythmias).

Some recent research suggests that a person who has a pattern of frequent, heavy drinking, especially over a lifetime, is much more likely to develop insulin resistance syndrome, a dangerous cluster of risk factors for heart disease (see page 107). Also, heavy episodic drinking is a harmful pattern. Studies support the guidelines recommending moderate alcohol consumption: if you do drink, it's much healthier to have one drink a day than to have seven drinks on the weekend.

If you enjoy drinking alcohol occasionally, the heart-healthy recommendation is straightforward: drink in moderation, which means no more than one drink a day if you are a woman, or two drinks a day if you are a man. One drink is defined as one 12-ounce can of beer; 1½ ounces of 80-proof liquor such as vodka, gin, Scotch, whiskey, and others; 1 ounce of 100-proof liquor; or a 4-ounce glass of wine. Drinking with food may be better, because food slows down the absorption of alcohol. A person who drinks alcohol with a meal usually drinks more moderately.

You may have read about findings that moderate consumption of alcohol, especially red wine, has health benefits. It now appears that all forms of alcohol are associated with these benefits. Studies have suggested that moderate drinking raises HDL cholesterol, helps prevent blood clots, reduces the risk of heart attack and the most common type of stroke (ischemic), and reduces blockages in the arteries in the legs, among other findings. Men over 50 years of age appear to derive the greatest cardiovascular benefit. Study is focused on certain components in red wine or dark beer called flavonoids and other antioxidant compounds, which may contribute to the effect on HDL cholesterol. A substance called resveratrol, found in red wine, may be the agent that reduces blood clot formation.

Alcohol is certainly not the only way to derive these benefits, however. Some of these substances can also be found in grapes or red grape juice, and antioxidants are found in many fruits and vegetables (see pages 85 and 95). Exercise increases HDL. Aspirin can reduce blood-clotting. Researchers are still not sure whether wine, beer, or liquor is more beneficial, and the interaction of other lifestyle factors is still in question. Even drinking in small amounts can dim your alertness and affect your coordination and reaction time, increasing the chances of accidents and falls. When you weigh the possible benefits of drinking alcohol against the many serious risks, there is no reason to start drinking every day if you do not already.

7

Overweight and Obesity

In the last 25 years or so, people in the United States have become pro-gressively more overweight and obese. Today, about 65 percent of Americans are considered overweight and about one-third are obese, and the numbers of obese and overweight people keep rising. To check if you are overweight or obese, see the body mass index table on page 101.

Also important is how one's body fat is distributed. A disproportion-ate amount of body fat, especially if it is distributed around your waist area, creates an even greater risk of developing a range of health prob-lems, including high blood pressure, high blood cholesterol, diabetes, heart disease, and stroke. Research shows that an overweight or obese person's heart muscle changes and pumps less effectively, even without evidence of heart disease.

Independent of any other factors, obesity seriously increases your risk of developing cardiovascular disease. Obesity is associated with high levels of "bad" LDL cholesterol and triglyceride levels, lower levels of "good" HDL cholesterol, higher blood pressure, and diabetes. It also harms your muscles and joints and increases your risk of certain kinds of cancers, including cancers of the breast, prostate, and colon.

Most people who are obese simply consume more calories than they burn off. It is most probably that combination of rich diet and lack of physical activity that has led to our epidemic of obesity in the United States. But other causes also contribute to the problem:

- Obesity tends to run in families. This is largely a result of shared lifestyle behaviors.

- Aging slows your metabolism, making it more difficult for your body to burn calories quickly, so you don't need as many calories to maintain your weight. As we get older, we need to be concerned about calorie intake.

- Men burn more energy when they are at rest than women do, so they need more calories to maintain their weight. After menopause, a woman's ability to burn calories decreases still more.

- Foods that are high in calories and fat but relatively low in nutritional value, served or purchased in excessively large portions, are a habit for many people.

- Lack of exercise is strongly related to obesity. More than two-thirds of Americans report no habitual physical activity.

- Childhood obesity tends to lead to adult obesity. Researchers think that the fat cells a person forms as a child remain into adulthood. Dieting in adulthood decreases the fat-cell size rather than the number.

- Some illnesses such as an underactive thyroid or depression can cause obesity, but this occurs only rarely.

Body Mass Index

A useful way to estimate your body fat is a formula called the body mass index (BMI). The BMI is an assessment of your weight relative to your height and is a good indicator of the proportion of fat in most people's bodies. You can calculate your BMI by multiplying your weight in pounds by 703, dividing by your height in inches, then dividing again by your height in inches. (For example, let's say your weight in pounds is 140, and you are 67 inches tall. Multiply 140 by 703 to get 98,420. Divide that by 67 to get 1,468.95. Divide again by 67 to get 21.92. This is your BMI value.) Since these calculations are fairly complicated, see the convenient chart of body mass index by height and weight on page 101. According to the National Institutes of Health:

- A BMI less than 18.5 is considered underweight.
- A BMI from 18.5 to 24.9 is considered normal. In this range you are at minimal risk of heart disease, provided you have no other risk factors.

- Some individuals are inappropriately classified as overweight or obese due to large muscle mass or frame size.
- A BMI from 25.0 to 30.0 is officially classified as overweight. In this range, your risk of cardiovascular disease increases slightly.
- A BMI of 30.0 or more is considered obese. Your risk level is high.

BODY MASS INDEX (KILOGRAMS PER SQUARE METER)
Height is measured in stocking feet, and weight is measured unclothed.

Height	Body Weight (pounds)													
4'10"	91	96	100	105	110	115	119	124	129	134	138	143	167	191
4'11"	94	99	104	109	114	119	124	128	133	138	143	148	173	198
5'	97	102	107	112	118	123	128	133	138	143	148	153	179	204
5'1"	100	106	111	116	122	127	132	137	143	148	153	158	185	211
5'2"	104	109	115	120	126	131	136	142	147	153	158	164	191	218
5'3"	107	113	118	124	130	135	141	146	152	158	163	169	197	225
5'4"	110	116	122	128	134	140	145	151	157	163	169	174	204	232
5'5"	114	120	126	132	138	144	150	156	162	168	174	180	210	240
5'6"	118	124	130	136	142	148	155	161	167	173	179	186	216	247
5'7"	121	127	134	140	146	153	159	166	172	178	185	191	223	255
5'8"	125	131	138	144	151	158	164	171	177	184	190	197	230	262
5'9"	128	135	142	149	155	162	169	176	182	189	196	203	236	270
5'10"	132	139	146	153	160	167	174	181	188	195	202	209	243	278
5'11"	136	143	150	157	165	172	179	186	193	200	208	215	250	286
6'	140	147	154	162	169	177	184	191	199	206	213	221	258	294
6'1"	144	151	159	166	174	182	189	197	204	212	219	227	265	302
6'2"	148	155	163	171	179	186	194	202	210	218	225	233	272	311
6'3"	152	160	168	176	184	192	200	208	216	224	232	240	279	319
6'4"	156	164	172	180	189	197	205	213	221	230	238	246	287	328
BMI	19	20	21	22	23	24	25	26	27	28	29	30	35	40

Key: Underweight (less than 18.5); healthy weight (18.5 to 24.9); overweight (25 to 29.9); obese (30 and above)

Adapted from the National Heart, Lung, and Blood Institute.

- A BMI of 40.0 is extreme obesity or morbid obesity. Your risk level is extremely high.

Waist Circumference

Another way to estimate body fat is by measuring your waistline. Your waist circumference is the measurement of your natural waist, just above your navel. A high-risk waistline is more than 35 inches for women and more than 40 inches for men, and indicates central obesity. Waist circumference is a means of determining whether you tend to store fat around your waist (for an apple shape) or around your hips and thighs (for a pear shape). Apple-shaped people tend to have higher levels of "bad" cholesterol and triglycerides that clog arteries and raise the risk of heart disease.

Strategies for Losing Weight

If you are overweight or obese, you and your doctor can start immediately to bring your weight down (see pages 83–98). It's not easy to contemplate making major changes in your eating and exercise habits, but

Body Composition and Disease Risk

This table shows you how your risk of disease (type 2 diabetes, high blood pressure, and coronary artery disease) increases with your body mass index (BMI) and your weight distribution.

		DISEASE RISK	
Weight Classification	BMI	Low Waist Measure[a]	High Waist Measure[b]
Underweight	less than 18.5	low	low
Healthy	18.5 to 24.9	low	low
Overweight	25.0 to 29.9	normal	increased
Obese	30.0 to 39.9	high	very high
Extremely obese	more than 40.0	extremely high	extremely high

[a]Less than 35 inches for women; 40 inches for men
[b]More than 35 inches for women; 40 inches for men

Adapted with permission from R. S. Lang and D. D. Hensrud. *Clinical Preventive Medicine*, 2nd ed. Chicago: AMA Press, 2004.

it is possible—and a positive attitude is a big help. Try to drink at least eight glasses of fluid a day; avoid calorie-laden soda, fruit juices, and alcoholic drinks. Also, eliminating extra calories by not putting sugar and cream into your coffee can help you lose weight.

Many dietary and exercise programs are available commercially. Some dieters have reported short-term success with a high-protein diet or a modified high-protein diet with additional vegetables, fruits, and whole grains. In general, though, be cautious about programs that eliminate entire groups of foods other than sweets or foods high in saturated fat or programs that require a very abnormal diet regimen that will be hard to stick to if you travel or are sick. Some diets may alter your body chemistry and change your cholesterol levels in unwelcome ways.

If you have been diagnosed with high blood pressure, diabetes, or heart disease, a long-term program of balanced eating is by far the best for your health.

You will be most successful at shedding excess weight and keeping it off if you think in terms of making permanent changes to become a healthier, more active person. Here are a few strategies:

1. Talk to your doctor or dietitian in detail about your eating habits—how you eat during a typical day and over the course of a week. Talk about the results of your previous efforts to lose weight. Think about what triggers that urge to overeat. Try to identify the problem areas, like that sweet roll in the morning, or crackers and cheese before dinner. Once you know your own patterns, you can start substituting healthier choices.

2. Develop an eating plan that reduces calories overall. A goal of about 1,200 to 1,600 calories per day is a good general target for weight loss. Think about how to cut down on energy-dense foods (like butter, sugar, meat, potato chips) that have lots of calories even in small amounts. Replace them with less energy-dense foods (like fruits and vegetables) that you can fill up on.

3. Set a realistic, measurable goal to get started. One or two pounds a week is a healthy rate at which to shed overweight. At first you may lose more weight, but then a plateau period will follow in which you are still being careful and yet not losing. Continue your program of eating less and exercising more. Remember that even a relatively modest weight loss (for example, 10 pounds if

you are overweight, or 10 percent of your body weight if you are obese) can have real health benefits.

4. Exercise, exercise, exercise! Burning off calories is the other half of the weight-loss equation. It is very difficult to lose weight by diet alone; as you reduce calories, your body slows its metabolism to compensate for that. Exercise prevents that from happening and helps your body burn more calories, even at rest. Develop an enjoyable exercise plan that fits into your life. Get a friend involved to make it more fun and to benefit both of you.

5. Become more active all day long—walk around while you talk on the telephone, take the stairs instead of an elevator, park your car in the space farthest from the supermarket, and start mowing your own lawn. Spend more time outside.

6. Set specific goals not just for the amount you want to lose, but for *how* you are going to lose weight. Make a point of eating one more serving of vegetables each day. Or, if you have not been exercising, start with one 15-minute walk each day. Using a pedometer to measure your steps will help you reach a target number every day; a minimum of 10,000 steps is recommended to keep you healthy.

7. Keep track of your progress with a food diary and a record of time spent exercising. You will be encouraged as you see your habits improve, and you can spot trouble areas or backsliding more easily.

8. About backsliding: we all do it. You can get back on track. When you feel the urge to overindulge, do something else for just 15 minutes to distract yourself. Better yet, take a brisk walk.

9. Allow occasional splurges into your life for special occasions as appropriate. The key is to consider your eating at birthday parties or weddings as an exception, not an everyday habit. The long-term key to healthy eating is moderation.

8

Controlling Diabetes

For a variety of reasons, diabetes is increasing in the American population at an alarming rate, even among younger people. Most authorities place most of the blame on the increase in overweight and obesity, along with a sedentary lifestyle. Diabetes is a serious disease in which the body does not produce or properly use a hormone called insulin. Produced in the pancreas, insulin is necessary to turn the sugars in the blood and in food into energy. In a person with diabetes, because insulin is deficient or not working well, sugars (glucose) build up to dangerously high levels in the blood.

There are two types of diabetes: type 1, also known as juvenile diabetes, and type 2, the most common form, usually diagnosed in adults. In a person with type 2 diabetes, the body does not use its supply of insulin efficiently—a condition called insulin resistance. At first the body can compensate by making more insulin. With time, however, the pancreas begins to fail and loses its ability to make enough insulin to overcome the body's resistance to insulin. Once this occurs, blood sugar levels rise to unhealthy levels. In this section, the focus is on type 2 diabetes and its role as a major risk factor in the development of cardiovascular disease.

The Link between Diabetes and Heart Disease

Diabetes can lead to many serious medical problems, but the most life-threatening of these is cardiovascular disease. Most people with diabetes—about two out of three—die of heart disease, stroke, or peripheral vascular disease. Treatment, through lifestyle changes and one particular medication (metformin), can help control diabetes and also reduce the risk of heart disease. With more people developing diabetes or its precursor, prediabetes (see below), it is important to get the message across that diabetes and heart disease are very strongly linked. The sooner you begin to control prediabetes or diabetes and reduce your risk of heart disease, the healthier and longer your life will be.

Diabetes appears to lead to heart disease through the process of atherosclerosis, which is a narrowing of the arteries caused by the buildup of plaque deposits, beginning with damage to the inner layer of the artery walls (the endothelium). The damaged walls promote the accumulation of lipids that develop into plaque, and the plaque buildup increases the likelihood of blood clots. Atherosclerosis can lead to a heart attack (when the blood supply to your heart muscle is cut off), coronary artery disease (when the blood supply to your heart is reduced), peripheral artery disease (when blood vessels in your legs are blocked), or a stroke (when a blood clot cuts off the blood supply to your brain). Although the entire disease process is not fully understood, diabetes may contribute to the initial damage to the endothelium, impair the ability of the artery walls to expand to accommodate blood flow, and render the body prone to make clots.

Some groups, including people of African American, Hispanic, or Native American descent, are at greater risk of developing diabetes because of their genetic makeup. Those with a parent or sibling with diabetes are at the highest risk. For reasons that are unclear, diabetes is more common and more severe in women than in men. But there is also a group of factors often typical of people with diabetes: obesity, physical inactivity, high blood pressure, and high cholesterol. All of these factors also contribute to the development of heart disease.

Prediabetes

As more of the U.S. population develops diabetes or the insulin resistance syndrome associated with it (see the box on page 107), doctors have become more aggressive about diagnosing and treating it, or preferably preventing it in the first place. A new term, *prediabetes*, has sprung up to identify people whose blood glucose levels are higher than normal but not high enough to be diagnosed as diabetes. Both the oral glucose tolerance test and the fasting plasma glucose test measure your blood glucose level (in milligrams per deciliter, or mg/dL) after you have fasted overnight. Either test can be used, but they result in different readings (see box on page 108).

If you are overweight and age 45 or older, ask your doctor to arrange a test for prediabetes at your next routine physical examination. If you are at a healthy weight and are 45 or older, you can ask your doctor if a test is appropriate. If you are younger than 45 and overweight, your doctor may recommend a test, depending on the presence of other risk factors such as a family history of diabetes, high blood pressure, or high cholesterol readings.

If you are in the prediabetes range, you can and should do something about it right away to prevent or delay the development of diabetes. Many people can return their blood glucose levels to normal with relatively small changes in lifestyle alone. You can benefit from even a

---

What Is Insulin Resistance Syndrome?

Insulin resistance syndrome, also called metabolic syndrome, is a combination of harmful health characteristics that dramatically increases the likelihood that a person will develop either type 2 diabetes, cardiovascular disease, or both. The syndrome is on the rise in the United States; more than one in four Americans has it. The underlying causes of insulin resistance syndrome and its increase in the U.S. population are overweight or obesity, a sedentary lifestyle, and some genetic factors. You are considered to have the syndrome if you have three or more of the following characteristics:

- An accumulation of fat around the waist (an apple shape, see page 102): a waist measurement of more than 40 inches for a man or 35 inches for a woman
- A high triglyceride level (see page 29): more than 150 mg/dL
- A low "good" HDL cholesterol level: less than 40 mg/dL for a man or less than 50 mg/dL for a woman
- A blood pressure level of 130/85 mm Hg or more
- A high fasting glucose level (see page 108), an indicator of insulin resistance: 110 mg/dL or more

modest weight loss of 5 to 10 percent of your body weight. If you can't get down to your ideal weight, even a loss of 10 or 15 pounds can make a significant difference. Similarly, increasing your level of activity to just moderate exercise (like walking) for 30 minutes a day is enough to make a difference. It's worth it to change your lifestyle at this early stage. Your doctor will also talk to you about other risk factors such as high blood pressure, high cholesterol, and smoking.

If You Have Diabetes

Having diabetes means that you are at much higher risk for developing heart and peripheral vascular disease (in your legs). You and your doctor will closely monitor your diabetes (by regularly measuring your blood glucose levels) and your blood pressure and cholesterol levels. Taking care of your heart will involve lifestyle changes including a healthful diet (see pages 83–98); losing weight or making sure you don't gain too much (pages 99–104); quitting smoking if you smoke now; keeping your alcohol consumption moderate, if you drink at all; and perhaps taking medication, also.

Preventing a Heart Attack

A major concern is to prevent coronary artery disease (the most common form of cardiovascular disease), which can lead to a heart attack.

Your doctor will work with you to make the lifestyle changes that will help you minimize your risk of heart attack. Your goal is to keep your blood glucose, blood pressure, and cholesterol levels appropriately controlled.

- Controlling your blood glucose level requires careful monitoring. Your doctor may show you how to check your blood glucose levels at home every day. Your doctor will also probably do a test called an HbA1C: a blood glucose test that measures the amount of sugar attached to the hemoglobin molecule. This estimates the average blood sugar level for the last 2 to 3 months and shows how well the blood sugar is controlled over time. Your target will be an HbA1C of less than 7, which means that throughout the day for the period being measured, your blood sugar levels averaged less than 150.

Taking Aspirin to Prevent Heart Attacks

Your doctor may recommend that you take a low-dose aspirin every day, in addition to any other medications you may take. A person with diabetes tends to form blood clots more easily than most people, and aspirin appears to keep red blood cells from forming clots.

Your doctor can recommend the lowest possible effective dosage for you, usually between 81 and 162 milligrams. Because some people experience irritation of the stomach lining from taking aspirin, you may prefer to take enteric-coated aspirin tablets. The coating enables the aspirin to pass through your stomach without dissolving. It dissolves in your intestine instead, reducing the risk of unpleasant side effects such as stomach pain or nausea.

Some people cannot safely take aspirin every day. You should not take it if you know you are allergic to it, you have a tendency to bleed easily, you have had bleeding from your digestive tract recently, you have liver disease, or you are under 21 years old (the effects of aspirin on younger people have not been fully studied). For those who cannot take aspirin, your doctor may prescribe an alternative such as clopidogrel.

- Controlling your blood pressure to a level below 130/80 mm Hg will ease the load on your heart and help preserve kidney function.
- Controlling your cholesterol involves target rates for each of three different types of blood lipids (fats): LDL, HDL, and triglycerides (see pages 26–29). For those with type 2 diabetes, the the goal is to achieve an LDL level of 100 mg/dL, or even better, less than 70 mg/dL.

Controlling High Blood Pressure

As many as two out of three people with diabetes have high blood pressure. The only way to know you have high blood pressure is to be tested. If you have diabetes, you should have your blood pressure checked every time you go to a doctor, or at least two to four times a year. Because both diabetes and high blood pressure are major contributors to cardiovascular disease, it is even more important that a person with diabetes keep blood pressure at a lower level (less than 130/80 mm Hg) than it is for others. In addition to diet, exercise, smoking cessation, and moderate alcohol consumption, your doctor may recommend one or more medications: diuretics, ACE inhibitors, beta blockers, angiotensin-2 receptor blockers, or calcium channel blockers (see pages 59–63 and 168–169).

Controlling High Cholesterol

Many people with diabetes have trouble keeping their levels of blood lipids (fats in the blood) at healthy levels. If you have diabetes, have a blood lipid profile (cholesterol check; see page 25) done at least once a year, more often if your doctor recommends it. People with diabetes are more likely than the average person to have low levels of HDL cholesterol and high triglycerides. They are more likely to have high levels of very high low-density lipoprotein (VLDL), a type of cholesterol particle that is particularly prone to forming plaque buildup.

It is extremely important for people with diabetes to keep their cholesterol and triglyceride levels low. Most people with diabetes need medications in addition to lifestyle changes to keep their blood lipid profile at target levels. Your doctor may prescribe one or more of several types of cholesterol-lowering drugs (see pages 33–36).

Target Cholesterol Levels for a Person with Diabetes

Type of Blood Lipid	Target Level (in milligrams per deciliter)
LDL cholesterol	Below 100
HDL cholesterol	Above 40 for men Above 50 for women
Triglycerides	Below 150

Source: American Diabetes Association.

Peripheral Artery Disease

Peripheral artery disease (PAD) occurs when the blood vessels in the leg are narrowed or plugged by the buildup of plaque. Atherosclerosis, the process that causes PAD, tends to start earlier in life and progress more rapidly in people with diabetes. In most people, PAD is symptomless in its early stages. If the disease progresses to a severe stage, however, the most common symptom is pain in the leg muscles—not the joints—when you exert yourself. This symptom, called intermittent claudication, means that the muscles in your legs and feet are not getting enough blood and oxygen when they are working. The pain of intermittent claudication comes on with activities such as walking and is relieved by rest or stopping the activity. Without treatment, PAD can progress to the point where the blood supply is so poor that it can lead to damage of skin and muscle tissue deprived of blood in your lower legs and feet. Surgery on the blood vessels or even amputation may be necessary in severe cases. A large number of amputations of toes, feet, or legs occurs in people with diabetes and PAD.

As many as one in three people with diabetes has peripheral artery disease, but they may not realize it if they have not experienced any signs. Your risk of having PAD is higher if you smoke, have high blood pressure, have high cholesterol, are overweight, are physically inactive, are over 50 years old, have a family history of cardiovascular disease, or have already had a heart attack or a stroke.

If you notice that your calves hurt when you exercise but stop hurting when you rest; if you often sense numbness, tingling, or coldness in your legs or feet; or if you have sores or infections on your feet or legs that don't heal, see your doctor right away to be tested for PAD.

If you have experienced neuropathy, a common diabetic symptom that is a burning sensation in the feet or thighs, you might easily confuse the two types of pain. Describe the pain as specifically as possible to your doctor. He or she may want to test for the condition even if you are not experiencing symptoms, especially if you have some of the risk factors in addition to your diabetes.

The most common test for PAD is checking the pulses in your ankles and feet. If you have PAD, your treatment will begin with lifestyle changes, including quitting smoking, controlling your diabetes, controlling your blood pressure, being more physically active, beginning an exercise program to improve blood flow, and eating a low-fat diet to control your cholesterol. Your doctor may also prescribe medications, such as drugs that treat your leg pain so that you can walk farther; antiplatelet agents, which help prevent blood clots; or statins (see page 34), which help lower your blood cholesterol.

9

Stress

In addition to the major risk factors for heart disease (high cholesterol, high blood pressure, physical inactivity, smoking, and diabetes), stress can be a contributing factor. The effects of stress on your heart health are difficult to study and quantify in part because people not only experience different levels of stress, but they also respond differently. Researchers have identified several ways that stress may adversely affect some people's hearts:

- Under stress, your body releases extra hormones (epinephrine and norepinephrine) that raise your blood pressure, which may over time injure the lining of your arteries. As the arteries repair themselves, they may thicken, which promotes the buildup of plaque.

- A stressful situation tends to raise your heart rate and blood pressure, so your heart requires more oxygen. In someone who already has heart disease, this oxygen shortage can bring on chest pain (angina).

- Stress increases the clotting factors in your blood, which increases the chances that a blood clot will form and block an artery, especially one already partially closed by plaque.

Then, of course, there are the ways that many people may choose to deal with stress—overeating, smoking, drinking excessively—that are damaging to the cardiovascular system.

The fact is that everyone is under stress of some kind at least intermittently and perhaps much of the time. You can usually recognize symptoms of your own stress in the form of aches and pains, difficulty fighting off mild infections like colds, sleeplessness, or feelings of anxiety or irritability. You also probably know when some of your less healthy coping mechanisms are escalating—as, for example, when you put on weight during a tough time, or start smoking more.

Learning to manage stress makes good sense for your overall health. But more research is needed before experts can reliably recommend specific methods of stress reduction as treatments for cardiovascular diseases. Generally, if you or your doctor believes that stress is having a harmful effect on your health, you can work on several strategies to manage its impact:

- Communicate with family and friends about the things that trouble you. Their support and love will help reduce your response to stressful situations.

- If you feel a sense of urgency because of competing demands on your time, consider time management techniques that will help you prioritize and set realistic expectations. Your workplace, library, or the Internet may offer specific methods. Also, be cautious about agreeing to take on new projects.

- Choose a relaxation technique, such as yoga, meditation, or biofeedback, and make time to master it and practice it regularly. Although there is no conclusive medical proof these techniques can lower blood pressure, there are some promising studies pointing in that direction.

- When you know that a specific problem is causing you anxiety, talk to your doctor or other health-care provider about a support group that focuses on that problem. These resources may be available through a community center, hospital, religious organization, or YMCA.

- Professional counseling or psychotherapy may help you through certain difficult periods. Your doctor can help refer you to an appropriate professional. If medications such as antidepressants are appropriate, your doctor or a psychiatrist can prescribe them and help you get essential counseling as well.

- Use commonsense therapy: eat a healthy diet, exercise regularly (see the box on page 80), limit alcohol and caffeine, and do not smoke.

Managing stress, or preventing stress in the first place, is especially important to people who have already had a heart attack or a stroke. Preventing another heart attack or stroke—called secondary prevention by doctors—is a key goal for the doctor-patient team. As noted repeatedly in this book, lifestyle changes are crucial to prevention or secondary prevention, and stress management should be a key focus of lifestyle changes that also include controlling your cholesterol level, controlling your blood pressure, losing weight if needed, exercising regularly, and stopping smoking.

Depression may be related to stress but is a disorder that needs treatment. It is natural to a certain degree to feel "blue" or be upset after a heart attack or a stroke. However, if you have persistent depression, it is important to note that it is treatable—that is, not just "something to live with" (see also "Depression after a Stroke," page 232). Depression symptoms include prolonged periods of feeling sad or unable to cope, strong feelings of guilt, strong feelings of pessimism or loss of hope, a loss of interest in normal pleasures (including sex), unusual weight changes (unintentional losses or gains), and difficulty relating to loved ones or coworkers. If you or a loved one has depression, seek treatment from your primary care doctor; he or she will make treatment suggestions, possibly including medications or talking therapy, or refer you to a psychiatrist or other mental health professional.

10

Physical Examinations and Diagnostic Tests

The best way to monitor your health is to see your doctor and work together as a team for your health. Many of the major risk factors (such as blood pressure and cholesterol) are apparent only with a medical examination. The earlier you can identify a problem area and start to work on it, the more likely you will be able to prevent the development of more serious disease. For instance, an evaluation of prehypertension (see page 43) or prediabetes (see page 106) gives you a head start on these risk factors. As you work on one risk factor (for instance, exercising more to lower cholesterol) you will very likely be improving others as well. Know all your risk factors from your medical history—not only high blood pressure, diabetes, and smoking, but also risks from menopause, aging, and lifestyle choices regarding food and exercise.

Evaluating a Heart Problem

If you experience any symptoms that might be indicators of a heart problem—such as chest pain, shortness of breath, or a pounding heart—see your doctor immediately. He or she will interview you thoroughly about your medical history and symptoms and then do a physical examination to try to detect what might be causing the symptoms. Depending on what the examination reveals, he or she may order further testing to diagnose the problem. If you know what to expect, you will probably feel more relaxed about the exam, and you can be better prepared to answer questions. It will be very helpful if you can bring in notes with specific details about when you experienced a symptom, how often it recurred, and how long it lasted.

Medical History

If you are seeing a doctor for the first time, he or she will ask some general questions about your medical history. If you are reporting a specific event, the questions will focus on that event. Here is a general outline of what to expect:

- **Questions about your chief complaint.** Your doctor will want to know what brought you into the office. He or she will ask specific questions such as how it felt, when it occurred, what you were doing when it occurred, or what seemed to relieve it. Be as thorough and specific as you can be. Do not hesitate to volunteer information beyond the questions.

- **Questions about your medical history.** Information about other medical conditions you have or have had can help indicate possible causes for your symptoms and rule out unnecessary tests or inappropriate treatments. Again, written notes may help you remember illnesses, tests, or surgery that you have had. If you

---

How Often Should I Be Tested?

	APPARENTLY HEALTHY		
	20–40 Years of Age	40–60 Years of Age	60 Years +
Checkup	Every 5 years	2–3 years	1 year
Blood pressure	2 years	2 years	2 years
Blood lipid profile	5 years	5 years	5 years

This chart shows the generally recommended intervals between examinations or tests by various age groups. Follow your doctor's instructions; your medical history and other risk factors may make it necessary to see your doctor or have tests more often.

are seeing a specialist, your other doctor or doctors may be able to send medical records and test results in advance of your appointment. If you are referred to a specialist, ask the referring doctor for pertinent test results to take with you to the appointment.

- **Medications.** Your doctor will want to review all the medications you are taking; bring a list that includes dosages to the appointment. It is important to include herbal preparations and nonprescription medications, because they may interact with other drugs. Also, know and remember your drug allergies.

- **Family history.** Be prepared to answer questions about the medical history of your parents, siblings, and children. This information gives the doctor clues about hereditary aspects of some conditions and your overall risk.

- **Lifestyle.** Information about habits such as smoking or drinking, diet, and exercise are important. Some of these factors may help explain a symptom; for instance, caffeine can cause an irregular heartbeat in some people. Do not worry about looking bad or being embarrassed by your habits. This information can help a great deal with diagnosis and treatment. You may also be asked questions about your workplace and about stress.

- **Other organ systems.** Your doctor may systematically review other body systems to make sure nothing is overlooked.

A Physical Examination in Detail

A cardiovascular physical examination will include taking your blood pressure (see page 43), measuring your heart rate and rhythm by checking your pulses, inspecting the veins in your neck, checking your body for swellings, and listening to the sounds of your breath, heart, and

> **WARNING!**
>
> ### Symptoms of a Possible Heart Attack
>
> If you have one or more of the following symptoms, call 911 or the emergency number for your area or go to a hospital emergency department immediately, and chew an adult (325 mg) aspirin:
>
> - Chest pain, fullness in the chest, or a squeezing sensation.
> - Shortness of breath or light-headedness with the chest pain.
> - Pain in the chest radiating to the neck or arm (usually the left arm).
> - Pain radiating to the jaw.
> - If you have diabetes, you may not feel sharp chest pains, but shortness of breath, light-headedness, nausea, and dizziness can be symptoms of heart attack.

blood vessels. You will probably be asked to change out of your clothes into a hospital gown and sit or lie on an examining table.

- **Measuring your heart rate and rhythm.** Your doctor will check the pulse at your wrist, in the carotid arteries in your neck, or in the femoral arteries in your groin. The pulses enable him or her to measure your heart rate and to determine if your heartbeat is regular, skips beats, or has extra beats. An absent or reduced pulse at one of the sites may indicate a blockage in a blood vessel.

- **Veins in your neck.** The doctor will look at (not feel) the jugular vein in your neck to observe the pulse. The location and size of the pulse indicates the pressure on the right side of the heart and the possible presence of excess fluid in your system.

- **Swelling.** Swellings in parts of your body such as your legs and ankles can indicate excess fluid or a blockage in a vein.

- **Listening to your breath.** Listening to your breath sounds by placing a stethoscope on your chest can reveal fluid building up in your lungs (which makes a crackling sound) or scarred tissue in your lungs. Thumping on your chest can help locate where the fluid is; a fluid-filled area sounds dull instead of hollow.

- **Listening to your heart.** Putting the stethoscope on four distinct sites over your heart, your doctor can listen to blood flowing through your heart and heart valves. A heart murmur is the sound of turbulence caused by a problem with a valve or another heart structure. You may be asked to stand up, squat, or lie back, because murmurs change when you are in different positions. Extra sounds, called gallops, or other types of sounds may indicate various types of heart problems. Some unusual sounds are completely harmless.

- **Listening to blood vessels.** Your doctor can evaluate blood flow in large blood vessels by listening at different points in your neck, abdomen, and groin. Turbulence in these vessels makes a sound called a bruit, which may indicate blockage.

Depending on what the doctor learns from this basic examination, or "cardiac workup," he or she may order blood tests, imaging procedures, or other tests of cardiac function in order to diagnose more specifically and plan treatment.

After a physical examination—including listening to your heart and lungs with a stethoscope—your doctor will need more detailed information about your heart. The doctor will ask questions about diseases you have been diagnosed with, any persistent symptoms you have noticed, and your family medical history. A variety of tests are available to examine the structure of your heart, how well it functions, whether it is damaged or diseased, and the nature or extent of the disease.

Which tests you take depend on your symptoms, your medical history, your general cardiac condition, and your doctor's assessment. Usually you will have some simple tests first, such as an ECG (an electrocardiogram, which records your heart's electrical activity), and then additional tests as needed to assess your particular problem. In addition to electrocardiography, other means of testing include blood tests; echocardiography (which uses sound waves to examine the heart valves and chambers); different types of stress tests (to study the heart while it is working harder); nuclear imaging (using safe amounts of radioactive materials to study heart function); other imaging techniques; and in some cases, more invasive tests that are done in a hospital setting.

The tests can reveal useful information specific to your heart symptom or problem that will help guide your treatment. Many of the tests

Questions to Ask about a Test

Your doctor or other health professional will be glad to answer any questions you might have about a test you are taking. Knowing what to expect will help put you at ease. Here are a few questions many people ask:

- Why do I need this test?
- How is it done?
- Who will perform the test?
- Will it hurt?
- Are there any risks?
- Are there any alternatives to this test?
- How soon will the results be ready, and how will I get them?

- What will the results tell us?
- Could the test bring on a heart attack or a stroke?
- Will my medications, pacemaker, artificial valve, or previous surgery cause problems?
- Do I need to prepare for the test in any way?
- Will I be sedated or anesthetized?
- Do I need someone to come with me or drive me home?
- Will I need more tests?

Source: Adapted with permission from the American Heart Association Web site.

are noninvasive, meaning that they do not involve a needle stick or the introduction of any catheters (tubes) into your body. Knowing how and why a test is performed will help you feel more comfortable, and understanding something about the possible results will help you learn about your heart along with your doctor. Don't hesitate to ask questions before or after any test. Many tests require your permission or informed consent, and your doctor should fully explain beforehand any risks from the tests.

Electrocardiography

Electrocardiography is a technique to study your heart's electrical activity by recording the path of an electrical impulse from its origin in the sinoatrial node through your heart as it causes the heart to contract (see page 11). The printout of this activity, an electrocardiogram, is a graph of the electrical activity of each heartbeat over time and the rhythm of successive beats.

Electrocardiogram

The electrocardiogram (ECG) is a safe, inexpensive way to get a wealth of information: it tells your doctor about your heart rate and heart rhythm. The ECG may also suggest whether a heart attack has occurred and whether there are potential problems with blood supply to the heart. It is a routine, painless test.

What to Expect

You do not have to prepare in any special way to have an ECG, except perhaps to wear clothes that you can take off easily. The ECG may be done in your doctor's office or in a hospital. For the test, you may be asked to change into a hospital gown and sit or lie on an examination table. In order to conduct the electrical impulse, electrodes will be attached to various parts of your body: your chest, back, wrists, and ankles. To ensure a good connection between your skin and each electrode, which is mounted on a sticky patch, the technician will clean these areas, perhaps shave areas of the chest on a man, and apply a conducting gel. Then he or she will hook up the electrodes and enter some data into the electrocardiograph machine. You will not feel anything during the testing, which usually lasts a minute or less. There is no electrical energy being passed into your body, and there is no danger of electrical shock. The ECG simply records your heart's activity.

What the Results Mean

In a healthy person, the electrical impulse during a heartbeat follows a regular, sequential path. The electrodes over different parts of your heart follow the path of the impulse and record it on the ECG. The most basic piece of information it gives is your heart rate, which is usually measured by your pulse, but the ECG can give a more accurate rate if your pulse is unusually irregular or hard to feel. Normal heart rates range between 60 and 100 beats per minute.

The ECG also indicates your heart rhythm, which should be regular. The test may reveal either an abnormally fast beat (tachycardia) or an abnormally slow one (bradycardia). It can also demonstrate an electrical blockage in the heart that alters the rhythm and causes an irregular ECG tracing. Each type of arrhythmia causes a distinctive type of tracing pattern.

In addition, the ECG may tell whether you have had a heart attack, because damaged muscle or scar tissue doesn't transmit the electrical impulse the same way as healthy tissue would. It can indicate approximately where the damage is in the heart ventricle. Often the ECG reveals evidence of a past heart attack that you didn't even know occurred. It can also indicate if you are having an attack during the test.

A component of the wave on the ECG can be affected by an inadequate supply of blood or oxygen to your heart, particularly if the test is obtained during chest pain symptoms. Further tests may be necessary to determine why this is happening and under what circumstances.

The ECG can provide information about structural abnormalities, the effects of medications on the heart rhythm and electrical conduction, hypertension, kidney problems, or hormonal problems that affect the wave pattern in specific ways. Although a normal ECG does not always exclude heart disease, it still is a reassuring finding. Also, if there is a heart problem, the ECG may give clues that indicate what type of testing is needed to further isolate and identify the problem.

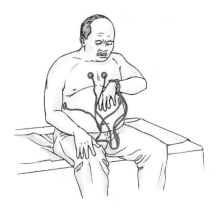

Wearing a Holter monitor

A Holter monitor is a portable recording device that provides a reading of your heart rate and rhythm over a period of 24 hours. While you wear the monitor, you will be asked to keep a log of your daily activities: what you did and at what time. This information helps your doctor determine the circumstances linked to your symptoms.

Holter Monitoring

Because a conventional ECG records only a brief period (6 seconds) of your heart activity, a continual recording over a period of 24 hours or longer may be useful to identify changes in your heart's rate or rhythm. To accomplish this form of ambulatory ECG, you will wear a battery-powered recording device called a Holter monitor. About the size of a small paperback book, the Holter monitor is portable enough to wear around your waist or on your belt. The monitor connects to electrodes placed on your chest via wires (leads) that pass under your clothes.

Being fitted for a Holter monitor is a painless procedure. It is a good idea to bathe or shower before you go to your doctor's office, because you cannot get the monitor wet once you are wearing it. The technician will prepare your skin just as for an office ECG. At least one electrode and lead may be taped down to secure it as you move around. You will wear the device usually for 24 hours, including while you sleep. You will also be asked to keep a log as you go about your usual day: what you were doing and whether you experienced any symptoms, and at what times. Every heartbeat will be recorded and analyzed for information.

After the designated monitoring period, you will return to your doctor's office to turn in the device. Having the electrodes removed might be uncomfortable, like tearing off a bandage. The tracings for the monitoring period will be analyzed, and correlations will be made between the Holter recording and the times of unusual symptoms or events in your log.

Event Monitoring

If you are having symptoms that are unpredictable or infrequent, you may have to use another ECG device called an event monitor or transtelephonic monitor, which records your heart rhythm. You are usually asked to use this monitor for one month. You can take it off to bathe, or for other brief periods, but it's best to wear it as often as possible. A small recorder is attached to a bracelet or finger clip. If you experience a symptom, such as light-headedness, you attach the recorder (if you are not wearing it) and push a button on the monitor that triggers a memory of what was recorded for several minutes before and after you pushed the button. This data can be transmitted over the telephone, or you can bring the monitor to the office. This helps identify any rhythm disturbances that occur while you have symptoms. If a dangerous rhythm problem is identified, you may be instructed to seek medical attention urgently.

Another type of event monitor, this one implantable, has been developed to capture your heart's activity during infrequent symptoms that occur only a few times a year. Called an implantable loop recorder, it is inserted in your chest, and you wear it for as long as 18 months.

Exercise Stress Testing

An exercise stress test is a continuous ECG that shows how your heart performs during exercise, when the body is demanding more blood and oxygen. It shows the adequacy of the blood supply to the coronary arteries and how well the heart muscle functions. You also might hear it called a treadmill test, an exercise tolerance test, or an exercise ECG. It is a common diagnostic tool for detecting coronary artery disease and the origin of symptoms such as chest pain, because it shows whether the blood supply in the coronary arteries is reduced. It can identify a safe level of exercise for any heart patient, checks the effectiveness of medications, helps predict the risk of heart attack, and checks the effectiveness of procedures done to improve circulation in a person with coronary artery disease.

The test is designed to place stress on your heart—about as much as a fast walk or a jog up a hill—in a carefully controlled environment with trained staff close at hand. During the test, the technician will carefully monitor your heart rate, breathing, blood pressure, heart rhythm, and how tired you feel.

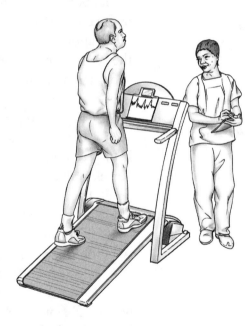

Having an exercise stress test
An exercise stress test is a type of ECG that shows how the heart performs when you exercise. Usually the test is done while you walk on a treadmill, and then the speed or slope are gradually increased to make your heart work harder. The test is like a carefully supervised workout, with a warm-up, a gradual increase in the level of exercise, and a cool-down period. A doctor or technician will watch you closely throughout the test.

The most typical stress test is done by having you walk on a treadmill or ride a stationary bicycle. If the test shows that your heart doesn't function normally during exercise, you may need to repeat the treadmill test combined with echocardiography (see page 132) or nuclear technology (see page 136) to better identify the problem. Often these tests are done with the initial exercise stress test to improve the accuracy of diagnosis, especially in women. If you are unable to exercise because of illness, you may undergo a chemical stress test (see page 128), for which you will be given a drug that mimics some of the effects of exercise on your heart rate while ECG tracings or nuclear images are made.

What to Expect

You will be asked not to eat for 12 hours before the test, because a meal can make you uncomfortable or nauseous. You can drink a small amount of liquid such as water, but no beverage such as coffee, tea, soda, or chocolate that contains caffeine. Be sure to ask your doctor about any medications you take and whether you should stop taking them before the test. If you have diabetes, you will be given specific instructions about taking insulin.

A technician will prepare your skin for the placement of electrodes, similar to the preparation for a regular ECG (see page 122). You will also be fitted with a blood pressure cuff. A resting ECG will be taken before you start exercising, and then you will get on a treadmill or a bicycle. The first 2 or 3 minutes you will exercise at a slow, warm-up pace. Then every 2 or 3 minutes, the speed or slope will be increased gradually to simulate going uphill. The doctor will probably encourage you to continue until you are too tired to go on, or until you have a symptom such as pain, dizziness, or shortness of breath. After this procedure, you lie down or sit quietly for about 10 minutes. Your doctor or technician will monitor your heart and blood pressure throughout this period. He or she will ask you questions about how tired or out of breath you feel. If the ECG reveals any potential problems, the doctor or technician will ask you to stop exercising. After the test is complete, you can return to your normal day.

What the Results Mean

The doctor reading the ECG may be able to tell you preliminary results immediately, but a complete analysis will probably take several days. If the test shows that your heart functions normally during exercise, the results can be used to help you plan a fitness program. If the results indicate that your heart functions abnormally during exercise, you may need to have more tests, such as an echocardiographic stress test (see page 133) or a nuclear stress test, to determine more precisely where the blood supply is being blocked. On occasion, you may go straight to having an angiography (see page 146). If you already have coronary artery disease, the test can reveal a new blockage or one that is worsening.

The choice of stress testing will depend in part on your medical history and your doctor's preferences. Exercise stress testing is less specific—and therefore, less helpful—than thallium or echocardiographic stress testing; however, exercise stress testing is much less expensive and thus is often used as a first step in screening for heart disease. Those who already have heart conditions that may influence the ECG result may need nuclear stress testing. Echocardiographic stress testing may be better for women because women, especially young women, are prone to false positives on ECGs.

Exercise Echocardiography

As with other stress tests, an exercise echocardiogram shows how your heart functions when it is working harder. It is most often done to confirm or rule out coronary artery disease. The moving image enables your doctor to see where blockages are occurring.

A stress echocardiogram may be done in a doctor's office or a hospital. The test has two parts. First, the technician does a resting echocardiogram (ultrasound of the heart) while you lie on a table. Then you get on a treadmill or a stationary bicycle and exercise until your heart is working to maximum (see page 133). A second echocardiogram is done while your heart rate is still high. The test will show if there are any exercise-induced changes in your heart in the results of the echocardiogram. For example, in areas of the heart where the blood supply is limited because of obstructions of the blood vessels to the heart muscle, that area may not contract as well as it should. In another example, an exercise-induced abnormality not present when the heart is at rest suggests reversible blood flow abnormalities and the need for treatment to prevent a heart attack.

Chemical Stress Testing

If a disability (for example, arthritis, back trouble, or a stroke) prevents you from exercising for a stress test, your doctor can use intravenous medication to increase your heart rate combined with an imaging technique such as echocardiography to see how your heart functions when it's working harder. This method is called chemical or pharmacologic stress testing. The medications most commonly used are dobutamine, dipyridamole, or adenosine.

The drugs are administered so that your heart rate increases gradually. If you are able to do some exercise, you may be asked to walk on a treadmill for a minute or so after the drug is injected. Trained medical assistants will monitor you throughout the test, and you should report any unusual symptoms. Dobutamine may cause a marked increase in blood pressure or an arrhythmia. Adenosine may cause a brief, passing slowing of the heart rate. Both adenosine and dipyridamole can cause wheezing and should be used cautiously, if at all, in people with asthma or chronic obstructive pulmonary disease. The drugs can be stopped at any time.

Preparation for a chemical stress test is similar to regular stress testing. You will be asked not to eat or drink anything for at least 3 hours before the test, in order to avoid nausea. If you take medications, be sure to talk to your doctor about what to do; you may need to stop taking them for an interval before the test. If you have diabetes and take insulin, you will need specific instructions. If you have any history of asthma, bronchitis, or emphysema, tell your doctor, because some stress-inducing medications may be harmful to you.

Chest X-ray

Even though far more sophisticated imaging techniques have been developed, the basic chest X-ray can occasionally be a useful tool to assess your cardiovascular system. The X-ray technique works by passing a small, relatively safe amount of radiation through your body and onto a piece of film. The chest X-ray gives your doctor an image of your heart and lungs that reveals the size and shape of your heart, the presence of calcium deposits within your heart, and the presence of congestion in your lungs. If your heart is enlarged, the shape of the enlargement may offer clues to the cause. For example, a narrowed heart valve causes a different shape than the enlargement due to congestive heart failure (see pages 233–254).

Calcium, which shows clearly on an X-ray, sometimes builds up in diseased or injured tissue. In the heart, calcium deposits may accumulate on a valve, an artery, or the heart muscle itself. The presence of these deposits will direct further testing.

X-rays also make a picture of your lungs and help your doctor determine whether your symptoms are caused by heart disease or lung disease. The presence of fluid in lung tissue (a sign called pulmonary edema) means that a weakened heart may have caused fluid to back up, thereby congesting the lungs (congestive heart failure).

Having an X-ray done is easy and painless. You will be asked to remove your clothes above your waist and to take off any jewelry that might interfere with the image. You will stand against the X-ray machine, hold your arms out, and hold your breath while the X-ray is being taken (to make your heart and lungs show up more clearly, and to help you hold still).

Blood Tests

Beyond routine blood tests that are done to assess a variety of conditions, some blood tests are specific to the diagnosis of cardiovascular disease. Blood tests can indicate the levels of lipids (cholesterol and triglycerides), cardiac enzymes (markers of cardiac damage), the oxygen content, and the amount of time it takes for your blood to clot (prothrombin time). Some newer blood tests detect injury to the heart muscle in a person who has had a symptom such as chest pain, shortness of breath, or light-headedness. These tests can be done quickly in an emergency setting for immediate detection of a heart attack.

For some types of blood tests, such as the lipid profile, you will be asked to fast overnight. For many heart-related blood tests, blood will be drawn from a vein or sometimes from an artery, rather than from a fingertip.

Lipid Profile

Measuring the cholesterol circulating in your blood is a common, routine test (see page 25). Called a lipoprotein profile, or sometimes a lipid panel, the test measures the levels of your total cholesterol, low-density lipoproteins (LDL, the "bad" cholesterol), high-density lipoproteins (HDL, the "good" cholesterol), and triglycerides (the most common form of fat in the blood). This is to determine whether you need treatment or to check if a treatment is working.

If these measurements are not precise enough, a more sophisticated test, called a nuclear magnetic resonance lipid test, can be done to more precisely measure and classify subparticles of HDL and LDL. Other new tests, which may help to further assess risk, include measuring apoprotein levels such as apoprotein B, a component of LDL, and apoprotein A-1, a component of HDL. The usefulness of these tests is uncertain; currently, they are used mainly to decide if people with borderline high LDL and HDL levels need drug treatment.

Cardiac Enzymes

Testing your blood for certain cardiac enzymes (proteins), which are sometimes called cardiac markers because they indicate heart muscle injury, can be a way to detect damage to your heart from a heart attack very early in the course of the attack. If you are having chest pains, your doctor may order these tests to see if damage is being done to your heart. If you go to an emergency room because of warning signs of a heart attack (see page 156), the doctor will probably do this analysis.

Small amounts of cardiac enzymes are found in the blood of healthy people. However, the heart muscle is rich in these enzymes, and they can leak into your blood in larger amounts if your heart is damaged by a heart attack. They may enter your bloodstream very early in an attack, before you realize you are having one, or before much heart tissue has been damaged.

One enzyme commonly measured to confirm the existence of heart muscle damage is creatine kinase (CK). Different types of CK are found in heart muscles and in the skeleton. The enzyme type that most accurately confirms heart damage is the form of CK known as CK-MB. The level of CK-MB found in the blood increases about 6 hours after the start of a heart attack and reaches its peak in about 18 hours. If you have had a symptom such as pain, testing for these markers can confirm whether a heart attack has occurred.

Other cardiac markers called troponins (including troponin I and troponin T) have a role in heart muscle contraction and are very sensitive indicators of heart muscle damage. Their presence in your blood can indicate very mild damage to your heart that tests for creatine kinase don't detect. Troponins increase in as little as 4 hours after the beginning of an attack and can remain elevated in your blood for 2 weeks.

Myoglobin is still another marker used to detect heart damage. It is a less specific marker of cardiac damage than one type of CK but has the advantage of being the very first of the cardiac markers to rise after a heart attack, as early as a couple of hours after the heart damage occurs. This makes a blood test for myoglobin useful in determining whether someone who is having chest pain is having a heart attack.

Homocysteine

Homocysteine is an amino acid in your blood. Doctors have studied homocysteine closely because high levels of it appear to place you at higher risk of cardiovascular disease, regardless of your age or other risk factors. Some evidence suggests that homocysteine might damage the lining of your arteries and promote blood clots, but no direct cause-and-effect relationship has been established. Although homocysteine levels were at first strongly linked to heart disease, more recently researchers have found that link not as strong as they first thought. The level of homocysteine in your blood may be partly hereditary, but it is also related to your diet. In some cases, an elevated level of homocysteine results from a vitamin B_{12} deficiency, so it is important that your doctor measure your level of vitamin B_{12} through a blood test.

Your doctor may test your homocysteine levels if you have a strong history of heart disease but you don't have the obvious risk factors such as high cholesterol, high blood pressure, diabetes, and others. Eating a diet rich in folic acid and B vitamins helps reduce homocysteine. Many doctors routinely recommend that those at risk for heart disease take folic acid and vitamin B complex. Other doctors recommend the supplements only if homocysteine levels are elevated; however, recent research suggests folate supplements may block the action of naturally occurring folates and vitamin B that you eat in your diet.

C-reactive Protein

Although high cholesterol is most often considered the major risk factor for heart attack because of its role in the accumulation of plaque in the arteries, not all people who have heart attacks have arteries that are blocked in this way. Doctors have been studying the role of inflammation within the arteries as a separate process that may contribute to the development of coronary artery disease. Inflammation may also explain why in some people, an artery recloses after a balloon angioplasty has been performed to open it.

Inflammation anywhere in your body causes swelling. If it occurs in your arteries, this swelling can reduce the blood flow to your heart. When inflammation occurs, your body produces a substance called C-reactive protein. The level of C-reactive protein in your blood (detected by a blood test) is a strong predictor of heart disease, especially in people who have had prior heart attacks.

No one is sure yet what causes the inflammation in the arteries. It may be a bacterial agent such as *Helicobacter pylori* (which also causes stomach ulcers) or a viral agent such as the herpes simplex virus. *Chlamydia pneumoniae*, another type of bacteria, has been studied as a possible predictor of heart disease but with no clear evidence that the bacteria is involved. Some research suggests that inflammation may damage the arterial wall in a specific way that increases the chance of blood clots that block the artery. Obesity and diabetes may also cause an increase in C-reactive protein levels. In fact, visceral or belly fat is the best predictor of an individual's high level of C-reactive protein. If you are at a moderate or high risk for cardiovascular disease, measuring your C-reactive protein may help guide your treatment (see page 154). You can lower your C-reactive protein with a heart-healthy diet and exercise to lose the belly fat, and also by quitting smoking.

Echocardiography

Echocardiography uses high-frequency sound waves (also called ultrasound) to produce a moving image of your heart. The sound waves are introduced into your body through a handheld device called a transducer. They bounce off the structures and fluids in the heart and return as echoes through the transducer. The echoes are converted into images on a monitor.

Echocardiogram

Using different types of echocardiography, your doctor can see the size, shape, and contraction of the heart muscle; watch the heart valves working; and see how blood is flowing through your heart and arteries. During one test, a two-dimensional mode looks at the heart's structures and function to see a larger picture, including a cross section; and a form called Doppler echocardiography to assess blood flow within the heart and to identify abnormal flow patterns.

In conjunction with a stress test, the echocardiogram may show that the wall of the heart does not move as well after exercise, suggesting that part of the heart may not get sufficient blood flow during exercise. That lack of blood can impair the heart muscle's ability to contract.

What to Expect

You can have an echocardiogram in a doctor's office or a hospital. You do not need to prepare in any special way. You will be asked to remove your clothes, and electrodes will be attached to your chest and back, as in the procedure for an ECG (page 122). The technician will spread a gel over your chest to help with transmission. He or she will move the transducer over your heart and chest, pressing firmly, and will ask you to lie in several different positions and breathe slowly, or hold your breath to improve the image. The entire procedure will take 45 minutes to an hour.

What the Results Mean

You may have to wait several days for the full results of the echocardiogram. If the test doesn't reveal anything unexpected, you may get the results by phone. The test will indicate to your doctor how the chambers or walls of your heart have been altered by conditions such as heart attack, high blood pressure,

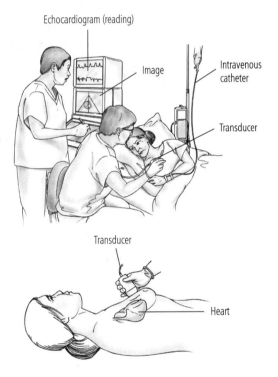

Echocardiogram (reading)

Image

Intravenous catheter

Transducer

Transducer

Heart

Having an echo stress test

If you are unable to exercise for an exercise stress test, your doctor can give you a drug (dobutamine) that makes your heart beat faster, just as exercise does, and then use echocardiography to image your heart. For an echocardiogram, sound waves (ultrasound) are introduced into your body through a handheld device called a transducer (see inset). The sound waves bounce off your heart and its structures and produce a moving image of its size, shape, and movement, as well as the blood flow in the heart.

previous heart damage, or heart failure. If you have had echocardiograms before, the doctor can compare the results of the tests to assess how effective treatment has been.

The test also allows the doctor to analyze the strength and nature of your heart's pumping action, which he or she may describe in terms of the "ejection fraction." A normal ejection fraction is about 55 to 65 percent, meaning that more than half of the blood in your left ventricle (the main pumping chamber) is squeezed out in a single heartbeat. If the percentage is significantly lower, the echocardiogram can show where the pumping action is weakened—for example, it may reveal an area of the heart weakened by a heart attack. The test may be especially meaningful for genetic conditions that can pose the risk of sudden death—for example, hypertrophic cardiomyopathy, which is an abnormal thickness of a heart muscle segment commonly observed in young athletes who die suddenly.

The echocardiogram also reveals the condition of each of the four heart valves and how well they are working. The use of the Doppler mode shows in real time how blood passes through the valves, which can indicate the nature of a valve problem; for example, backward flow may indicate a leaky valve. The echocardiogram also gives information about the volume of circulating blood, which might be affected by treatments such as diuretics. The echocardiogram answers questions about how several factors are interacting on your heart, how treatment can be tailored to address a specific type of malfunction, and how best to maintain the heart's ability to pump blood.

Transesophageal Echocardiography

Your doctor may order a transesophageal echocardiogram (TEE), a form of echocardiography that overcomes some of the limitations of a regular echocardiogram. As the name implies, a transesophageal echocardiogram involves threading a small probe (less than half an inch wide) down your esophagus (the tube from your throat to your stomach). Instead of viewing your heart through your chest wall, the transesophageal echocardiogram transmits images from within your esophagus, which is much closer to the heart. It may be necessary if your weight, body shape, or other considerations make conventional echocardiographic techniques less useful.

You should not eat after midnight on the day of the test. However, if the test needs to be done urgently, it is best not to have eaten for 4 hours so that you are less likely to feel nauseous or vomit. Discuss with your doctor any medications you are taking, and whether you should take them before the test.

The test will probably be done in a hospital. Because you will be given a sedative, you should make arrangements to get a ride home. First you will lie on a table and an intravenous (IV) line will be inserted into your arm to deliver a sedative. The technician will place electrodes on your chest that will be hooked up to an electrocardiographic machine to monitor your heart rhythms throughout the test.

After numbing your throat with an anesthetic spray, the technician will gently insert a probe with the transducer at the end into your throat and down your esophagus. This part of the procedure is the most uncomfortable, and you may feel like gagging. Once the transducer is in place, you will not feel any pain. You will be partially awake for the procedure, because you may be asked to hold your breath or strain as if you were having a bowel movement, which puts your heart under some pressure and may help reveal problems.

When the test is over, the transducer and IV will be removed and you will be disconnected from the electrocardiographic equipment. You may feel sleepy from the sedative, and the doctor will want to make sure that your heart rate and blood pressure are normal, so you may remain in the hospital for a few hours. Most often you will be advised to wait at least 2 hours before you eat or drink anything, because your throat may still be numb. After the anesthetic wears off, your throat may be sore for a day or two. It's best not to drive for 24 hours, to be sure that the anesthetic is entirely out of your system, so arrange for a ride home from the test.

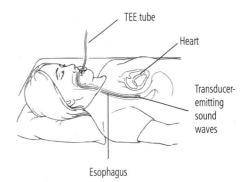

Transesophageal echo testing

In some instances, doctors insert an echocardiography transducer down the esophagus, instead of moving it over the chest. The transesophageal echocardiogram (TEE) transducer can get closer to the heart using this method, so the image is clearer. The person is conscious but sedated, so he or she does not feel discomfort.

Nuclear Imaging

Nuclear imaging, or scanning, techniques produce highly accurate pictures of your heart and its function by introducing a small, safe amount of radiation into your body. Trace amounts of radioactive material, called radionuclides, are injected into your bloodstream. The radionuclides tag your red blood cells and circulate with them into your heart and heart muscle. A specialized gamma camera, which reacts to the radiation by emitting light, constructs an image that is displayed on a monitor. Your doctor can study both your heart muscle and blood flow. Nuclear imaging techniques are often done in combination with a stress test and an injection of thallium. The nuclear isotope flows in the blood and may not appear on areas of the heart where there is a decreased blood supply; this is called a cold spot, or a perfusion (flow) defect.

Thallium Stress Test

A thallium stress test shows how well blood is flowing to the heart muscle during exercise. It can show any decreased blood flow to specific parts of the heart due to blockage of a coronary artery, the aftereffects of a heart attack, the effectiveness of procedures done to open coronary arteries, and other causes of chest pain. This test is also called a perfusion scan (perfusion is the flow of blood through a specific organ or tissue) or an isotope stress test (thallium and technetium are the two most common isotopes, or radioactive substances, used for these tests).

As with other nuclear scanning techniques, thallium or another tracing substance injected into your bloodstream travels to your heart and enters heart muscle cells. The images produced by the scan show how much blood is getting to different parts of your heart. If the supply appears reduced to a certain area, it indicates a coronary artery blockage. If no blood is getting to some tissue, it is probably dead (scar) tissue from a previous heart attack. The flow is compared at rest and after medication-induced stress. The test should not be performed during pregnancy.

What to Expect

You prepare for a thallium stress test like any other stress test. Do not eat or drink anything for 3 or 4 hours before the procedure, and wear clothing and shoes that will be comfortable during a treadmill exercise test—for example, athletic shoes or running shoes. Ask your doctor about whether you should take your usual medications before the test, particularly if you have diabetes and are taking insulin. For people who cannot exercise, this test can also be performed after medication is injected to simulate the effects of exercise. Ask how long the test will take; it may take several hours.

At the time of the test, a technician will apply electrodes to your chest and back that are attached to an ECG (electrocardiography) machine. Your heart rate and blood pressure will be measured, and then you will get on a treadmill. You will continue on the treadmill at a gradually increasing pace, until you are at or near your maximum level of exercise. You will be injected with the thallium (or other tracing material). Your heart rhythm is monitored continuously, and your blood pressure is checked periodically. You will then lie down on a table with a gamma camera over it, and the technician will take images of your heart while it is still working hard. You may need to hold a position for several minutes with your arm raised over your head.

After the exercise portion of the test is over, you can leave the office or laboratory for 3 or 4 hours. You may get something to eat and drink, as long as it does not contain caffeine or chocolate. When you return, you will lie down on the table under the gamma camera for images of your heart at rest. The thallium has moved through your body and can now be seen. It is important to lie still during this part of the test, which may last from 10 to 20 minutes. Some people find it challenging to lie in one position on a hard table, but there is no actual pain. When the test is complete, you can return to your usual activities and eat or drink anything you like.

Some laboratories choose to do the resting scan first and then the exercise scan. This test should not be performed during pregnancy.

What the Results Mean

You will probably get the full results in a few days. Generally, the results of a thallium stress test are as follows:

- If your results are normal during both exercise and rest, the blood flow through your coronary arteries to your heart muscle is adequate.
- If the blood flow is normal during rest but not during exercise (which your doctor may call a perfusion defect), then your heart is not getting enough blood when it is working harder. An artery is probably blocked.
- If your blood flow is reduced during rest and worsens during exercise, a portion of your heart is undersupplied at all times.

- If no thallium is present at all in some of your heart muscle both during and after exercise (the so-called fixed effect), you have probably had a heart attack and some tissue is dead; it is now scar tissue.

Multiunit Gated Blood Pool Scan (MUGA)

A multiunit gated blood pool scan (MUGA) is an assessment of how your blood pools in your heart during rest or exercise, or both. The test shows how well the heart pumps blood and whether it has to compensate for blocked arteries. It also reliably measures your ejection fraction, which is the percentage of your blood pumped out of your ventricles with each heartbeat. The ejection fraction normally increases during exercise.

What to Expect

If you are having only a resting scan MUGA, no special preparation is necessary. You should check with your doctor whether you need to stop taking any heart medications for a day or two beforehand. If you are having an exercise MUGA, you should not eat or drink anything other than water the night before the test. Depending on the extent of the testing, you should allow 2 to 4 hours for its completion. For the test, you will usually be asked to change into a hospital gown, and a technician will attach electrodes to your chest. The electrodes will be wired to a nuclear imaging computer. Then the technician will draw a small amount of your blood and mix it with the radioactive tracing material. About 10 minutes later, he or she will inject the prepared blood back into your arm. Then you will lie down on a table while the technician takes a number of images of your heart with the gamma camera. If you are having only a resting MUGA, the test is complete and you can go home.

If you are having an exercise MUGA, you will move to a different table with pedals at the foot. While you lie on the table, you will pedal as if you were on a bicycle, and the technician will take images. You will pedal through a warm-up stage, and then the exercise will be gradually increased until you are tired. You will be carefully monitored throughout the test.

After your MUGA, you may feel tired, but you can return to your usual activities. The harmless radioactive substance will leave your body in 2 or 3 days. This test should not be performed during pregnancy.

What the Results Mean

The full results of your test will be ready in a few days. In addition to the images produced, the computer also calculates the size and shape of your ventricles and measures the amount of blood in them. A low ejection fraction may be due to blockages in your coronary arteries or a problem with a heart muscle.

Other Imaging Techniques

Still more advanced technologies can be used to study your heart's structure and function. These procedures include computed tomography (CT), magnetic resonance imaging (MRI), magnetic resonance angiography (MRA), and positron emission tomography (PET). Such techniques are used to get more detailed information or to avoid more invasive procedures. These scanners are not available at all hospitals or diagnostic centers and are used only when needed to answer specific questions your physician may have.

Computed Tomography

CT scanning is an advanced X-ray technique that can take cross-sectional images of your heart. To have a CT scan done, you lie on a movable table that slides into the tubular CT scanner. Many images are taken from all sides of your body. A computer combines these images to construct a detailed cross section of a structure. Your doctor can assess images of your heart, lungs, or major blood vessels. CT scans are often used to see if calcification, a natural reaction to injury, has occurred in your blood vessels as a result of atherosclerosis (see page 152), or in your heart muscle as a result of a heart attack. As with other X-ray techniques, CT scanning passes some radiation through your body, but it is a minimal, safe amount that does not remain in your body after the test.

Allergy to Iodine Dye

For many tests, an iodine-based dye is used as a contrast medium to highlight various organs. The dye is given through injection, usually through a line placed in your arm. Tell your doctor beforehand if you know you are allergic to iodine; if so, you are more likely to react to the dye. Your doctor may prescribe a corticosteroid to take just before the test to help reduce the possibility of an allergic reaction. In rare cases, people experience tongue swelling, throat swelling, or difficulty breathing. If you have a marked reaction to the iodine dye during a test, you will be treated at the hospital. Be sure to report any previous allergic reactions before starting the test or during the test.

In some cases, a contrast agent (iodine-based dye) is injected into your bloodstream to get a clearer image. If you are not being injected with the dye, you will be told not to eat for about 2 hours before the test. If you are being injected with the dye, you should not eat for about 4 hours beforehand. In some people, this contrast agent causes hot flushing and other allergic symptoms, but this reaction is rare (see the box on page 139).

You will be asked to put on a hospital gown and lie down on the table. If a contrast medium is being used, an intravenous line will be placed into your arm. The table will be moved slowly into the scanner. The technician will start taking pictures, and you will be asked to lie still and hold your breath briefly as each image is taken. After the test, you may resume your usual activities.

Electron Beam Computed Tomography

Electron beam computed tomography (EBCT or fast CT) is a faster form of CT scanning that takes images in about one-tenth of a second (compared to 1 to 10 seconds for a conventional CT scan). Because the heart is always in motion, a conventional CT sometimes creates a blurred image. EBCT is fast enough to avoid this problem. EBCT enables your doctor to detect calcification in your arteries. EBCT is sometimes used for "whole body screening" for healthy people, but there is no evidence it is effective for that purpose.

Spiral Computed Tomography

Spiral computed tomography (or spiral or helical CT) is another form of fast CT scanning. For a conventional CT, you rest on a table while the scanner is moved slightly for each picture; with spiral CT, you lie on a table that moves slowly through the scanner while it takes images nonstop. These scanners are particularly helpful in finding aneurysms (ballooning in the wall of a weakened artery) and blood clots in the lungs (pulmonary emboli).

Multidetector CT Scans

A type of CT scanner with more detectors than a conventional CT machine can be used to provide the same kind of information about the coronary arteries as an angiogram reveals (see page 146). Because having a CT scan is easier and less expensive than an angiogram, the multidetector CT scan might be used more frequently in the future. A recent application is CT angiography, in which dye is injected and images are made of the coronary arteries that may detect both calcified and noncalcified deposits. CT angiography is being used as a screening tool in high-risk people and as a diagnostic tool in some hospital emergency departments with specialized chest pain centers. Medical experts are working on standards to guide the use of the new multidetector scanners.

Magnetic Resonance Imaging

MRI is another technology that uses magnetic fields and radio signals to form an image. Briefly, the MRI scanner surrounds your body with a magnetic field that reacts with magnetic elements in your body (such as hydrogen). The reaction causes radio signals from which a computer can construct an image. MRI scans produce images that are similar to those from a CT scan, but no radiation is used, and the MRI shows slightly different tissues. The test is painless, does not involve any injections, and does not pose any known risks. People who have pacemakers or other internal metallic devices cannot have an MRI, but people with artificial heart valves that are not magnetically active can have one safely. This test can be performed safely in the second half of pregnancy.

You do not need to prepare in any way for an MRI. You will change into a hospital gown and lie on a table that will be placed in the scanner, which is a long, narrow tube. Some people with claustrophobia may find the scanner uncomfortable. However, many scanners are now made with open ends that eliminate this problem. If you are concerned about being inside the scanner, talk to your doctor before the test is done; a sedative may be administered to help you relax through the test.

When you are inside the scanner, you may be asked to hold your breath briefly while images are taken. You may hear loud noises inside the scanner. Sometimes you can listen to music through headphones while you are inside the scanner, but the technician's instructions will also be transmitted via the headset. After the test, you can go about your usual activities.

Magnetic Resonance Angiography

MRA uses an MRI scanner to analyze the blood vessels leading to the brain, kidneys, and legs. This type of scan is done using different settings on the scanner, so the procedure is the same as for an MRI from your point of view. Usually, an MRA is done using gadolinium, a magnetic contrast agent to which virtually no one is allergic. This contrast agent is given as an injection, usually in your arm, before the scanning is done.

Positron Emission Tomography

PET scanning uses information about the energy released by subatomic particles in your body to form an image. A radioactive substance is injected into your body that will travel to damaged or malfunctioning tissues. These tissues have increased or decreased metabolic activity. The PET scanner detects and measures the radioactive substance in these areas of your body, and a computer constructs images. A PET scan is highly accurate because it shows your heart tissue at work. The uses for this technology are still developing, but it has the potential to show how your heart uses energy at a cellular level. Currently, PET scans are used mainly in research rather than in patient care or diagnosis of heart disease.

You do not need to prepare for a PET scan in any way. You will be asked to remove your clothes from the waist up, and a technician will place a ring of detectors around your chest. You will lie down on a table that will be moved into the PET scanner. The scanner is shaped like a large funnel, and your body will be in the tube. The technician or doctor will take a picture of your heart before the radioactive substance is injected. You need to keep your arms above your head during this part of the test, which takes about 15 to 30 minutes. Then the radioactive material will be injected, usually in your arm. You will have to wait about 45 minutes for the substance to move into your heart. Again, you will be asked to keep your arms over your head while the images are being taken. After the test, you may resume your usual activities.

Cardiac Catheterization

Cardiac catheterization is a technique doctors use to perform many tests and procedures on the heart and blood vessels. Catheterization is an invasive procedure in which a catheter (a long, thin tube) is inserted into your body. For cardiac catheterization, a small puncture is made, usually in your groin, to access directly the underlying vein or artery. The catheter is guided through a blood vessel into your heart. A number of tests and some treatments can be accomplished by injecting substances (such as dyes) or guiding instruments into the catheter.

Typically, cardiac catheterization is the method by which iodine-based dye is introduced for a coronary angiogram (imaging of the inside of your blood vessels, such as your coronary arteries; see page 145); a ventriculogram (imaging of the interior of your ventricles, done for some types of heart valve diseases or diseases of the heart muscle); or electrophysiology studies (an assessment of your heart's electrical activity; see page 147). Specialized types of angiograms can be done via catheterization to get information about your peripheral blood vessels and the arteries in your lungs (pulmonary angiography). Cardiac catheterization can also be done to study congenital heart defects and to assess the pressures of the blood within the heart.

Less invasive and less expensive tests (such as echocardiography or nuclear scanning) can provide a great deal of information, but only cardiac catheterization can detect some types of problems such as blockage in the artery. Cardiac catheterization may be done after other tests, in order to confirm or build on those results. Doctors can also do a biopsy (obtaining a sample of tissue) of heart muscle via a cardiac catheter, to detect inflammation or to check for tissue rejection after a heart transplant (see page 250).

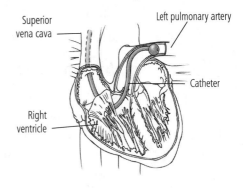

Cardiac catheterization

Doctors can image the heart or even treat some conditions by using cardiac catheterization. The doctor inserts a catheter (a thin tube) into a blood vessel (often in the thigh) and then gently threads it into the heart. In this instance, the right side of the heart is seen. Substances or instruments can be introduced into the heart via the catheter.

Elective Cardiac Catheterization

If you are having cardiac catheterization done for a diagnostic test such as an angiogram or other nonurgent reason, you will probably go to a hospital, but often it is an outpatient procedure. Cardiac catheterization is a relatively common procedure, but because it is invasive it does carry some risk. Your doctor may still recommend it because he or she thinks that the benefit from the information the test can provide is greater than the risk. Talk to your doctor beforehand and ask any questions that concern you. Some people experience problems such as bruising, temporary numbness, or bleeding at the site of the catheter insertion, but these reactions are infrequent. Some people have allergic reactions to the iodine-based dye that is used as a contrast medium (see the box on page 139).

More serious complications such as inducing a heart attack, stroke, or an arrhythmia are even rarer and usually occur only in people who are already seriously ill. Remember that you will be carefully monitored and sterile procedures will be followed throughout the test.

What to Expect

Before having cardiac catheterization, talk to your doctor about any medications you are taking, because he or she may want you to stop taking them—especially blood thinners or anticoagulants—for several days before the procedure. It's a good idea to make a written list of your medications, including dosages, and bring it with you to the procedure, so that any doctors and technicians present know exactly what you are taking.

You will be told not to eat or drink anything after midnight before having cardiac catheterization. If you have diabetes, talk to your doctor beforehand about your food and insulin intake. If you are allergic to iodine dye, you will receive steroids the day before the test and another medication just before the test (see also the box on page 139.)

On the day of the cardiac catheterization, you can expect that the preparations and the procedure together will take 2 to 3 hours, with several more hours spent in a recovery room. You will probably have blood tests, an ECG (see page 122), and a chest X-ray done first. The procedure itself will be done in a catheterization laboratory, or cath lab. You will be attached to an ECG machine and will wear a blood pressure cuff. An IV will be inserted into your arm, and you will receive a mild sedative to relax you throughout the procedure.

The doctor or nurse will prepare the area of your groin where the catheter will be inserted by cleansing it and shaving it if necessary. He or she will inject your groin area with a local anesthetic so that you will not have any pain, but you will be awake so that your doctor can tell you what is happening and what he or she will do next throughout the procedure. Then the doctor will puncture the skin to enter the artery or vein into which the catheter will be inserted, using a specialized needle, and he or she will thread the catheter into the blood vessel toward your heart. You should not feel any pain during this process.

The doctor will thread the catheter through your artery and up into your heart. Then whatever test or procedure you are having will be performed via the catheter. The doctor may guide more than one catheter into different areas of your heart. A variety of instruments can be inserted to guide the tip of the catheter, draw blood samples, inject dye, take pressure readings in the chambers of the heart, and perform other testing procedures. Depending on what you are having done, you may feel sensations such as flushing, brief nausea, or your heart skipping a beat. These feelings are normal, so don't worry if they occur. Ask your doctor beforehand what you might expect. If you feel any chest pain, tell your doctor right away.

When the procedure is complete, the catheter and the IV will be removed. To stop any bleeding, the doctor or nurse will press very firmly on the insertion site, which may be uncomfortable, and then will put on a bandage.

You will be moved to a recovery room, and pressure will be applied on the insertion site for another 15 minutes or so. In some people, stitches or a closure device like a plug are needed to close the artery. You should try to lie still and keep your leg straight for several hours. A nurse will continue to monitor your heart rate and blood pressure. You will be free to leave when the sedative has worn off and any bleeding is controlled.

Someone else should drive you home. At home, plan on resting with your leg (or arm, if that was the insertion site) still for 6 to 8 hours. You should not strain or lift heavy objects for 48 to 72 hours, but you can probably resume normal activities after that. You may be told to take plenty of fluids to flush out the dye. Most people can walk in about 6 hours or so.

What the Results Mean

Cardiac catheterization can be used both as a diagnostic tool and for treatment. The most common diagnostic use is to help show clearly the anatomy of your heart and in particular the blood vessels of your heart. Through imaging during cardiac catheterization, doctors can detect if there are blockages in your blood vessels and also the sizes and locations of the blockages. Treatment options include management with medications and a healthy lifestyle, surgery, or treatment done during catheterization. For example, your doctor may perform balloon angioplasty (see page 176) as part of the cardiac catheterization if he or she sees plaque inside the arteries that needs to be compressed against the walls of the blood vessels to allow for improved circulation of blood. In addition, the doctor might place a stent to improve blood flow through a blocked artery. If after catheterization it appears that your blood vessels will need surgical repair, the doctor will discuss with you the possibility of a cardiac artery bypass graft (see page 180). The information from the pictures taken during the catheterization helps the surgeon in planning the procedure. See also "Considering Your Options," page 165.

Angiography

Angiography is an X-ray examination in which a contrast dye outlines the heart or blood vessels. To perform an angiogram, your doctor will insert a cardiac catheter (see page 143), positioning the tip of the catheter either into your left ventricle or at the opening of each of the coronary arteries. Then an iodine-based contrast agent (dye) will be injected so your doctor can watch the blood flow through these structures. Some people are allergic to the iodine-based dye (see the box on page 139 for information on what to do if you are allergic). When the dye is in your ventricle, you may feel warm.

The angiogram shows how well the heart is pumping, its shape and internal parts, and whether there is any faulty valve action that causes leakage or backflow. If the dye is in your coronary arteries, the angiogram shows whether any narrowing or blockages are restricting or cutting off blood supply.

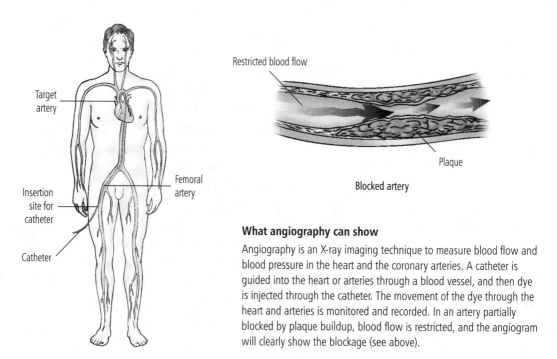

Target artery

Insertion site for catheter

Catheter

Femoral artery

Restricted blood flow

Plaque

Blocked artery

What angiography can show

Angiography is an X-ray imaging technique to measure blood flow and blood pressure in the heart and the coronary arteries. A catheter is guided into the heart or arteries through a blood vessel, and then dye is injected through the catheter. The movement of the dye through the heart and arteries is monitored and recorded. In an artery partially blocked by plaque buildup, blood flow is restricted, and the angiogram will clearly show the blockage (see above).

The diagnostic catheterization and angiogram will probably take about 1 hour, but you should allow most or all of the day for the entire procedure. After the test, you will rest until the sedative has worn off. You can drink lots of liquids to help rid your body of the contrast agent.

Electrophysiology Studies

For some people with problems related to their heart's electrical activity, such as arrhythmias (irregular heartbeats), an ECG or other tests do not give enough information. Electrophysiology studies are tests that require cardiac catheterization to enable doctors to send controlled electrical impulses into the heart to determine where the problem is and how it might be corrected.

To perform electrophysiology studies, the doctor inserts a cardiac catheter (see page 143) and then passes a type of electrode into the chambers of your heart. This electrode catheter will relay impulses into your heart to make it beat at different speeds. Your doctor can follow the impulses and map your heart's electrical conduction system and its reaction to the impulses. You might be given a medication through the catheter to cause an arrhythmia, or you might be given medications designed to stop the arrhythmia in order to see which ones work best in you.

Tilt-table testing is another type of electrophysiology test. You will not feel pain, but you will feel your heart changing speeds, and this feeling might be uncomfortable or even alarming. In the course of the studies, the table you are lying on may be tilted to bring you into an upright position, because your heart rhythm or blood pressure might change when you are upright. Straps around your chest will hold you securely. This test is usually done on people who have unexplained light-headedness. Because the studies may involve both diagnosing your condition and testing some drugs, the procedure may be lengthy. Depending on what is being done, the studies may take 1 to 4 hours.

After the studies are done, your recovery period will be similar to that for any cardiac catheterization (see page 145). The risks involved in electrophysiology studies include the risks of any catheterization procedure. In addition, even though the electrical stimulation of your heart is very carefully controlled, there is some risk of severely abnormal heart rhythms occurring. The laboratory in which the studies are done is equipped with a defibrillator (a machine that stops abnormal heart rhythms with electric shock). If such an emergency occurs, you may lose consciousness and the doctors will use the defibrillator and resuscitate you if necessary. If you do remain conscious, you will be given a fast-acting anesthetic before the defibrillator is used.

The Testing Process

Very probably, your doctor will need to do several tests to gather enough information to diagnose your condition and decide on the right course of treatment. The series of tests your doctor recommends for you will not necessarily be the same as for someone else with a similar problem. The results of one test might yield information that requires more testing to fully understand your unique situation. You also might need to have the same test several times to determine how your heart is responding to any medications, surgical procedures, or other treatments. Your personal medical history is also a factor in determining which tests are appropriate.

Don't hesitate to ask your doctor why a specific test is required at this time and what information he or she hopes to derive. Ask the doctor directly about the pros and cons of any procedure, and discuss thoroughly how you feel about any risks versus benefits of having the procedure.

You can also ask what different results might indicate about the next steps in your treatment. If you have any questions or concerns, you always have the option of seeking a second opinion. Remember that you are in charge of your own health and should make sure you have enough information to make an informed decision about any test or treatment.

If you decide to get another opinion, either to confirm a diagnosis or to get more information about your options, tell your doctor that you plan to do so. Your primary-care physician or local medical society can help you find another qualified doctor. Never feel guilty about getting a second opinion or think this will hurt your doctor's feelings.

When you go to see a doctor for a second opinion, bring a complete set of your records and copies of any tests that have been done. If you get a different recommendation from a second doctor, it doesn't necessarily mean that one is right and the other is wrong. There is room for legitimate differences of opinion, especially concerning a complicated problem or major treatment decisions.

You are the most important decision maker. Your confidence in the choices made and your priorities about how treatments for your heart condition affect your life are extremely important factors to consider. Your overall treatment will be most successful if you and your doctor or doctors are working together to make decisions that positively affect your life.

11

Heart Attack

A heart attack occurs when a blockage in the coronary arteries—those that supply the heart itself—shuts off the flow of oxygen-rich blood to heart muscle tissue. Without oxygen and nutrients, the heart muscle will begin to die. Prompt medical attention can restore blood flow and limit the extent of damage, but dead tissue cannot be restored. The lack of blood supply, called ischemia, can weaken your heart or stop it altogether. If there is a prolonged decrease in blood supply, tissue dies, so this is an urgent matter. The severity of the heart attack depends on how much tissue is damaged and where in your heart the damage occurs.

Several different mechanisms can cause a heart attack:

- Atherosclerosis, in which the walls of the arteries thicken and accumulate fatty deposits called plaque, can narrow or block one or more arteries supplying a section of heart muscle.

- A blood clot can form within the artery and stick to the walls of the narrowed coronary artery, already thickened with plaque, and stop the blood flow.

- A blood clot also can form in the coronary artery itself, as a result of atherosclerotic plaque that cracks open, emptying its cholesterol and other components into the bloodstream.

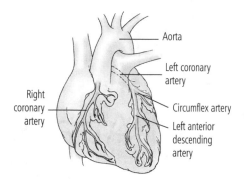

Healthy coronary circulation

The coronary arteries supply nourishing blood to the heart muscle itself—separate from the blood that passes through the heart to the rest of the body. Two main coronary arteries, left and right, branch off from the aorta and extend over the surface of the atria and ventricles. The circumflex artery, branching off from the left coronary artery, goes around the back of the heart.

- A coronary artery can temporarily spasm, narrowing the artery and restricting or stopping blood flow. These spasms most commonly occur in a blocked artery but may occur in a normal one.

The most common mechanism begins when a fracture develops within atherosclerotic plaque, exposing the inside of the plaque. This causes platelets to stick to the site of the rupture, triggering a cascade of events resulting in the formation of a blood clot that blocks the artery. This explains why aspirin, which helps reduce stickiness of platelets, is effective in reducing the risk of heart attack.

Every year in the United States, about 1.2 million people have heart attacks, and more than 40 percent of those people die before they reach a hospital. As scary as these numbers may sound, they are substantially lower than the figures of 25 years ago. Today, many Americans are doing a better job of reducing their own risk of heart attack. Doctors have made major advances in treatment, so that a person who gets medical help quickly is much more likely to survive a heart attack. A heart attack survivor has a much better chance of getting fully rehabilitated than ever before. The survival rates for men after a heart attack have improved in recent years, but this has not yet occurred for women. See also chapter 16, Women and Heart Disease.

Atherosclerosis

Most coronary artery disease leading to heart attack results from the process of atherosclerosis, the stiffening and narrowing of arteries. Early changes are seen in people as young as their twenties. A healthy artery is highly elastic, responding readily to changes in the amount or pressure of the blood flowing through it. As you age, the walls of your arteries tend to become somewhat thicker and stiffer, causing some resistance to the pumping action of the heart. This loss of flexibility in the arteries, which tends to accelerate as you get older, is the cause of higher blood pressure in older people and contributes to several forms of heart disease.

Apart from or in addition to these effects of aging, atherosclerosis is a disease process affecting the interior walls of the major arteries, including the coronary arteries that supply the heart. The inner walls of the arteries become inflamed and irregular and begin to accumulate fatty materials, cholesterol, and other debris that together form plaque. The plaque gradually builds up until it significantly narrows the channel through which blood is flowing. This unhealthy process of atherosclerosis is not fully understood, although a high-fat diet, high levels of cholesterol, smoking, and other known risk factors (see pages 19–22), along with genetic background, are major contributing causes. As plaque builds up, it can form accumulations (called atheromas or plaques) that ultimately shut off the blood flow. A blood clot traveling through the bloodstream can lodge on an accumulation of plaque and block the already narrowed channel altogether.

When a coronary artery is temporarily blocked, it can deprive some portion of the heart of oxygen and nutrients, resulting in a condition called myocardial ischemia. Prolonged ischemia can damage or destroy tissue anywhere in the heart, leading to an infarction (or death of tissue), depending on what part of the heart the affected artery supplies. Extensive damage to the left ventricle, the main pumping chamber of the heart, will affect a person's long-term health and activity level.

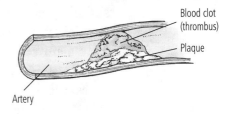

Atherosclerosis and blood clots
A coronary artery affected by atherosclerosis can be blocked by two means: plaque buildup and blood clots. As plaque (fatty materials, cholesterol, and other debris) accumulates on the inner artery wall, it narrows the channel and restricts blood flow. A blood clot (thrombus) passing through the artery can be easily snagged on the accumulated plaque, completely blocking off the blood supply to part of the heart.

The Role of Inflammation

Scientists now know that inflammation is a major component of the process of atherosclerosis. Just as inflammation of bones and joints can, over time, lead to arthritis, an inflammatory process inside blood vessels can lead to coronary artery disease or stroke.

Research has not yet pinpointed what causes the low-grade inflammatory process that may contribute to or even cause atherosclerosis in some people. In the future, a specific bacterial or viral infection may be identified, and treatment for coronary artery disease may include antimicrobial or antiviral agents, just as treatment for stomach ulcers now involves antibiotics for the bacteria that is known to be the cause.

In many people who have heart attacks, inflammation has caused the artery wall itself to absorb fat particles to form a type of plaque sometimes called "soft" or "vulnerable" plaque. This plaque, buried in the wall of the artery, is not the same as the plaque that builds up in the channel of an artery. Soft plaque is composed of fat-filled cells contained in a thin shell. If the shell containing the soft plaque breaks open, the plaque spills into the bloodstream, and a blood clot forms at the site of the rupture—the body's usual response to injury. This blood clot—rather than the plaque—may be the blockage that shuts off the blood supply. The inflamed and swollen artery may be less elastic as well. This process, starting with a type of inflammation and leading to a blood clot, may explain heart attacks in some people who do not have the traditional risk factors for coronary artery disease, such as high cholesterol.

A marker of the inflammatory (or immune) response is the presence of a substance called C-reactive protein (CRP) in the blood. Everyone's body makes CRP, but in different amounts, depending in part on genetic factors and in part on lifestyle. The same factors that tend to contribute to increased risk of heart attack—smoking, overweight, high blood pressure, lack of exercise—contribute to high levels of CRP. A person's CRP levels can be elevated early in the development of plaque in the arteries, and at the time of a rupture. When a heart attack occurs, CRP levels rise dramatically. As a result, measuring CRP levels in a person's blood is a good predictor of the development of coronary artery disease and the risk of future heart attacks, as well as a good indicator in an emergency department that a heart attack has occurred.

Nowadays, CRP is measured through a relatively simple test that can be done in a doctor's office. An elevated CRP level may be as reliable a predictor of heart attack risk in some people as a high level of LDL (low-density lipoprotein, the harmful cholesterol; see page 132). Research suggests that in some people, high levels of CRP are a significant risk factor for heart disease, independent of high cholesterol. It may be a better predictor in women than in

WARNING!

Signs of Cardiac Arrest

A person in cardiac arrest:

- Loses consciousness
- Stops breathing
- Lacks a pulse

Respond immediately:

- Call 911 or the emergency number for your area.
- If you are trained in CPR, use it to help keep the person alive until emergency help arrives to perform defibrillation.
- Look for automated external defibrillator (AED) equipment to use on the person. See also the box on page 155 on using an AED.

men. Other factors may raise the CRP level in the blood, however. At present, there is no specific treatment for high CRP levels, except for treating any underlying conditions.

Recognizing Symptoms of a Heart Attack

Clearly, knowing the signs of a heart attack and responding quickly are important. If people live long enough to reach the hospital, their chances of dying are dramatically reduced. Treatment to open clogged arteries is most effective within the first 60 to 90 minutes after symptoms (such as chest pain) occur. If the blood flow is completely shut off, permanent damage to heart muscle occurs in about 20 minutes. So every minute counts, both to save your life (or someone else's) and to improve the quality of life after the attack.

Calling 911 or the emergency services (fire department or ambulance) in your area should be your first step, before doing anything else. Paramedics can begin treatment immediately, even before you reach the hospital. If your heart actually stops beating, paramedics have the knowledge and equipment to begin advanced life support and to restore a heartbeat. Also, a heart attack victim who arrives by ambulance gets faster treatment at the hospital, because emergency medical technicians begin treatment as soon as the ambulance arrives.

Take an aspirin if you have one on hand. Chew it; don't swallow it. If you're unsure whether you personally should take aspirin, wait until the paramedics arrive. If you're alone, unlock your door, then sit down or lie down while you wait for the ambulance.

What to Do If Symptoms Occur

Many people delay going to a hospital, sometimes for as long as 2 hours after they first notice symptoms. Some

Using an Automated External Defibrillator

An automated external defibrillator (AED) can be used by people who are not doctors or nurses—for example, firefighters and flight attendants. Increasingly, AED units are being installed in workplaces and other public places where a person with some training on the device can save lives. The AED detects and measures the person's heart rhythm and automatically determines the appropriate amount of electrical current needed to restore normal rhythm.

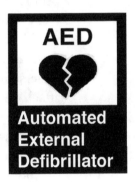

Locating an AED

Prompt use of an automated external defibrillator (AED) most effectively increases a person's chance of surviving a heart attack if it is used within 3 minutes of the person's collapse. When you are in any public place where people gather or where the incidence of heart attack might be high—for instance, an airport, a train station, a nursing home, or a health club—look for signs similar to this one indicating where an AED is placed.

Warning Signs of Heart Attack

Heart attacks may start with relatively mild symptoms. Call 911 or the emergency medical services in your area if you experience any of these symptoms for as much as 5 minutes:

- **Chest discomfort.** An uncomfortable feeling—such as pressure, squeezing, or a sensation of fullness—in the center of the chest that lasts for a few minutes or that goes away and then comes back. The feeling may not be truly painful.

- **Discomfort in other parts of the upper body.** The uncomfortable feeling or pain may spread to one or both arms, the back, the neck, the jaw, or maybe the stomach.

- **Shortness of breath.** Difficulty breathing often occurs with or just before chest discomfort. It may be the only sign of a heart attack.

- **Light-headedness, cold sweats, nausea, or indigestion.** Some people, particularly women, experience these symptoms, and some report having a sense of impending doom.

If you have heart attack symptoms and for some reason cannot call 911 (or the emergency number for your area), have someone else drive you to the nearest hospital immediately. Never drive yourself unless you have absolutely no other choice.

people are just hoping the symptoms will disappear, some don't want to feel embarrassed by a false alarm, some think that a "real" heart attack would be dramatic and unmistakable, and some don't realize the enormous advantage of immediate treatment. Although these feelings are understandable, doctors urge you to seek help at the first signs of a heart attack, so that effective treatment begins as soon as possible.

It's easier to respond quickly to symptoms—either your own or someone else's—if you have thought through the steps you will take before an emergency arises. First, of course, you have to learn the warning signs (see box). Talk to your doctor about your personal risk of a future heart attack and how you should respond—for example, whether you should take aspirin or use nitroglycerin (see page 166). If you are at risk, talk with your family, friends, and coworkers about the warning signs and the best response. Find out who, if anyone, knows cardiopulmonary resuscitation (CPR) and alert him or her to the possible need for it. If 911 services are not available, keep the numbers for your area's emergency medical services (fire department and ambulance) next to the telephone. Find out which hospitals nearby have 24-hour emergency cardiac care.

When you arrive at the emergency room, a doctor or other staff may ask you questions about your symptoms. If you are able to respond, the information you give them will help guide your treatment. Questions may include:

- When did you first notice symptoms?
- What were you doing at the time?
- Were the symptoms most intense right away, or did they build up gradually?
- Did you notice any symptoms other than the first or most intense ones?
- On a scale of 1 to 10, how would you rate the discomfort you felt?
- What medicines have you taken today?
- What medicines do you usually take?

Chest Pain

Most people would probably name chest pain as the symptom they associate most closely with heart attack. But very often the symptom that a person experiences from a blockage in the coronary arteries is not a sharp or stabbing pain. People who have experienced a heart attack often go to great lengths to say that the sensation they had was not exactly pain, but rather an uncomfortable feeling of squeezing or pressure (angina pectoris; see page 158–160).

The somewhat confusing fact is that chest pain may be caused by a heart condition other than heart attack, and it can also result from problems having nothing to do with the heart, such as gallbladder disease, a muscular disorder, or a digestive problem. The most important distinguishing feature of pain caused by coronary artery disease is probably a link to some sort of stress, either physical or emotional—an indication that the heart's increased need for oxygen is not being met. Chest pain at rest deserves immediate medical attention, especially in a person with risk factors for heart attack. The first episode of chest pain in a person's life may be the sign of an impending heart attack, so don't delay seeking medical help.

For reasons that are not at all clear, women with heart disease are more likely to experience symptoms other than chest pain—such as shortness of breath, indigestion, or fatigue—making diagnosis more complex. People with diabetes also may not experience typical chest pain. Some people may have jaw pain or arm pain that for them is the

Calling for Emergency Help

If you or someone you know might be having a heart attack, call 911 or the emergency services number for your area. More than 90 percent of the United States now has 911 service, but in some communities the emergency number is that of the fire department, police department, or town hall. Keep the number handy at home for all family members. If you call for emergency services from a cell phone, be sure to mention the location you're calling from because the location can't be traced quickly, as it can from a landline. Also, if you use cable or broadband service for Internet-generated calls, find out whether your service will give you access to a 911 service or to some other administrative service office that does not handle emergency calls.

equivalent of chest pain—a sign of a heart attack. If you have experienced symptoms of heart attack before, the important point is to learn to recognize them when they occur so that you can respond without hesitation.

A form of chest pain related to heart disease may also be caused by inflammation of the outer surface of the heart, the pericardium. Like inflammation anywhere in the body, an inflamed pericardium swells and causes pressure on nerve endings that may result in pain when you breathe in, when you move in certain ways such as leaning forward, or when you lie down. Even though not all chest pain indicates a heart attack, you should still get medical help if you experience any kind of a chest pain that lasts for as long as 5 minutes. It is definitely better to be safe than sorry.

Angina Pectoris

Angina, or angina pectoris, is the term that describes the typical chest discomfort or pain that signals an inadequate flow of blood to the heart, most often the result of a blockage in the coronary arteries. Many people who have experienced angina struggle to characterize it, but they often describe it as a constricting pressure or fullness; a squeezing, crushing, or burning sensation; or a dull pain in the center of the chest. It may radiate out to the arms, shoulder, back, neck, or jaw. But it may also be confined to a small area of the chest, and it can last several minutes. Alternatively, it goes away and returns over a period of minutes. However, pain that lasts less than 30 seconds or more than 30 minutes is usually not anginal pain.

Angina usually occurs when the heart demands more blood for a variety of reasons: physical exertion, such as walking uphill or having sexual intercourse; mental or emotional stress, including fright or anxiety; cold temperatures; or even eating a meal that triggers digestive activity. When pain brought on by exercise is relieved by rest, angina is suspected by your doctor. Many people have "stable angina"—that is, they have episodes of angina that occur in a fairly predictable pattern. This is the reason behind stress testing as a way to reproduce a person's chest pain symptoms during exercise: to help diagnose coronary artery disease. Usually, a person with stable angina can relieve the symptom with rest or nitroglycerin (see page 166), or both.

Unstable angina is a form of chest discomfort that occurs for the first time in that person or occurs when the person is at rest. It can be more severe and prolonged than stable angina. The blockage in the arteries that brings on unstable angina may be atherosclerosis, a blood clot, inflammation, or infection. The experience of unstable angina is an emergency situation. If you have new, unpredictable, or increasingly severe chest discomfort, go to a hospital emergency department immediately for evaluation.

A variant form of angina, sometimes called Prinzmetal's angina, differs from other types because it is not related to physical or emotional stress. It usually occurs when the person is at rest or asleep, often between midnight and 8 o'clock in the morning. Variant angina is a

Heartburn or Heart Attack?

It's not always easy to distinguish between the chest discomfort of a heart attack and the burning sensation of heartburn (acid reflux). About one out of ten people who go to an emergency department complaining of chest pains has heartburn. Either symptom occurs in the general area of the chest, may have a burning quality, and may occur after a big meal. The location of the pain may be a clue: heart attack pain is likely to radiate from the chest into the shoulder, arm, or neck, especially on the left side, while heartburn usually stays more centered and travels into the neck or throat. But don't take any chances. Remember that most of the damage done by a heart attack occurs in the first hour or so. Get to an emergency department quickly if you have any doubt about the nature of your discomfort.

symptom of coronary artery spasm (see page 161), which may occur in an open artery or in an artery already blocked by atherosclerosis. The spasm occurs close to the blockage and obstructs blood flow to the heart muscle.

Angina can occur more rarely as a symptom of other heart conditions such as valve disease, cardiomyopathy (disease of the heart muscle; see page 162), or extreme high blood pressure. Angina may be treated with nitroglycerin or other medication (see page 166).

Shortness of Breath

Shortness of breath is another common symptom of a heart attack that can be difficult to differentiate and describe. Difficulty breathing can take the form of feeling unusually breathless with exertion; experiencing rapid or shallow breathing; or feeling short of breath at rest. Some people report that they feel conscious of the need to draw breath.

Of course, it is normal to feel short of breath for a while after strenuous exercise. Anxiety can cause hyperventilation, a form of rapid or shallow breathing. An overweight person may breathe more heavily just from the exertion of carrying extra weight, or someone who is out of shape may feel short of breath with even limited exercise. You are the best judge of when your shortness of breath feels abnormal.

If you feel short of breath at what for you is a moderate level of exercise, or if you become short of breath while at rest, or if your breathlessness occurs with chest pain, don't hesitate to get medical help.

Light-headedness and Other Symptoms

Some people feel light-headed—like they might pass out—as a symptom of a heart attack. (This sensation is different from dizziness, which makes you feel as if you or your surroundings are whirling.) Light-headedness can also signal other heart conditions, such as heart rhythm problems or problems unrelated to your heart.

Women are more likely than men to have atypical or more vague symptoms of heart attack such as light-headedness, nausea or queeziness, or fatigue, rather than chest pain. Researchers have only relatively recently recognized this gender difference, and the reasons for it are not yet clear. Genes, hormones, or lifestyle differences may be at work. Both women and their doctors need to be aware of the nature of a woman's symptoms and respond quickly to the possibility of heart attack. It is vital to keep in mind that heart disease is the leading cause of death for women, just as it is for men.

Silent Ischemia

A person can have an episode of ischemia (lack of blood to the heart) without angina or other symptoms, a phenomenon called silent ischemia. If the ischemia is severe or lasts too long, it may cause a heart attack with all the attendant dangers of heart damage or cardiac arrest, even if there is no chest pain. For many people the first sign of heart disease may be a cardiac arrest. Cardiologists estimate that 3 to 4 million Americans have silent ischemia every year. The resulting damage to the heart muscle is a leading cause of heart failure (when the heart's pumping action is inadequate). Most people who have episodes of angina or chest pain are likely to have episodes of silent ischemia, too. Although there is no way to know when silent ischemia occurs, an exercise stress test (see page 125) indicates how the blood flow in your coronary arteries is affected by exercise, and Holter monitoring (see page 124) records an episode of silent ischemia if it occurs while you wear the monitor.

Treatment for silent ischemia is aimed at improving the flow of blood to your heart and reducing your heart's need for oxygen—just like the treatment for any other symptoms of coronary artery disease. Your doctor will recommend lifestyle changes, medications, or perhaps ultimately surgical procedures such as angioplasty to reach these goals.

Coronary Artery Spasm

Chest pain may result from a spasm of the artery. Some people's coronary arteries have a tendency to go into spasm periodically (doctors are not sure why). The spasm, called a vasospasm, temporarily constricts the passageway and blocks blood flow to the heart. A spasm usually occurs in a coronary artery that is already blocked by atherosclerosis, but it can occur in an otherwise healthy vessel.

The spasm is temporary, but it can cause a heart attack, irregular heart rhythm (arrhythmia), or even sudden cardiac death. The major symptom of coronary artery spasm is a variant form of angina (see page 158) that is particularly painful and often occurs at the same time each day. To treat coronary artery spasm, your doctor may prescribe a medication called a calcium channel blocker (see page 168), which relaxes the smooth muscle in the artery walls and eases the discomfort of angina. In some cases, a nitrate may be prescribed also.

Outcomes of a Heart Attack

Lack of blood flow to the heart (myocardial ischemia) usually causes symptoms such as angina, a sensation of pressure in the chest; shortness of breath; or light-headedness. Ischemia may lead to a heart attack (myocardial infarction), as some part of the heart is deprived of blood for a period long enough for the heart muscle tissue to die. It is important to recognize these symptoms and seek medical help urgently, especially if you have any risk factors for coronary artery disease. Prompt medical help, in which the blocked arteries can be opened quickly with medications or a procedure such as angioplasty (which compresses the plaque on the artery walls), can minimize damage to heart tissue.

Insufficient blood supply can also cause cardiac arrest—when the heart stops abruptly. Cardiac arrest most often occurs when a person's heart rhythms are disturbed. The electrical impulses that control heart rhythms become either too fast (tachycardia), chaotic (fibrillation), or in rarer cases, extremely slow (bradycardia). A person in cardiac arrest is in extreme danger. To reverse cardiac arrest, the person's circulation should be maintained by cardiopulmonary resuscitation (CPR), and the heartbeat must be restored with an electrical shock (defibrillation). Brain death begins in just 4 to 6 minutes after a person's heart stops.

In some people the main effects of a heart attack are seen in the pericardium, the layer of protective tissue around the heart (see "Pericarditis," page 163).

The worst possible outcome of a heart attack is sudden cardiac death. Any form of heart disease can cause sudden death. But in most victims (about 90 percent) two or more major arteries are blocked by plaque, and the heart also shows scars from previous attacks. Sudden cardiac death can occur without a warning sign.

Ischemic Cardiomyopathy

Cardiomyopathy is a term for disease of the heart muscle (see page 7) that results from a condition that impairs the muscle tone of the heart and reduces its ability to pump blood. One form of the disease, called ischemic cardiomyopathy, starts as a result of damage from blockage in a coronary artery supplying a portion of the muscular walls of the heart. This damage leads to the inefficient pumping that is characteristic of cardiomyopathy. Frequently, cardiomyopathy is diagnosed by an echocardiogram (see page 132). The echocardiogram measures the ejection fraction, which is the amount of blood pumped with each heartbeat. In people with cardiomyopathy, this number is low, meaning that not enough blood is being pumped. Often the heart will dilate (widen) to compensate, so people with cardiomyopathy often have an enlarged heart.

Treatment for ischemic cardiomyopathy focuses on restoring the heart's pumping ability with medications and opening the blocked arteries to improve blood supply to the heart. Other types of cardiomyopathy include a viral cardiomyopathy, in which the heart is damaged by a virus, and toxic cardiomyopathy, in which the heart is damaged by some outside agent—for example, alcohol. If the heart has been severely and irreparably damaged by the disease, doctors may recommend a heart transplant (see page 250).

Pericarditis

Pericarditis is an inflammation of the pericardium, the membrane surrounding your heart. The pericardium actually has two layers, one of which is attached to the heart's muscular walls and the other which lines the cavity of the chest in which the heart is located. Fluid between the two layers enables the heart to move as it beats, yet stay in position. When pericarditis inflames the membrane, the amount of fluid increases and the heart's movement (particularly its ability to fill with blood) can become restricted. About 10 percent of people who have had a heart attack develop pericarditis, as a result of the death of tissue. Pericarditis occurs more often in men than in women. Infection, often due to a virus, is a common cause of pericarditis, especially in young adults. In many cases the causes of pericarditis may be unknown. Other causes of pericarditis include cancer or radiation therapy for cancer, injury to the chest, prior chest surgery, autoimmune disease, kidney failure, or use of medications that suppress the immune system.

The most common symptom of pericarditis is a sharp, stabbing pain in the center or the left side of the chest, and it sometimes radiates to

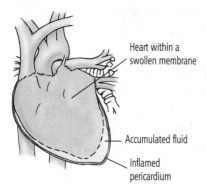

Inflammation of the pericardium

The pericardium is a thin, fluid-filled cushion surrounding the heart. In a person with pericarditis, the pericardium is inflamed and excess fluid builds up between the two layers of the membrane. The swelling puts pressure on the heart and restricts its movement.

the neck or shoulder. It can easily be mistaken for a symptom of a heart attack. Your doctor can begin to diagnose pericarditis by listening to your description of the pain and how it began. He or she can also listen with a stethoscope for characteristic rubbing sounds in your chest, which sometimes can be heard when the inflamed layers of the pericardium rub against each other as the heart beats. A chest X-ray may show an accumulation of fluid around your heart, which can be confirmed by an echocardiogram (see page 132). An electrocardiogram can show changes that indicate pericarditis. Occasionally, periocardiocentesis—a procedure in which a sample of fluid is withdrawn and analyzed—is needed to help determine the cause of the pericarditis.

Pericarditis is usually treated with pain relievers and anti-inflammatory medications such as aspirin or ibuprofen. When the condition is the result of a heart attack, pericarditis usually responds well to treatment and you are likely to recover in 1 to 3 weeks.

However, if the condition causes an accumulation of fluid around your heart that is seriously restricting your heart's filling ability (a rare but life-threatening disorder called cardiac tamponade), your doctor may perform pericardiocentesis (either with a needle or as minor surgery) to remove the excess fluid. Examination of the extracted fluid can help determine the cause of the cardiac tamponade. Repeated accumulations of fluid may require surgery.

Complications of pericarditis are rare, but the infection can cause arrhythmias or even a heart block (when the electrical impulses triggering heart rhythm fail to perform).

Constrictive pericarditis can also develop, in which the inflammation causes the pericardium to thicken and develop scar tissue (adhesions) between the pericardium and the heart. The pericardium becomes inflexible, and heart failure can result. In such cases, surgical removal of part or all of the pericardium is the only remedy.

There are other complications after a heart attack, depending on where the damage is located in the heart and how severe it is. The heartbeat may slow markedly, requiring a pacemaker. Arrhythmias (see page 255) or heart failure may also occur.

Considering Your Options

If testing shows that you have blockages in your coronary arteries, if you have angina, or if you have a heart attack, your physician may recommend treating your condition with lifestyle changes, medications, or procedures such as angioplasty or bypass surgery. In making a treatment recommendation, he or she will consider the overall pumping strength and electrical stability of your heart, as shown by testing, and also the severity of your symptoms. Deciding which treatment or combination of treatments is best for you is complex, but you and your doctor may discuss these strategies:

- **Lifestyle changes.** Lifestyle changes such as eating a healthy diet, getting regular exercise, and quitting smoking are proven to be beneficial in reducing the risk of heart attack, improving angina, or slowing the progression of disease after a heart attack. These factors are essential to support any other treatments you may receive. Your doctor will provide you with information and support, but only you can follow through.

- **Medications.** Medications such as beta-blockers, calcium channel blockers, ACE inhibitors, or statins (cholesterol-lowering drugs) can improve your heart's function and treat contributing factors such as high blood pressure and high cholesterol. They may relieve symptoms such as angina and may play an important role in controlling inflammation and preventing the plaque ruptures (see page 151) that lead to some heart attacks. They also may be prescribed after surgery to support your heart during recovery.

- **Angioplasty.** If one or more of your arteries is substantially blocked, angioplasty (see pages 175–180) will clear the blockage and restore blood flow. If you are having a heart attack, angioplasty at the time of the heart attack may help minimize heart damage. It is a considerably less invasive, less risky, and less expensive procedure than bypass. But some arteries are not suitable for angioplasty because they are too small. Other blockages are too dense or too large to penetrate with angioplasty. During angioplasty, a stent may be placed in an artery in an attempt to keep it from closing up (see also pages 177–180).

- **Bypass.** Bypass grafting (see pages 180–185) is the best approach for some people with severe angina or extensive blockages. Your doctor may recommend bypass surgery if your left main coronary artery, which supplies the left ventricle (the major pumping chamber), is significantly blocked, because any problem with angioplasty could cause serious damage to the heart muscle; if you have several major coronary arteries blocked; or if you have had previous angioplasty procedures. Bypass also may be necessary if you have another condition such as heart failure or diabetes.

Medications for Angina or Heart Attack

If you experience angina, medications are certain to be a part of your treatment. Because angina is an indication that your heart needs more oxygen (usually because of a blocked coronary artery), treatment includes drugs that either reduce your heart's oxygen requirements or increase blood flow to your heart so that it gets more oxygen. The goal of treatment with medications is to prevent or ease the discomfort of this symptom.

If you have a heart attack, you may be given medications (thrombolytic agents) at the hospital to dissolve blood clots that may have formed in an artery already clogged with plaque. This step limits the extent of damage to heart muscle and may save tissue before it is beyond repair.

Nitroglycerin

If you have angina, your doctor is likely to prescribe nitroglycerin, which is a vasodilator, meaning that it expands blood vessels to increase blood supply. Used properly, it relieves angina in as little as 2 minutes by reducing the return of (depleted) blood to the heart and thereby easing its workload, and by relaxing the coronary arteries to allow more oxygen-rich blood to reach your heart. It's important to remember that angina alone does not mean that you are having a heart attack or that heart muscle is being damaged—it is a temporary decrease in blood to the heart because of restricted supply and increased demand. Nitroglycerin provides a "quick fix" that allows you to be more active and free of pain.

Nitroglycerin is inexpensive and not at all habit-forming. You can take it several times a day without harm. It works best if you take it at the very earliest sensation of discomfort. Better yet, doctors advise people with stable angina to learn to recognize the conditions (exertion, excitement, or deep emotion) that are likely to lead to the pain and take nitroglycerin preventively. Many people experience angina in predictable circumstances, such as walking outdoors on a cold, windy, or humid day; carrying parcels or heavy items and hurrying; getting exercise after a heavy meal; working under deadline pressure; speaking in public; engaging in sexual activity; or feeling angry, worried, or tense. Being able to "head off" angina or keep an episode short is an excellent way to take control of your heart condition.

How to Use Nitroglycerin

Nitroglycerin is easy to take and fast-acting: it works in 2 minutes or less.

- Put the tablet under your tongue and let it dissolve, which takes only 20 to 30 seconds. (You can chew it, but it will not be as effective.)

- The medication works best in a moist rather than dry mouth.

- Keep several tablets in a handy pillbox so that you can take them promptly. The tablets are good for 3 or 4 months if they are kept in a tightly closed container.

- If three nitroglycerin pills taken 5 minutes apart do not relieve your chest pain, go immediately to the nearest hospital emergency department. If you are taking nitroglycerin in a different form (see the box on page 167), follow instructions on when to seek help.

If your doctor prescribes nitroglycerin, ask for directions about how to take it (see box) and talk to him or her about any concerns you have about using it. If you feel uncertain about it, ask to take a nitroglycerin tablet in your doctor's presence. You will probably feel a slight tingling sensation under your tongue, your face may flush, or you may have a sensation of fullness in your head as the medication works in your blood vessels, but more troublesome side effects (light-headedness or headache) are rare. Once you are accustomed to taking nitroglycerin freely, you can derive the full benefit of the relief it provides.

Beta-blockers

Beta-blockers (or beta-adrenergic blocking agents) are a group of drugs that reduce the heart's workload and decrease its need for oxygen. They are commonly prescribed for angina, high blood pressure (see page 62), irregular heartbeat, cardiomyopathy (disease of the heart muscle), and heart failure. (They are also used to treat non-heart-related conditions such as migraine headaches and glaucoma.)

A beta-blocker works by interfering with the body's natural response to stress. When your body is responding to stress, it releases hormones called catecholamines (norepinephrine and epinephrine) that stimulate an increase in heart rate, heart muscle contraction, and blood pressure. A beta-blocker diminishes the effects of the catecholamines, thereby modifying the heart's response to stress. Numerous beta-blockers are available that act selectively on different aspects of the action of catecholamines.

If your doctor prescribes beta-blockers for angina, the effects of the drug will enable your heart to work longer during exercise or other stress before the angina occurs. You will need to take the beta-blockers daily, in addition to other drugs such as nitroglycerin. Even if you have no symptoms, doctors will often prescribe beta-blockers, since studies have shown they can reduce the risk of a second heart attack.

If you experience a heart attack, your body will produce high levels of catecholamines that cause your heart to work harder. Doctors may give you a beta-blocker to ease your heart's activity and limit the injury done to heart tissue. After the heart attack, beta-blockers can help prevent another one from occurring. You may take the drugs indefinitely to reduce your risk of another heart attack.

Although beta-blockers are a well-established remedy for heart conditions, some people who take them experience muscle fatigue after exercise, light-headedness, or fainting. If you have a lung condition such as asthma, beta-blockers can cause a spasm of the bronchial muscles and thus interfere with passage of air into the lungs, resulting in shortness of breath or wheezing. Some people with diabetes may have light-headedness if the drug interferes with their recognition of when their blood sugar levels are too low. If you experience any side effects from beta-blockers, notify your doctor immediately. A different beta-blocker or an adjustment in the dosage may resolve the problem. However, do not stop taking the drug suddenly, and try not to miss any doses because that could worsen any cardiac symptoms. If you are taking other medicines or herbal remedies, be sure to tell your doctor to avoid a harmful drug interaction.

The following are some commonly prescribed beta-blockers, listed by their generic names: acebutolol, atenolol, betaxolol, bisoprolol, carvedilol, metoprolol, nadolol, pindolol, propranolol, sotalol, and timolol.

Calcium Channel Blockers

A group of drugs called calcium channel blockers, or calcium antagonists, relax the arteries and increase the supply of blood to the heart, while reducing its workload by decreasing blood pressure, heart rate, and muscular contraction. Chemically, calcium channel blockers work by preventing an essential step in the process of muscle contraction—the movement of calcium into muscle cells—in the heart and blood vessels. As a result, the heart and blood vessels relax. Calcium channel blockers may be prescribed for high blood pressure (see page 61) or angina and may also be used to prevent migraine headaches. Calcium channel blockers are also very effective for the treatment of coronary spasm and the variant angina it causes (see pages 159 and 161).

There are many calcium channel blockers, including both short-acting and longer-acting types. Calcium channel blockers are often used in combination with beta-blockers. Possible side effects vary with different types of the drug, but some people experience headache; tenderness, swelling, or bleeding of the gums; drowsiness; constipation; or a slow pulse rate (less than 50 beats per minute). Talk to your doctor immediately about any side effects, but do not stop taking the medication abruptly.

The following are some frequently prescribed calcium channel blockers, listed by their generic names: amlodipine, bipridil, diltiazem, felodipine, isradipine, nicardipine, nifedipine, nisoldipine, and verapamil.

ACE Inhibitors

ACE (angiotensin-converting enzyme) inhibitors are a group of drugs widely prescribed to treat high blood pressure and are now also given to many people after a heart attack to improve heart function. After a heart attack, some heart muscle is damaged and weakened, and it may continue to weaken over time. By lessening the workload of the heart and arteries, ACE inhibitors slow down this weakening.

As antihypertensives (drugs that lower blood pressure), ACE inhibitors reduce the workload on the heart caused by hypertension, and help prevent damage to the blood vessels of the heart, brain, and kidneys. Controlling high blood pressure reduces the likelihood of stroke, heart failure, kidney failure, and heart attack.

ACE inhibitors appear to work by blocking an enzyme (protein) in the body that helps produce angiotensin, a substance that makes the blood vessels contract. By inhibiting this process, the drugs relax blood vessels, the vessels expand, blood pressure goes down, and the workload for the heart decreases.

If your doctor prescribes ACE inhibitors after a heart attack, you will probably take the drugs for the rest of your life. These drugs also control blood pressure and preserve kidney function in people with diabetes.

ACE inhibitors tend to increase the level of potassium in your blood, so it is particularly important that you remind your doctor if you are taking potassium, salt substitutes (which often contain potassium), or low-salt milk (which can increase potassium levels). Talk to your doctor about any other medications you are taking, and check with him or her before using any over-the-counter medications or supplements.

Some people taking ACE inhibitors experience side effects including dizziness, light-headedness, or fainting; skin rash; fever; or joint pain. If you experience any of these effects or others, check with your doctor as soon as possible. A high potassium level often has no symptoms or very nonspecific symptoms such as nausea, weakness, malaise (feeling list-less), palpitations, irregular heartbeat, or a slow or weak pulse. Tell your doctor if you experience these symptoms. However, high potassium levels usually cause few symptoms until they are dangerously high, so your doctor may periodically monitor the potassium level in your bloodstream.

The following are commonly prescribed ACE inhibitors, listed by their generic names: benazepril, captopril, enalapril, enalaprilat, fosino-pril, lisinopril, perindopril, quinopril, ramipril, and trandolapril.

Angiotensin-2 receptor blockers (ARBs) may be prescribed. ARBs differ from ACE inhibitors in that ARBs inhibit the effect of angio-tensin, rather than blocking it in the first place (see also page 61).

Medications to Treat Blood Clots

Blood clots often play a prominent role in cardiovascular disease. In a healthy person, specialized blood cells called platelets have the capacity to form a clot in response to injury, as a way to limit loss of blood. How-ever, in a person with cardiovascular disease, a blood clot that forms abnormally in an artery leading to the heart can cause a heart attack (myocardial infarction), and one that travels to an artery leading to the brain can cause a stroke (cerebral infarction; see chapter 13).

In a person with coronary artery disease, the plaque that builds up in the coronary arteries can be destabilized by factors such as high blood pressure, high blood sugar, or the toxic ingredients in tobacco. A type of plaque called soft plaque (see page 154) can rupture, and the platelets respond as they would to an injury, by forming a clot over the damaged area. A blood clot in an already clogged artery can block the blood flow completely, causing a heart attack.

Thrombolytic Agents

Thrombolytic agents ("clot busters") dissolve clots in the arteries, restoring blood flow to heart tissue. Their use has substantially reduced disability and death from heart attacks and strokes. These drugs (including streptokinase, urokinase, and tissue plasminogen activator, or tPA, used for strokes) can be given as soon as you have been diagnosed as having a heart attack or stroke, either because of your symptoms or in response to the results of an electrocardiogram. If you get to a hospital immediately and the thrombolytics go to work within 4 to 6 hours of the onset of your symptoms, you are very likely to have only minimal damage to your heart function. If too much time passes before the thrombolytics are given, the damage is already done and restoring blood flow will not revive the tissue.

Emergency department personnel administer thrombolytic agents intravenously. The most serious drawback of these drugs is that they do not distinguish an abnormal blood clot from a useful one. You cannot receive them if you have a condition that might cause a bleeding problem, such as a stomach ulcer, a recent injury or surgical procedure, or a recent stroke.

Antiplatelets

Antiplatelet drugs interfere with platelet function and the formation of blood clots. Platelets are the elements within the blood that stick together and form clots. Some drugs (such as aspirin) are used to prevent clot formation in people at high risk of heart attack. Some types are given if you are having uncontrolled chest pain (unstable angina) or during or immediately after a heart attack to reduce recurrence. Antiplatelets are also given after an angioplasty, insertion of a stent, or bypass surgery to prevent clots from forming inside the vessel.

Clotting is a chemically complex process, and different antiplatelet agents disrupt specific stages of clot formation. They are used alone or in combination to treat different types of heart attacks or under various circumstances.

Aspirin is the most familiar antiplatelet drug (see page 173). Because it is inexpensive, effective, and easy to take by mouth, it is often the first treatment given at the onset of heart attack symptoms, even before you get help from emergency medical services (see page 174).

Taking aspirin right after a heart attack may improve survival rates by as much as 20 percent. At the hospital, other antiplatelets (such as clopidogrel or glycoprotein inhibitors) may also be given, either orally or intravenously. Doctors are learning more all the time about how to use these drugs to benefit more patients.

Because all antiplatelet drugs interfere with normal blood clotting, the main risk of taking them is bleeding. The bleeding is usually very minor, such as skin bruising or nosebleed. In people who are being treated in a hospital for heart attacks, the most common sites of bleeding are where catheters have been inserted— for example, in the groin where an access catheter is inserted for angioplasty. This type of bleeding is usually easily controlled by applying pressure to the site. Rarely, bleeding occurs from another source such as a stomach ulcer.

Anticoagulants

Anticoagulants are used to prevent the forming or growth of a blood clot by interfering with the clotting process. But they do not dissolve an existing blood clot, as a thrombolytic agent does. Although they are commonly called blood thinners, they do not really thin your blood; they just reduce the blood's ability to clot. These agents, such as warfarin, are stronger than the antiplatelet medications. Therefore, your doctor's office will need to do careful and frequent monitoring—in the form of a blood test—of the clotting factor in your bloodstream. This is vital to prevent bleeding complications and to ensure adequate clotting effect.

If you have had a heart attack, you are at greater risk of developing a blood clot near the site of a clot that was dissolved by a thrombolytic agent. If severe damage occurred in your left ventricle, a clot could also form there, where it can cause serious complications, and your doctor may prescribe warfarin. Also, if you are in bed for a long time after a heart attack, blood clots can develop in your legs. Anticoagulants help prevent all these possibilities.

Heparin, which is administered intravenously in the hospital, is a powerful and well-established anticoagulant for heart attack patients. If

COX-2 Inhibitors and Heart Disease

Many people with arthritis pain have turned to a group of drugs called COX-2 inhibitors for relief. COX-2 inhibitors reduce pain and inflammation but cause less stomach damage than some other anti-inflammatory drugs (including aspirin).

Recently, rofecoxib, one of the best-selling COX-2 inhibitors, was taken off the market because studies showed that the drug increased the risk of heart attack and stroke in some people. Several studies showed that COX-2 inhibitors appear to affect the cardiovascular system adversely. All COX-2 inhibitors are being carefully reevaluated for their effect on the heart, since there is debate about whether only some drugs in the class or all of them increase the risk of heart attack and stroke.

Valdecoxib was voluntarily withdrawn from the market by its manufacturer, and celecoxib stayed on the market, but with a strong warning of possible heart damage. In the meantime, if you have been relying on one of these drugs, talk to your doctor about how to relieve pain while minimizing your risk of stomach or heart problems. For some people (such as those with severe arthritis pain and no risk factors for cardiovascular disease), the benefits of these drugs may outweigh the risks, so be sure to consult with your doctor.

You may need to consider combining other drugs to get relief while still protecting your stomach. You can also try nondrug alternatives such as heat wraps, ice packs, physical therapy, acupuncture, or massage. If you have no history of heart disease, diabetes, or high blood pressure—particularly if you are under 60—you may be able to take another COX-2 inhibitor. If you are over 60, you may be better off taking nonsteroidal anti-inflammatory drugs (NSAIDs), because your risk of heart disease and stroke increases with age.

Some doctors recommend checking your blood pressure once a month if you are taking either an NSAID or a COX-2 inhibitor. If your blood pressure starts to creep up, or if your ankles start to swell, see your doctor immediately. Some people report pain relief from taking glucosamine-chondroitin, a nutritional supplement, but there is no conclusive medical proof that this works.

you undergo a procedure such as angioplasty, heparin will be administered to prevent clots from developing at the site of the procedure. The dosage must be carefully adjusted and its use must be monitored closely. A new type of heparin, called low-molecular-weight heparin, has been developed that is injected and does not require as much monitoring. Any form of heparin can cause unintended bleeding as a side effect. After an angioplasty, stronger clot-preventing medications such as clopidogrel may be prescribed.

Aspirin for Heart Disease

For some people, taking aspirin regularly is a means of preventing the recurrence of certain types of heart symptoms or events. Your doctor

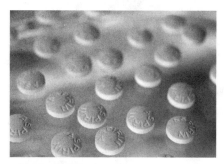

Taking aspirin for your heart

Your doctor may prescribe aspirin to help prevent heart attack, stroke, or chest pain. Aspirin is a type of drug known as an antiplatelet, which stops blood from clotting and reduces inflammation in arteries. Taking aspirin regularly is different from taking it occasionally, so talk to your doctor about what dosage to take and when to take it (morning or evening).

may recommend aspirin if you have had a heart attack, a transient ischemic attack (TIA; see page 214), or an ischemic stroke (see page 216), or if you have had trouble with recurring angina (chest pain; see page 158). Some studies even suggest that aspirin may help prevent a first occurrence of some of these events. Aspirin helps ensure adequate blood flow and may reduce the likelihood of clot formation. Aspirin works by slowing down the work of platelets in your bloodstream; when platelets are less sticky, clots are less likely to form. Aspirin may also help protect against the inflammation of arteries that occurs with atherosclerosis and may help prevent heart attacks in people with diabetes.

Taking aspirin regularly is different from taking it occasionally for something like a headache, and it poses some risks. You should not start taking aspirin for your heart without talking to your doctor first. In evaluating whether aspirin therapy is right for you, your doctor will consider your medical and family history; other drugs you may take, including vitamin or herbal supplements; allergies; the likelihood of certain side effects such as stomach

---

WARNING!
Aspirin during a Heart Attack or a Stroke

If you are having warning signs of a heart attack (such as chest pain), the most important thing to do is to call 911 or the emergency number for your area. Do not take an aspirin to see if it will relieve the pain before calling 911. Although aspirin will not treat a heart attack by itself, many experts recommend chewing one adult aspirin if you think you may be having a heart attack. Of course, if you are allergic to aspirin or have a condition that prevents you from taking aspirin, then wait until you get advice from a doctor. The 911 emergency operator may ask you about allergies and then recommend that you take an aspirin, or the emergency medical technicians may give you one in addition to other treatments. A single adult aspirin may reduce the chance of dying from a heart attack by about 20 percent, making it one of the most cost-effective life-saving measures in medicine.

If you or a family member is having a stroke, do not take or administer an aspirin, because not all strokes are caused by blood clots. The emergency department is best qualified to make a judgment about whether aspirin might be effective for the particular type of stroke.

bleeding; the relative risk versus benefit; and what dose is right. If you have some medical conditions such as bleeding disorders, asthma, ulcers, or kidney disease, aspirin may not be a safe choice. (See page 109 for information about aspirin and heart disease if you have diabetes.)

If your doctor recommends aspirin, it's important to take it exactly as he or she directs so that you get the desired benefit, and the chance of side effects is minimized. The instructions on the aspirin bottle are intended for general use, not for heart patients, so do not follow them. But read the label on the product you buy to be sure that it contains aspirin in the correct amount recommended by your doctor. Check the drug facts label for "active ingredients: aspirin" or "acetylsalicylic acid." If you experience any adverse effects after you start taking aspirin—such as stomach pains, indigestion, cramps, or black tarry stools (a sign of internal bleeding)—tell your doctor immediately.

Angioplasty

Medications and lifestyle changes are not always enough to prevent a heart attack. A person who comes to the hospital with severe angina or a heart attack probably has one or more coronary arteries that are completely blocked. The first priority is to restore blood flow immediately, and the next concern is to reduce the risk of another heart attack. Your risk is especially high if your heart's pumping ability has been compromised by damage, if you have blockages in three or more arteries, or if one of the blockages is in the left main coronary artery, which supplies the powerful left ventricle. Angioplasty, or balloon angioplasty, is a procedure that opens a blocked artery by compressing the plaque against the walls of the artery to clear a wider channel.

Angioplasty is also called percutaneous (through the skin) transluminal (in an artery) coronary angioplasty (PTCA). The procedure is done by inserting a catheter into an artery, usually in the groin, to pass it through the aorta to the heart. When the balloon reaches the site of the blockage, it is inflated to compress the plaque.

By opening an artery, angioplasty effectively relieves the pain of angina and minimizes damage to the heart. It may be done as an emergency procedure when a person arrives at the hospital in the midst of a heart attack. Angioplasty may also be performed on a nonemergency basis, to relieve angina symptoms or to try to prevent a heart attack. In

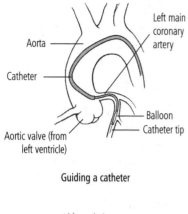

Aorta

Catheter

Aortic valve (from
left ventricle)

Left main
coronary
artery

Balloon

Catheter tip

Guiding a catheter

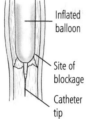

Inflated
balloon

Site of
blockage

Catheter
tip

Compressing blockage

Balloon angioplasty

To perform angioplasty, a doctor threads a balloon-tipped catheter through a blood vessel and into a blocked coronary artery, and then inflates the balloon at the site of a blockage to compress plaque against the arterial walls. This procedure quickly restores blood flow to the heart at relatively low cost and low risk.

the United States, more than 1.2 million angioplasties were performed in a recent year in people with coronary artery disease.

In most cases (70 to 90 percent) of angioplasty procedure, the doctor will insert a stent into the artery (a device to support the walls from the inside). Some stents are covered with medications that help reduce the risk of clot formation. The reason that stents are not placed in some people is the location and the type of lesion.

The main purpose of a stent is to reduce the possibility of the artery narrowing again in the same place, a process called restenosis (see page 178). Restenosis occurs in about 40 percent of people with angioplasty alone, and only about 20 percent of people with angioplasty and stenting. For reasons that are unclear, people with diabetes are at increased risk for restenosis.

If your doctor recommends that you have an angioplasty, you will probably have a chest X-ray, an electrocardiogram (see page 122), and blood tests before the procedure. You and your doctor can thoroughly discuss why you are having the angioplasty, how it will be done, and what you can expect afterward. Be sure to talk about any medications you are taking; your doctor may ask you to stop taking them—particularly antiplatelet or anticoagulant drugs—before the procedure. You will also be asked not to eat or drink anything after midnight before the procedure. If you have diabetes, talk to your doctor in detail about your medications and your food intake, because either of these factors affects your blood sugar levels.

How Angioplasty Is Done

An angioplasty is usually done in a catheterization laboratory, often called the cath lab. Electrodes will be placed on your chest and you will be connected to an electrocardiogram machine to monitor your heart during the procedure. You do not need a general anesthetic, but you will receive an intravenous sedative. The area of your leg (or sometimes the arm) where the catheter will be inserted will be anesthetized, then cleansed and shaved. After this area is numbed, you will not feel any pain during the procedure, but you will be awake.

The doctor will locate the appropriate artery and insert a catheter (a thin tube) through the skin. He or she will guide the catheter through the artery up the aorta and into your heart, watching its path on a monitor. When the catheter is at the opening of the coronary artery, a dye is injected so that the doctor can take an image of the arteries (an angiogram; see page 146) and see on the monitor if there is a blockage of blood flow within the artery. After studying the size and extent of the blockage, he or she may insert a tiny balloon-tipped device, guide it to the site of the blockage, and then inflate the balloon, which will expand against the walls of the artery. The inflated balloon is kept in place for up to 2 minutes and then deflated. The doctor can inflate it several times if necessary to shape the inside of the artery. When the results are satisfactory, the deflated balloon and catheter are removed.

Laser Angiography

In some medical centers, angioplasty can be done using laser technology. A laser-tipped catheter is guided through the artery and into the blockage, and then pulsating beams of light vaporize the blockage. The procedure can be done alone, or in combination with conventional angioplasty. Laser technology is not used very often because of the effectiveness of other techniques. The decision about whether to treat you with balloon angioplasty, stenting, or laser angioplasty—or coronary artery bypass—depends on where the blockage is, how many blockages you have, and the extent of the blockages. Discuss your options with your doctor so that you fully understand the treatment your doctor recommends.

How Stents Are Placed

A stent is a piece of tubing made of springy wire mesh. It is placed over the balloon on the tip of the catheter and guided into position in the cleared artery. Then the balloon is inflated and the stent expands, locks in place, and props the artery open, with the compressed plaque behind it. The balloon is deflated and removed, and the stent remains permanently. Within a few weeks, new tissue forms over the surface of the stent so that the interior passageway is smooth. Stenting can be done alone, but is usually done in combination with angioplasty. The surgeon can work on several blocked arteries during one procedure.

After the Procedure

An angioplasty procedure is likely to last from 45 minutes to more than 2 hours. After the procedure is done and the catheter is removed, the doctors or nurses will stop the bleeding by applying pressure, either manually or with specially designed pressure devices, for 20 minutes or more over the place where the catheter was inserted, and then will bandage the area. You will feel sleepy until the sedative wears off. You will be asked to lie very still during the recovery period for up to 8 hours. A nurse will monitor your heart and blood pressure and will check the incision site frequently for signs of excessive bleeding or damage to the blood flow through the artery. You will probably spend from 1 to 2 days in the hospital.

You will have to arrange to have someone drive you home, and you should not drive for several days afterward, while the incision is still healing. Your doctor will ask you not to bathe, or stand and walk for long periods of time, for at least 2 days after the procedure. Once you get home, call your doctor promptly if you see any bleeding or swelling at the site of the incision or if you have a fever, which is a possible sign of an infection. If you have a stent, you should probably avoid exercising vigorously for about 30 days. However, there are many cases on record of people returning to work or exercise sooner than that; ask your doctor what is best for you.

Your doctor may prescribe medications such as nitroglycerin (see page 166) to relax the coronary arteries, calcium antagonists to guard against coronary artery spasm (see page 161), or aspirin and other antiplatelet drugs (see page 171) to prevent blood clots in the area of the blockage. If you have a stent, you will have to take blood thinners (such as aspirin) indefinitely. You will also take an antiplatelet such as clopidogrel (see page 172) at least one month after a bare-metal stent is placed in your artery and two or more years after a drug-eluting stent is placed in your artery. Because of the presence of the metal stent, you should not have magnetic resonance imaging (MRI) for at least 4 weeks without checking with your doctor first. But you can go through a metal detector at an airport without a problem.

Restenosis

Restenosis (renarrowing or constriction) can occur in the same area of the blood vessel where your angioplasty was done, often within about

6 months of the original procedure. Although placement of a stent greatly reduces the likelihood that this will happen, restenosis can occur in an artery with a stent (in-stent restenosis). The artery becomes blocked again because, in addition to the healthy new tissue that forms over the stent, scar tissue can develop under the surface that becomes so thick it obstructs the blood flow again. People with diabetes have a higher risk of restenosis, but it can occur in other patients as well, depending in part on the location of the blockage and the pattern of scar tissue growth.

If a restenosis occurs, the person is likely to experience the same types of symptoms (chest pain after exertion) that he or she felt before the first angioplasty was done. (A patient with diabetes may have fewer or less typical symptoms.) Fortunately, restenosis very rarely causes a heart attack. Your doctor will be watching closely to detect restenosis and to check for blockages in other arteries by monitoring your symptoms and having you take a follow-up exercise stress test. Be sure to report promptly any symptoms that you experience after your angioplasty. If a restenosis does occur, another angioplasty or bypass surgery may be required to correct the blockage.

Of course, doctors are searching for ways to prevent restenosis. A major advance has been the development of drug-eluting stents—that is, devices that are coated with slow-release medications that penetrate

Chelation Therapy

You may hear about chelation therapy as an alternative to conventional treatments for coronary artery disease. Chelation therapy involves injections of a synthetic chemical called EDTA (ethylenediamine tetraacidic acid). EDTA is used to treat metal (lead or mercury) poisoning because it binds to metals in the bloodstream and promotes their passage from the body in urine. Some practitioners advocate taking EDTA for coronary artery disease, on the theory that it can remove calcium (a component of plaque) from the body, causing the plaque to break up and dissolve.

Some patients claim to feel better as a result of chelation therapy. Many practitioners also recommend positive lifestyle changes that may in part account for the anecdotal successes.

No scientific evidence validates chelation therapy, and insurance companies and Medicare will not cover its use for cardiovascular disease. Also, taking EDTA poses serious risks of kidney failure, harmful effects on bone marrow, and heart arrhythmias, among other reactions. The National Institutes of Health is currently conducting a major clinical trial to accumulate data about the safety and effectiveness of chelation therapy for heart disease patients. In the absence of data, a person with heart disease needs to think carefully about pursuing this form of therapy, especially if it is in place of proven treatments.

the surrounding tissue to prevent the growth of scar tissue. Drug-eluting stents appear to substantially improve the long-term success of angioplasty procedures, though they also increase the short-term risk of clot formation. If you have a drug-eluting stent, you will need to take clopidogrel for at least two years and aspirin indefinitely. Before surgery, ask your cardiologist if a bare-metal stent or drug-eluting stent is best for you.

Doctors at some medical centers are working with a procedure called brachytherapy, which uses radiation to stop tissue growth around a stent. A catheter with a radioactive tip is threaded into the blockage around a stent and a dose of radiation is administered. Although the radiation lasts only about 10 minutes, it inhibits long-term growth of tissue. Brachytherapy is not widely available, however, and needs study.

You can help protect yourself from restenosis by leading a heart-healthy lifestyle after angioplasty. Quit smoking, eat a low-fat diet, get regular exercise, take your medications, and follow up regularly with your physician to contribute to the success of your angioplasty. A cardiac rehabilitation program will offer advice and support to help you incorporate these vital changes into your life (see page 185).

Coronary Artery Bypass

Coronary artery bypass, which creates new routes for blood to flow around or bypass a clogged artery, is a major surgical procedure to restore adequate blood supply to the heart. To perform a bypass, a surgeon removes part of a vein from the person's leg or thigh, or an artery from the chest wall or arm, and grafts the segment to a blocked coronary artery to form a detour around the blockage. You may sometimes hear the operation called CABG (coronary artery bypass grafting, or "cabbage") or CAB (coronary artery bypass). Doctors may recommend bypass surgery as an aggressive strategy to treat coronary artery disease for a variety of reasons: when medications and lifestyle changes are not enough to prevent severe angina or heart attack, when blockages are numerous and extensive, or when a medical condition such as diabetes or heart failure make other treatments such as angioplasty less workable. (See "Considering Your Options," page 165.)

In the United States, more than 500,000 people had bypass surgery in a recent year. Bypass surgery requires dividing the sternum (breastbone) in order to expose the heart. The operation usually requires putting the person on a heart-lung machine throughout the procedure, meaning that the person's heart is stopped and not moving while the surgeon works on it.

A person may require more than one bypass to provide adequate blood to the heart. The number of arteries bypassed is not totally indicative of how severe your condition is, however. The location and extent of the blockages are significant as well.

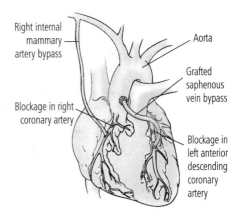

Coronary artery bypasses

Instead of opening a blocked coronary artery, a surgeon can create a bypass around the blockage. He or she grafts a section of blood vessel from elsewhere in the body onto the artery so that blood flows around the blockage and reenters the artery below it.

What to Expect

Most coronary artery bypass operations are scheduled surgeries, rather than being done as an emergency measure. If your cardiologist recommends a coronary artery bypass, you will have the opportunity to discuss why he or she wants you to have the surgery, what the risks are, what your alternatives are, and what your family needs to know about your surgery and recovery period. If you decide to proceed with the surgery, be sure to remind your doctor about any medications you are taking, including over-the-counter drugs and supplements. Make a list of your medications and bring it with you to the hospital when the surgery is scheduled. As the day of the surgery approaches, tell your doctor about any changes in your health. It is especially important to be aware of symptoms of a cold or flu, such as fever, chills, coughing, or a runny nose. Even minor infections could affect your recovery.

You will probably be admitted to the hospital the morning of the surgery, or perhaps the night before. You will be asked to bathe before arriving. You will be asked not to eat or drink anything after midnight before the surgery, to prevent regurgitating the stomach contents and choking on them. (If you do have something to eat, be honest and tell the doctor or nurse about it.) Be sure to ask whether you should take medications at home—with a very small sip of water—that you normally take each morning. You can expect to have an electrocardiogram (ECG), blood tests, urine tests, and a chest X-ray. Then a nurse will give you a sedative to relax you before you go to the operating room. The areas that will be operated on (your chest and leg or arm) will be washed, sterilized, and shaved if necessary.

How Bypass Is Done

In the operating room you will be wired to an ECG machine to monitor your heart (see page 122). You will be given a local anesthetic before an intravenous (IV) line is placed in your arm, and then you will be given a general anesthetic. The surgery will probably take 4 to 6 hours, depending on the number and complexity of the blockages. When you are completely asleep, a breathing tube (endotracheal tube) will be inserted through your mouth and down your trachea to help you breathe and to enable nurses to clear secretions from your lungs. Another tube will be inserted through your nose and down your throat to your stomach to prevent liquid or air from entering your stomach, so that you will not feel nauseous or bloated after you wake up. A catheter (a thin tube) will be placed in your urethra (the passageway to your bladder) to collect urine during and after the procedure.

You will be given an anticoagulant medication (see page 172) such as heparin to keep your blood from clotting. Then you will be connected to the heart-lung machine (see the box on page 183), which will take over your heart's pumping action and oxygenate your blood during the surgery, so that your heart is still and not full of blood while the surgeons work.

The number of vessels bypassed during surgery depends on how many coronary arteries and their main branches are blocked. Your surgeon can construct a bypass in different ways. He or she may remove a piece of a long vein in your leg (the saphenous vein) or the radial artery in your arm, neither of which is crucial to the circulation in those areas. The surgeon will stitch one end of the vessel onto your aorta (the large artery leaving your heart) close to where the coronary arteries originate, and graft the other end to the affected coronary artery below the blocked area. In effect, a new artery has been created to route blood around the blockage.

In many cases, at least one bypass will be created using a segment of one or both of the two internal mammary arteries, located behind your breastbone on your chest wall. These arteries originate from the aorta, so the surgeon does not have to entirely remove a piece of the artery. He or she can detach one end of the artery from the chest wall and reattach it to the coronary artery below the blockage. Remaining arteries are able to supply the chest wall with adequate blood. These arteries are used frequently because they may have less of a tendency to develop blockages after the surgery.

The Heart-Lung Machine

One of the most fascinating aspects of heart surgery is the heart-lung machine, or cardiopulmonary bypass machine. This equipment, which takes over the functions of your heart and lungs, enables surgeons to stop your heart while they perform a coronary artery bypass, valve repair or replacement, or heart transplant. It would not be practical for a surgeon to do the delicate work that is needed on a beating heart. While the heart is stopped and is not receiving blood, it is kept cool so that it needs less oxygen and tissue is not damaged.

At the beginning of the procedure, your heart is cooled down by one of several techniques so that it slows and then stops. The heart-lung machine goes to work, diverting oxygen-poor blood (returning from your body to your right atrium) before it enters your heart and bringing it into an oxygenating unit. In the oxygenator, oxygen is bubbled up through the blood so that the red blood cells pick it up, as they would do in your lungs. Then the air bubbles are removed from your blood and it is pumped back into your aorta, downstream from your heart. The oxygenated blood then moves throughout your body as usual.

The heart-lung machine can work for hours at a time, monitored by a specialist called a perfusionist. When the surgery is complete, the surgeon starts your heart again with an electrical shock and the heart-lung machine is shut off. Your heart and lungs resume their pumping and oxygenating functions.

When the operation is complete, the surgeon makes sure that your heart is adequately supplied, that blood is not leaking, and that the area is soft to the touch. Also, an angiogram while you are still on the table verifies that your arteries are not leaking internally. Then the surgeon restarts your heart with an electrical shock. The heart function is transferred from the heart-lung machine back to your heart.

Recovery in the Hospital

After surgery you will probably spend the first 1 to 3 days in the intensive care unit, where the staff will monitor your heart function closely. You will have a breathing tube and be connected to a ventilator for at least several hours, and you will have temporary drainage tubes in your chest to remove excess blood and fluids. (Some people, especially those with underlying lung disease, will need to be connected to a ventilator for a longer period of time.) You will have a catheter in your neck or under your clavicle in the chest to permit monitoring of your heart function and pressure. You will also have pacemaker wires attached to the heart muscle that come out of the chest and are attached to a pacemaker generator. You will receive intravenous fluids to keep you hydrated, and you will be given pain medications.

Some hospitals offer pain pumps that allow you to control the delivery of pain medications into your vein. A small catheter is placed in your chest incision that can deliver a local anesthetic directly to the area of your surgery. You can activate the pump by pushing a button at your bedside. Studies show that when patients control their own pain medication, the pain is better controlled but also people tend to use less medication. Self-administered pain relief allows people to recover faster and more comfortably.

The breathing tube is removed within hours. Most patients can get out of bed within 24 hours of bypass surgery and can walk in 1 or 2 days. When your doctor is satisfied that your heart has stabilized, you will be able to leave the intensive care unit, and the other catheters and tubes may be removed. Some people experience a rapid, irregular heart rhythm after the surgery, but this condition can be treated with medications. Or there may be slowing of the heart and if necessary, a pacemaker is installed. You will probably be strong enough to leave the hospital in 5 to 7 days.

Complications of bypass surgery may include pneumonia, urinary tract infection, or stroke. Anemia is common after the surgery, but the body usually recovers over time. Heart rhythm disturbances may occur and require treatment with medication or the installation of a pacemaker.

Recovery at Home

Subsequent recovery at home generally takes several weeks until you get back to your usual self. Some people experience loss of appetite and constipation. You may feel easily tired, moody, or depressed, and it may be difficult to sleep. Some people experience swelling in the area from which a blood vessel was removed, such as the lower leg, and you may have some muscle pain in your shoulders and upper back. These effects are normal and will probably disappear in 4 to 6 weeks. A full recovery may take several months, in part because your breastbone must heal, which may be painful. Don't hesitate to tell you doctor about bothersome side effects.

Your doctor can help you determine how quickly to get back to your daily routines. He or she will probably recommend that you gradually work your way back to normal activities such as walking, going out with friends, doing light housework or yard work, and climbing stairs.

Results of Bypass Surgery

A coronary artery bypass operation improves symptoms such as angina for most people (about 90 percent), and it may prolong life in certain high-risk cases. Most people can return to work or to the same activities they enjoyed before surgery and remain free of symptoms for many years. But bypass surgery does not cure coronary artery disease. New blockages can form in different places in the arteries, and the grafted routes can become clogged. Some branches of arteries are too small to be corrected by a bypass, and blockages in these small arteries can cause angina. Statistically, about 40 percent of people who have bypasses show signs of a new blockage in the bypass grafts within 10 years of surgery.

Controlling the risk factors that lead to blockage is the most important way that you and your doctor can manage your coronary artery disease. It is more important than ever to maintain normal weight or lose weight if necessary, quit smoking, eat a heart-healthy diet, and get regular exercise. Your doctor will work with you to achieve good control of high cholesterol, high blood pressure, and diabetes. Your cardiologist will want to see you every 1 to 3 months at first, and then at least annually to monitor your condition.

You will almost certainly be advised to take aspirin indefinitely. Your doctor may also prescribe medications such as ACE inhibitors, beta-blockers, or cholesterol-lowering drugs to help control your disease and improve your heart function.

Cardiac Rehabilitation

A cardiac rehabilitation program, often available through a community hospital, is a medically supervised program to help you learn to live with heart disease. This program provides you with the resources to get any kind of help you need to ease your transition back to a full, satisfying life. It involves a commitment of time, but it probably speeds your way to a full recovery. The trained staff can work with you to tailor your steps toward recovery to suit you, your medical condition, and your work and family demands. Exercise in a supervised setting, with skilled medical personnel available, usually provides a level of security that helps many people achieve exercise targets more easily and sooner than they would on their own. Many insurance plans cover cardiac

Living with Heart Disease

After you have had a heart attack, or after you have had a procedure such as angioplasty or bypass surgery, you need to step back and reassess your lifestyle to figure out how you can lessen the likelihood of another attack. Your goal for recovery will certainly involve returning to your normal activities. The nature of your recovery will depend on how active you were before your heart attack, how severe and damaging the attack was, how your body responds to it, and what kind of treatment you had. In the weeks and months after your heart attack, you will recover more quickly if you avoid stress, extremes of temperature, and specific circumstances that place a load on your heart. You may be able to resume some activities with modifications that lessen either the physical or the emotional stress on your heart.

It's important to talk to your doctor about your situation, but here are some guidelines:

- **Driving.** Driving involves sitting at attention; it may involve sudden movements and tensing; and it can be unpredictably stressful. After a heart attack, your doctor may recommend that you avoid driving for a week or more. If you have had bypass surgery, you can probably expect to drive again in about 4 to 6 weeks, although at first it may be advisable to limit yourself to short trips and familiar areas.

- **Work.** How soon you return to work depends in part on the physical and emotional demands of your job. Most people go back to work within 4 weeks to 3 months after a heart attack. After bypass surgery, if you have an office job, you may be able to return to work in 4 to 6 weeks. If your job involves heavy lifting or other strenuous physical exertion, you need to recover for 3 months. You may need to talk to your supervisor about ways to reduce either physical or psychological stress by changing assignments temporarily, or even taking a new job that is not so hard on your heart. People with white-collar jobs are more likely to return to work than are blue-collar workers whose jobs are physically demanding.

- **Sex.** There is no reason not to resume sexual activity as soon as you are physically ready for it. After a heart attack, you can probably start making love again in 3 to 4 weeks. You may need to start out slowly, by trying different positions or using pillows for support, and gradually working your way back to your usual patterns. If you have had surgery such as a bypass, your sternum (breastbone) will not be fully healed for about 3 months. During this time, you will need to avoid activity that puts pressure on your arms and shoulders. But you don't need to be afraid of sex. It is not true that having sex will bring on another heart attack. The often quoted statement by doctors is that once you can walk up two flights of stairs, you can usually have sex safely. After a heart attack, sex is easier with a longtime partner.

On an emotional level, if you are feeling discouraged or depressed during or after a heart attack or a major procedure, these feelings will probably diminish as your recovery progresses. Don't hesitate to talk about your feelings with your partner. If you or your partner have any concerns, discuss them with your doctor.

rehabilitation. Your cardiologist can give you information about programs near you.

A rehabilitation program usually lasts for the first 3 months or so after your heart attack. It is generally organized in four phases: hospitalization; early recovery (2 to 12 weeks after you go home); late recovery (6 to 12 weeks or more); and maintenance. The maintenance "phase" extends for the rest of your life, as your lifestyle changes become permanent and you resume your normal activities.

A cardiac rehabilitation program will help you:

- Gradually adjust your level of physical activity to strengthen your heart, monitoring your progress so that you can safely maximize your capacity for exercise
- Adjust your cooking, snacking, and eating styles to focus on a low-fat, low-cholesterol diet
- Work out a plan to balance your diet and exercise needs to control your weight
- Get counseling or other help to quit smoking
- Get advice about the impact of your job on your heart, and how you can take steps to protect yourself
- Learn about techniques (such as yoga, meditation, or massage) to manage stress on and off the job
- Deal with the emotional and psychological sides of the changes in your life
- Talk to other people who are facing the same challenges and making the same kind of changes in their lives

Minimally Invasive Heart Surgery

Cardiologists in some medical centers are exploring two alternatives to coronary bypass surgery in efforts to find less invasive and less expensive ways to treat coronary artery disease. Both of these alternatives are promising, but the results and long-term outcome are still being evaluated.

Port-Access Coronary Artery Bypass (PACAB or PortCAB)

For this procedure, your heart is stopped and a heart-lung machine assumes its function. The surgeon makes small incisions, called ports, in

Q. I've heard about an alternative to bypass surgery called TMR. What is it?

A. Transmyocardial revascularization (TMR) is an experimental procedure that uses lasers to treat severe angina in people who have no other treatment options.

Q. How is it done?

A. The surgeon makes an incision over the person's heart, then uses a laser drill to create 20 to 40 tiny channels in the wall of the heart. He or she applies pressure over each hole long enough to stop bleeding and seal it from the outside. More blood flows into the heart muscle through the channels from the inside, but does not leave the heart itself. Although the mechanism is not fully understood, TMR may work because the laser stimulates new blood vessels to grow to supply the heart muscle. Or it may destroy nerve fibers, making the person's angina painless.

Q. Why don't more people have TMR?

A. Surgeons don't know yet how long the treatment will last, and little follow-up data is available. Candidates for TMR now might include a person who has already had bypass surgery or angioplasty and cannot withstand another such procedure, a person whose blockages are too diffuse to be treated with bypass, or a person with a heart transplant who develops blockages in the arteries.

your chest and may remove part of the rib over your heart. He or she performs bypass grafting through these ports, viewing the work on video monitors rather than directly.

Minimally Invasive Coronary Artery Bypass (MIDCAB)

This procedure is done without the heart-lung machine, while your heart is still beating. It is used only when one or two arteries are being bypassed. The surgeon creates the small ports described above, and also makes a small incision directly over the blocked artery, so that he or she can view the work area directly, instead of on a monitor. Usually, an artery from the chest wall is used for this procedure.

12

Heart Valve Problems

The four valves that control the one-way flow of blood through the chambers of your heart open and close with your every heartbeat. These delicate structures deep inside your heart are critical to the measured passage of about 100 gallons of blood every hour. Responding to pressure changes behind and ahead of them, the leaflets (or cusps) of each valve must open fully and close tightly to keep blood moving properly (see pages 8–10).

If the valves are malformed or not fully functioning, two types of problems can interfere with the one-way flow. If a valve fails to open fully, impeding the forward flow of blood, the condition is called stenosis. Since the narrowed heart valve may limit blood flow, this can cause symptoms from inadequate circulation. Stenosis is usually the result of the leaflets thickening, stiffening, or even fusing together. Over time, the heart has to work harder to push blood through the valve, which can damage the heart muscle and enlarge the heart chamber.

If a valve cannot close completely to seal off back-flow, the problem is called regurgitation (also known as insufficiency or incompetence). Because blood is leaking backward, the heart chamber behind the valve tends to enlarge and may pump less efficiently.

Your heart has remarkable ability to adapt to and compensate for valve problems. Often a doctor can detect an abnormality in one of your valves by listening to your heart sounds through a stethoscope. The disruption in flow causes some audible blood turbulence, called a heart

The heart valves

The four heart valves open and close with each heartbeat, controlling the one-way flow of blood through the heart's four chambers. Blood from the body enters the heart through the right atrium, then flows through the tricuspid valve into the right ventricle. From the right ventricle, it flows through the pulmonary valve into the lungs. It returns to the heart through the left atrium, goes through the mitral valve into the left ventricle, and then is pumped through the aortic valve into the aorta, from which it is distributed throughout the body.

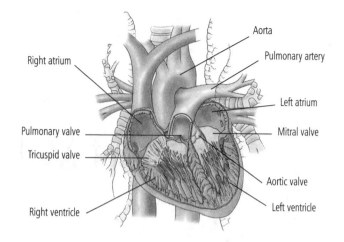

murmur. Because the heart has adapted, you may not have any symptoms and your heart may function quite normally for decades. But if, over time, your heart can no longer compensate, then symptoms such as shortness of breath can develop. It is important to have the problem diagnosed so it can be treated before permanent damage is done to heart muscle.

How Valve Problems Occur

Any of the four heart valves (mitral, aortic, tricuspid, or pulmonary) can be defective or become diseased in a variety of ways. The most common problems occur in the mitral and aortic valves, on the left side of the heart. The most typical causes of valve problems are:

- Congenital defects, meaning that a person is born with an abnormal heart valve
- Infectious disease, usually bacterial endocarditis, which can damage the valve with scar tissue
- Rheumatic fever, now uncommon
- Changes in valve structure or function that occur with aging
- Coronary artery disease, a heart attack, or heart muscle dysfunction that leads to problems with the way valves work, because of structural changes in the heart or a decrease in blood flow to the muscle that controls the valve's functioning.

The symptoms of valve problems can be subtle and gradual. They differ depending on which valve is involved and what type of malfunction is occurring. (For detailed information about specific valve disorders, see below and pages 192–203.)

Congenital Valve Defects

Some people are born with a defective valve but may never experience symptoms or may not have problems until later in life. Then the abnormal valve may be more vulnerable to calcium deposits that occur as a result of aging or abnormal functioning. If the defect is severe, the symptoms may occur earlier in life.

A valve defect that is congenital (present since birth) also increases a person's risk of endocarditis, an infection of the lining of the heart (endocardium) or heart valves (see page 192). Small amounts of bacteria may enter your bloodstream but are usually removed by your body's defense system. However, these bacteria are somewhat more likely to lodge on an abnormal valve, where they can cause an infection that can damage your heart valve. For this reason, if your doctor determines that you have a defective heart valve, to prevent infection you may need antibiotics to kill the bacteria before you have certain dental or surgical procedures (see page 194).

Innocent Heart Murmurs

If you are a parent, your doctor may tell you that your child has a heart murmur. This term just describes the sound that the blood makes as it flows through the heart. It does not mean that there is anything wrong. Because a child's heart is close to his or her chest wall, a murmur is often audible and may get louder or softer if the child is excited or has a fever.

Your child's doctor may call the sound an innocent, or functional, heart murmur, meaning that the sound will not cause any problems. There is no reason to worry or restrict your child's activities in any way.

If the doctor needs other tests to ensure that the murmur is innocent, he or she may order the tests or may refer you to a pediatric cardiologist. To help determine whether a heart murmur is innocent or is a sign of heart disease, initial tests include a chest X-ray, electrocardiogram, or echocardiogram. If the tests do not detect a problem, the murmur is in fact innocent, and your child's heart is absolutely normal and healthy.

Adults may also have murmurs that do not represent serious heart disease. The initial evaluation is similar to that for children and includes a chest X-ray, electrocardiogram, and echocardiogram. Murmurs may sometimes be heard in adults because the flow of blood across a normal valve is excessive. For example, in people with severe anemia, the heart may have to pump more blood to compensate for the body's decreased ability to transport oxygen.

Infective Endocarditis

Infective endocarditis is an infection of the lining of the heart chambers (endocardium) or the heart valves. It is caused by microorganisms—usually bacteria, but sometimes fungi or other types of microorganisms—that enter your bloodstream and lodge in your heart. These microorganisms occur naturally and harmlessly in other parts of your body, such as your mouth or urinary tract, and may enter your bloodstream from any tiny cut or breakdown of tissue (see box, page 194). The presence of bacteria in your bloodstream (which is called bacteremia) does not necessarily lead to infection, and not all bacteria are even capable of causing endocarditis. It is a relatively uncommon disease.

When endocarditis does occur, the microorganisms in the bloodstream stick to the surface lining of the heart or abnormal valves, perhaps aided by microscopic blood clots that have formed at the site. Your body responds by sending in immune cells and fibrin (a clotting material) to trap the organism. A clump of cellular material, called a vegetation, forms over the organism. Vegetations can interfere with a valve's function, or they can break off and block a blood vessel in a vital organ.

You are more likely to get endocarditis if you have existing valve disease, if you have had heart valve surgery, if you have a congenital heart defect, if you had rheumatic fever as a child that scarred your heart valves, or if you have an artificial heart valve or other foreign material in your body. Drug addicts who share needles or use dirty needles are also at risk for endocarditis.

Symptoms of endocarditis are variable, but they usually include fever. Many people report other flulike symptoms, too, such as muscle aches and pains, fatigue, night sweats, and loss of appetite. If you have chronic endocarditis, also known as subacute endocarditis, the symptoms can be subtle and last for months before the diagnosis is made. Sometimes symptoms of heart failure such as shortness of breath and confusion are the first sign of a problem. You or your doctor may also notice changes in your skin and nails, such as red spots on the palms of your hands or the soles of your feet, painful

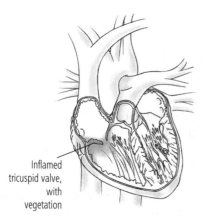

Inflamed
tricuspid valve,
with
vegetation

Infective endocarditis

Endocarditis is an infectious disease that affects the surface lining of the heart or heart valves. On a valve, the smooth lining becomes inflamed and a deposit forms, made up of the infecting bacteria, immune cells, and tiny blood clots. This deposit, called a vegetation, can interfere with valve function, or it can break off and lodge elsewhere in a blood vessel.

sores on the tips of your fingers and toes, or dark lines (tiny hemorrhages) under your nails that resemble wood splinters. Endocarditis can cause additional problems such as anemia and blood in the urine.

Your doctor may initially suspect endocarditis by your symptoms, especially if you are at known risk because of congenital heart disease, rheumatic fever, or valve disease. He or she will listen to your heart sounds with a stethoscope and may report a new heart murmur (the sound of turbulence in the blood flow through your heart) or a change in an old one. From blood samples that are sent for cultures, your doctor can identify if there is an infection and which microorganism is causing the infection. Only rarely are blood cultures negative (that is, falsely suggesting no problem) in people with endocarditis. An echocardiogram (see page 132) will often confirm the diagnosis by showing vegetations on the heart valve. The echocardiogram will also show the size of your heart and indicate how well the valves and heart wall are functioning.

To treat endocarditis, you will need to take intensive doses of antibiotics for 2 to 6 weeks to kill the infecting microorganisms in your bloodstream and to sterilize the heart valve. At first, you will need to be hospitalized so that the antibiotics can be given intravenously. In some people who respond well to the initial treatment, the full course of antibiotics may be completed at home or in a long-term-care facility. Your doctor will want to do regular blood tests to ensure that the medication is working.

In some people, endocarditis seriously damages a heart valve (natural or artificial). Endocarditis can also cause heart failure, the infection can extend into the heart, or the vegetations can repeatedly break off and travel throughout the bloodstream. Surgery may be necessary to remove infected tissue and repair or replace the valve (see pages 204–209).

Rheumatic Fever

Rheumatic fever was once the most common cause of heart valve problems. This inflammatory disease, which can develop as a result of untreated strep throat in children more commonly than in adults, occurs in some people when the body's immune response to fight the strep infection mistakenly attacks connective tissue (such as joints or the heart) instead. The affected tissue, often the heart valves, swells and develops scars. On a valve, the scar tissue may interfere with either opening or closing of the valve leaflets.

Taking Antibiotics to Prevent Endocarditis

In some cases, your doctor may recommend that you take antibiotics before some dental and surgical procedures, including professional teeth cleaning, to help prevent infective endocarditis. If you have a serious case of a condition associated with an increased risk of endocarditis (an abnormal valve, previous valve surgery, an artificial heart valve, endocarditis, or some congenital heart diseases), there is an increased risk that these procedures could introduce bacteria into your bloodstream that could lodge in your heart or valves.

Current medical guidelines recommend that only those people with serious underlying conditions take preventive antibiotics before these procedures, performed in parts of the body where bacteria are normally found:

- Dental procedures likely to cause bleeding, including teeth cleaning

- Tonsillectomy or adenoidectomy

- Bronchoscopy, an examination of the respiratory passages with a viewing instrument (bronchoscope)

- Some types of surgery done on the respiratory passageways, the digestive tract, or the urinary tract

- Gallbladder or prostate surgery

You can help prevent endocarditis by practicing good oral hygiene to keep your mouth healthy; telling your dentist about your heart or valve condition; giving your dentist your doctor's phone number so that they can discuss your case; and following instructions from your dentist and doctor about taking antibiotics before a procedure. You can also carry an endocarditis wallet card, available from the American Heart Association.

These measures cannot entirely prevent endocarditis, because it is not always possible to predict how or when microorganisms enter the bloodstream, to identify people at risk before procedures are performed, or to isolate the specific organism that might be involved. Doctors are very concerned about antibiotic use that might contribute to resistance to antibiotics. Ongoing research is investigating the most effective ways to prevent endocarditis.

Fortunately, the use of penicillin and other antibiotics to treat strep throat has almost eradicated rheumatic fever in the United States. But rheumatic fever remains a concern throughout the world. Without antibiotic treatment, anyone who gets strep throat can develop rheumatic fever, but it is most likely to occur in children from 5 to 15 years old. There is probably a genetic factor involved that makes some people more susceptible to rheumatic fever. The damage to heart tissue can last a lifetime, although it may not be noticeable for years after the illness.

If you have had rheumatic fever, even decades ago, you are more susceptible to heart attacks and valve disease. Although rheumatic fever rarely affects adults, you are more susceptible to it if you had it in childhood. Be sure to tell your doctor if you know that you have a history of rheumatic fever; you may need to take preventive antibiotics.

To protect yourself against the rare occurrence of rheumatic fever, it is important to get prompt treatment for a strep throat (caused by *Streptococcus* bacteria). Symptoms of strep throat include a sore, red throat; difficulty swallowing; a sudden fever; swelling in the glands in the neck; and sometimes a rash. If you experience these symptoms for 3 days, see your doctor to be tested for a strep infection. With antibiotic treatment, the symptoms are likely to disappear within a few days. It is essential that you continue taking the antibiotics as long as your doctor instructs, even after the symptoms are gone, to reduce the risk of rheumatic fever (though only a small percentage of strep infections result in rheumatic fever).

Symptoms of rheumatic fever can occur in 3 days to 1 month or more after an untreated strep infection. The symptoms include fever; joint pain or swelling in your wrists, elbows, knees, or ankles; nodules under the skin on your elbows or knees; a raised rash on your chest, back, or stomach; or weakness or fatigue.

See your doctor immediately if you experience these symptoms. He or she will do a throat culture (take a swab of material from your throat for analysis) and may order a chest X-ray or electrocardiogram.

If you have a strep infection that leads to rheumatic fever, your doctor will probably prescribe anti-inflammatory medications, including aspirin, to reduce swelling. You may also need to take a diuretic to get rid of excess fluids. Your doctor may prescribe antibiotic treatment monthly or even daily for life, to prevent reinfection.

If your heart has been damaged by rheumatic fever, you may need to take specific antibiotics if you undergo certain dental or surgical procedures (see box on page 194). Surgery to repair or replace a damaged valve may be necessary (see page 204).

Fen-phen and Heart Valve Problems

In the late 1990s, some women who had been taking fen-phen (a combination of fenfluramine and phentermine, two prescription appetite suppressants used to treat obesity) developed thickening and regurgitation in their heart valves. As a result, fenfluramine and a similar drug called dexfenfluramine were withdrawn from the market. Since that time, major studies have shown that most people who took fen-phen will not have valve problems. But if you took fen-phen at any time in the past, it's a good idea to tell your doctor and be examined carefully. If you develop any symptoms of a valve disorder, including a heart murmur, your doctor may order an echocardiogram.

Phentermine is still on the market, because no one has developed valve problems from using this drug alone. The original approval by the Food and Drug Administration was for each of the three drugs used separately; the fen-phen combination was never approved.

Mitral Valve Problems

The mitral valve regulates the flow of blood from the left atrium to the left ventricle, the main pumping chamber that pumps blood out into the arteries (see page 7). It is composed of two leaflets supported by a fine structure of stringlike tissues attached to the heart muscles. The mitral valve may be affected by prolapse, regurgitation, or stenosis.

Mitral Valve Prolapse

About 2 percent of the U.S. population have mitral valve prolapse, meaning that one or both of the flaps of the mitral valve are enlarged and the supporting muscles are too long. As a result, the leaflets do not close tightly and they billow into the atrium as the left ventricle contracts. Sometimes a small amount of blood leaks back into the atrium (regurgitation). Although there may be a variety of causes, many forms of prolapse are probably inherited. It occurs more frequently in women than men, often in very slender people who may have minor chest wall irregularities or scoliosis (a curvature of the spine). But it may be more severe in men.

In the vast majority of people, mitral valve prolapse is completely harmless and does not cause any long-term problems. Some people experience symptoms and seek treatment for them; symptoms include chest pain, palpitations (the sensation of feeling the heart beat), an irregular heartbeat, fatigue, shortness of breath when lying down, trouble breathing after exercise, or coughing.

Your doctor may detect mitral valve prolapse when listening to your heart through a stethoscope, because the billowing leaflets can cause a characteristic click, followed by a murmur. If necessary, he or she can confirm the diagnosis with an echocardiogram (see page 132) and assess the degree of regurgitation.

If you have little or no regurgitation and an otherwise normal heart, you will not need treatment. But if significant regurgitation develops, or if other illness is present, you may be at risk of a serious problem, infection of the valve.

Symptoms of mitral valve prolapse may improve with regular exercise, a decrease in caffeine consumption, and adequate fluids. Or you may be prescribed beta-blockers (see pages 62 and 167) to alleviate symptoms such as palpitations.

Mitral Valve Regurgitation

A mitral valve that fails to close completely when the powerful left ventricle contracts allows blood to "regurgitate" back into the atrium, undermining the one-way flow. Mitral valve regurgitation may be caused by damage to the valve from rheumatic fever (see page 193), infective endocarditis (see page 192), or a heart attack that damages the part of the muscle attached to the valve. The regurgitation can also result from enlargement of the left ventricle, possibly brought on by coronary artery disease or untreated high blood pressure, which stretches the perimeter of the mitral valve so that the leaflets do not close completely.

Many people have no symptoms; in others, symptoms develop over a period of years because the heart compensates for the problem. But over time, the extra effort can cause the left ventricle to enlarge or pressure to build up in the lungs as the blood leaks backward. The symptoms of regurgitation may come on slowly and can include shortness of breath or rapid breathing, fatigue, heart palpitations, or cough.

To relieve the symptoms of mitral valve regurgitation, your doctor may prescribe medications to lower your blood pressure (see page 59) or diuretics to rid your body of excess fluids. He or she may also recommend that you take antibiotics before some dental or surgical procedures to prevent infection of the valve (see page 194).

If surgery is necessary to restore valve function, your doctor will time the surgery carefully to be sure that your heart muscle does not become too weak to withstand the operation. The surgeon will repair your valve if possible, but in some people, an artificial valve is the best solution (see pages 206–207). After surgery, the long-term outlook for most people is very good.

Mitral Valve Stenosis

Mitral valve stenosis is a narrowing of the mitral valve. The narrowing or obstruction causes an increase in the pressure behind the valve in the left atrium. In most people, this type of damage to the valve was caused by a case of rheumatic fever in childhood (see page 193). Because the use of antibiotics has dramatically decreased the occurrence of rheumatic fever, mitral valve stenosis is becoming rare in the United States. It may occasionally occur in older people as a result of calcium deposits on the perimeter of the mitral valve, combined with the degenerative aging process that affects the tissues of the heart.

Many people with mild mitral valve stenosis do not experience symptoms, and treatment is not required. If the condition does cause symptoms to develop, they may develop slowly. Symptoms may include trouble breathing at night or after exercise; coughing, perhaps with traces of blood; fatigue; or chest pain that gets worse with exertion. There is risk of abnormal heart rhythms in the left atrium (atrial fibrillation), which can cause blood clots to form in the heart. The clots can dislodge and travel to the brain, increasing your risk of stroke.

A person with mitral valve stenosis may need to take antibiotics before undergoing certain medical or dental procedures to prevent infective endocarditis (see page 192) in the valve. Medication to slow the heart rate may help some people feel better. In some people with moderate stenosis, a balloon valvuloplasty (a procedure to open the valve with a balloon; see page 204) may be an option. For a person with a severely diseased valve, particularly an older person, surgical repair or replacement of the valve (page 206) may be necessary.

Aortic Valve Disease

The aortic valve, which has three crescent-shaped cusps (leaflets), regulates blood flow from the left ventricle into the aorta, where it then circulates to the rest of the body (see page 8). Either stenosis (narrowing) or regurgitation (backward leakage) can disrupt the blood flow. The valve can be damaged by rheumatic fever or infection. But some people are born with a bicuspid aortic valve—a valve with two leaflets instead of three. A bicuspid valve may be less efficient and more prone to infection or calcification with aging. The aorta may be abnormal, too, in people with bicuspid aortic valves, regardless of the severity of the valve disease.

Aortic Valve Regurgitation

When an aortic valve does not close completely, blood leaks or regurgitates back into the left ventricle. The condition occurs more commonly in men, often between the ages of 30 and 60. The most typical causes of mild regurgitation are structural abnormalities of the valve (such as a bicuspid valve), damage from rheumatic fever, high blood pressure, or calcification on the valve as a result of aging. In the most serious cases, the valve may suddenly start leaking as a result of infective endocarditis that actually makes holes in the leaflets or from a tear or severing of the aorta above the valve.

As with other heart valve problems, a person may not experience symptoms for years. But if the regurgitation forces the left ventricle to work harder over a long period, it may enlarge. Left untreated, irreparable damage to the left ventricle—the heart's main pumping chamber—could take place.

Symptoms, if or when they occur, include shortness of breath, chest pain with exercise, swelling in the ankles, fatigue, and a rapid pulse. Even if you do not have symptoms, your doctor may detect aortic regurgitation by listening to your heart sounds through a stethoscope. He or she will confirm the diagnosis and assess your heart function with tests, including a chest X-ray, echocardiogram (see page 132), and electrocardiogram (see page 122). You may be advised to take antibiotics before some dental and surgical procedures to prevent endocarditis (see page 194). Medications to treat high blood pressure and reduce the heart's workload may help reduce symptoms. Your doctor will evaluate you periodically by monitoring changes in your symptoms, your physical examinations, and tests such as echocardiograms.

Your doctor may recommend surgery to replace the aortic valve (see page 206) and limit damage to the heart muscle. As with surgery for mitral regurgitation, the procedure will be carefully timed to correct the problem before the heart is substantially weakened. If the problem is corrected before damage occurs, you are very likely to be able to return to a normal lifestyle.

Aortic Stenosis

If your aortic valve (which regulates the blood flow between your left ventricle into the aorta) becomes narrowed, your heart must work harder to force blood through the valve. As a result, the left ventricle enlarges and thickens. Over time, the heart may be unable to maintain the workload, and fluid may back up in the lungs.

Today the most common cause of aortic stenosis is a degeneration of the valve that occurs with aging. Calcium, a mineral found in the blood, can build up on the valve over the course of your lifetime. Some calcification may not cause any trouble, but in some people, calcium deposits

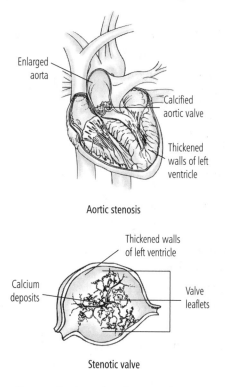

Aortic stenosis

Thickened walls
of left ventricle

Calcium
deposits

Valve
leaflets

Stenotic valve

Damage from aortic valve stenosis

Calcification on the aortic valve, usually as a result of aging, can fuse the leaflets of the valve so that it cannot close completely and blood cannot flow smoothly from the left ventricle into the aorta. As pressure builds in the left ventricle, its walls thicken. The aorta enlarges to try to keep blood moving.

and scarring develop that deform or even fuse the valve leaflets so that they do not close tightly. Another frequent cause, particularly in people diagnosed before the age of 50, is a congenital (from birth) defect in a valve, for example, the bicuspid valve, which may calcify it. Very high levels of LDL (low density lipoprotein) cholesterol also promote increased calcification (forming of calcium deposits) around the heart valve. Aortic stenosis is more common in men.

Aortic stenosis may not cause symptoms, and your doctor may first detect it by just listening to the heart with a stethoscope. An echocardiogram (see page 132) will confirm the diagnosis. But if the problem becomes more severe, a person may experience shortness of breath, chest pain (angina), dizziness, or fainting. Your doctor may recommend that you avoid vigorous exercise. Because your valve is abnormal, you are at greater risk of infective endocarditis (see page 192), and you may need to take antibiotics before some dental or surgical procedures to reduce that risk.

If the stenosis is severe, replacement of the valve (see page 206) may be required. After surgery, most people are able to resume a normal lifestyle. Balloon valvuloplasty (inserting a balloon-tipped catheter; see page 204) of the aortic artery is a temporary solution in adults if they are not able to have surgery when the stenosis is diagnosed. In some young adults or children, valvuloplasty will open the valve.

Tricuspid Valve Problems

The tricuspid valve is on the right side of the heart, regulating the blood flow between the right atrium and the right ventricle (see page 8). Disease in this valve is fairly rare. However, regurgitation (backward leakage of blood through the valve) may occur as the only valve problem or may occur with other problems. Stenosis (narrowing of the valve opening) is most often congenital (from birth) and rarely occurs in adults.

Tricuspid Regurgitation

If the tricuspid valve fails to close fully, blood leaks back (regurgitates) from the right ventricle into the right atrium. Instead of the blood moving forward through the right ventricle to the lungs to pick up oxygen, it backs into the major veins. It most often occurs if the right ventricle becomes enlarged or stiffened from another disorder, such as high blood pressure within the lungs and right side of the heart (pulmonary hypertension). Tricuspid regurgitation may also result from infective endocarditis (see page 192), rheumatic fever (see page 193), or cardiomyopathy (see page 249).

A person with tricuspid regurgitation usually does not have any symptoms, or the symptoms may be mild enough to live with for years, and no treatment is necessary. If you have high blood pressure in the lungs, as well as tricuspid regurgitation, you may develop symptoms of heart failure such as swelling in the stomach, liver, feet, and ankles; weakness and fatigue; and decreased urine output. Treatment with medications such as diuretics may relieve the symptoms. If tricuspid regurgitation is due to pulmonary hypertension, calcium channel blockers may be prescribed. In some people, surgery to replace the tricuspid valve (page 206) may be necessary.

If you have tricuspid regurgitation because of an abnormal valve, you are at increased risk of infective endocarditis, and you will need to take antibiotics before some dental and surgical procedures (see page 194).

Tricuspid Stenosis

If the tricuspid valve is narrowed or blocked, blood flow from the right atrium to the right ventricle slows down. The atrium may become enlarged and the blood flow to the right ventricle may be impaired. Tricuspid stenosis, which is rare, may be congenital (from birth) or the result of rheumatic fever. If rheumatic fever is the cause, other valves of the heart are usually involved.

Generally, the only symptoms of tricuspid stenosis are fatigue and the pain pressure in the liver (which you are likely to feel in your upper right abdomen). Often these symptoms, as well as some shortness of breath and fluid retention, are caused by disease in another valve. Treatment is likely to focus on the other valves. If your tricuspid valve is severely damaged, surgery is possible. As with other valve disorders, you are at increased risk of infective endocarditis, and your doctor may advise you to take antibiotics before some dental and surgical procedures (see page 194).

Pulmonary Valve Problems

The pulmonary valve controls the blood flow between the right ventricle and the pulmonary artery leading into the lungs (see page 14). Although disease is rare, the pulmonary valve can develop regurgitation (backward leakage) or stenosis (narrowing).

Pulmonary Regurgitation

Pulmonary regurgitation is a condition in which some blood is allowed to leak back from the pulmonary artery into the right ventricle. It is usually caused by congenital (present since birth) disease or pulmonary hypertension (high blood pressure in the lungs and right side of the heart). It is often associated with congenital heart disease affecting other parts of the heart. Very rarely, infective endocarditis (see page 192) damages the valve.

Many people with some pulmonary regurgitation do not have symptoms of the condition. Your doctor will monitor your heart regularly to ensure that the right ventricle is not becoming strained or enlarged. You will probably not need to limit your physical activities. If you have a valve that has been malformed since birth, you are at greater risk of infective endocarditis and may need to take antibiotics before dental or surgical procedures (see page 194).

If the regurgitation becomes serious, it causes the right ventricle to start to fail. Then you may experience symptoms such as shortness of breath, especially during exercise; fatigue; chest pain; or leg swelling. Arrhythmias may occur. Ask your doctor about any exercise restrictions. You may require surgery to repair or replace the valve (see pages 204–209).

Pulmonary Stenosis

Pulmonary stenosis is a condition in which the pulmonary valve (or the artery just beyond the valve) is narrowed, reducing the flow of blood into the lungs. It is usually present at birth and may progress in childhood or not until later in life. If it occurs later in life, it may have been caused by rheumatic fever (see page 193), congenital heart disease, or infective endocarditis (see page 192).

Pulmonary stenosis can be very mild or moderate, and it usually does not cause severe symptoms. Your doctor will check your heart regularly, watching for signs of strain on your right ventricle. You may not need to limit your physical activity, but you are at greater risk of infective endocarditis, so you will need to take antibiotics before having some dental and surgical procedures (see page 194).

If the condition is severe, it may cause symptoms such as shortness of breath, especially during exercise; fatigue; chest pain; or rarely, a bluish skin tone. Severe stenosis could cause life-threatening failure of the right ventricle. Sometimes surgery to repair the valve is done early, during the preschool years of a child's life. In an older person, balloon valvuloplasty is usually needed to open the valve, or rarely, valve replacement (page 204) may be necessary.

Medications for Valve Disease

Although medications cannot "fix" a diseased valve, they can help ease your symptoms, reduce the load on your heart as it works to compensate for a damaged valve, and regulate your heart's rhythm if it is disturbed by abnormal blood flow.

Digitalis (digoxin) is frequently prescribed for a person with valve disease to strengthen the contraction of the heart muscle and slow the heart rate. It is also used to treat congestive heart failure and some types of arrhythmia such as atrial flutter or atrial fibrillation. Derived from the foxglove plant, digitalis is a powerful drug that has been used medically for more than 200 years. Your doctor will discuss with you exactly how much digitalis you are to take, and it is important to follow instructions carefully. Other medicines you take can interact with digitalis, so be sure to tell your doctor about all other prescription and over-the-counter drugs you use. Also, be sure your doctor knows about any allergies you have or other medical problems such as diseases of the thyroid, liver, lung, or kidney. (For more information about digitalis, see page 243.)

Your doctor also may prescribe diuretics (water pills), which promote the removal of fluids by the kidneys. This medication decreases blood pressure and eases the workload on your heart. Blood tests may be needed to check for electrolyte loss from the diuretics.

Anticoagulant medications (see page 172) help prevent blood clots, particularly if you have an irregular heart rhythm (atrial fibrillation) or have had heart valve surgery and have a mechanical replacement valve (see page 207). Beta-blockers (see page 167) can regulate your heart rate and lower your blood pressure. Calcium channel blockers (see page 168) alter the muscular contractions of your heart and lower your blood pressure. By easing the workload on your heart, these drugs may help postpone the need for heart valve surgery, or enable you to avoid it altogether.

Repair or Replacement of Heart Valves

The vast majority of procedures to repair or replace heart valves are done on the mitral and aortic valves on the left side of the heart. The mitral valve controls inflow and the aortic valve controls outflow for the hard-working left ventricle that pumps blood to the rest of the body. These two valves are more prone to disease, and they are also more critical to the overall function of the heart.

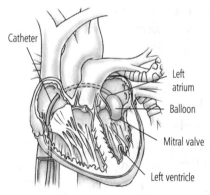

Valvuloplasty on a mitral valve

To open a stiffened or immobilized mitral valve, the surgeon inserts a balloon-tipped catheter into a vein and up into the heart. The catheter pierces the atrial septum (the membrane between the two atria) and is guided into the narrowed valve opening. Then the surgeon inflates the balloon, compressing calcium deposits (if any are present) and widening the valve opening.

The progress of valve disease in any one person can be unpredictable, so the course and timing of your treatment involves individualized decision making. If you are not having symptoms, or if your valve irregularity is not affecting your heart's function negatively, your cardiologist may choose just to watch your condition carefully.

For badly damaged and narrowed valves, valvuloplasty (opening a valve with a balloon-tipped catheter), or surgical repair or replacement may be necessary. A valvuloplasty is a less invasive procedure, because the repair is done using a catheter threaded into your heart through an artery. Other types of repair or valve replacement almost always involve open-heart surgery, meaning you are given a general anesthetic, the breastbone is divided, and a heart-lung machine (see page 183) takes over the function of your heart during the procedure.

Usually, your cardiologist and a thoracic (chest) surgeon will work together to determine what type of procedure is required, and when to do it. Even if you don't have any symptoms, these procedures are sometimes necessary to prevent damage to your heart.

Valvuloplasty

Valvuloplasty, which uses a balloon catheter to open a valve, is most often done to correct moderate to severe mitral valve stenosis. It can also be done on the tricuspid and pulmonary valves, and rarely, the aortic valve. The procedure is done in a catheterization laboratory rather than an operating room and is similar in many ways to balloon angioplasty done on coronary arteries (see page 176).

You will be given a local anesthetic at the site where the catheter will be inserted, usually in the groin. The surgeon makes a small incision and threads a balloon-tipped catheter (a thin tube) into an artery or vein. To open a mitral valve, he or she guides the catheter up into the right atrium of the heart, piercing through the atrial septum (the wall that separates the right and left atria), and through the left atrium into the mitral valve. He or she inflates the balloon, which opens up the stiffened or fused valve leaflets, pushes aside and compresses any calcium deposits, and stretches the valve opening. Then the balloon is deflated and the catheter is removed. The hole in the atrial septum will heal by itself.

There is some risk that the valve will close up again or leak somewhat after the procedure. But after a successful valvuloplasty, you can probably enjoy a lifestyle as active as your lifestyle before the procedure, if not more so.

Other Types of Valve Repair

Other types of valve repair are open-heart surgical procedures. A surgeon may fix a valve in several ways:

- Commissurotomy is a procedure to open a narrowed (stenotic) valve by cutting between thickened or fused leaflets along their natural edges (called commissures).
- Annuloplasty reshapes and strengthens a regurgitating (leaking) valve by inserting a ring device that supports the valve opening and enables it to close tightly. The valve is also surgically repaired.

- Cutting out part of a leaflet and then sewing the remaining tissue back together may enable the valve to close more tightly. Sometimes holes or tears in a leaflet can be patched.
- Repairing supporting muscles (chordae tendoneae) that are torn or stretched may allow the leaflets to close fully.
- Removing calcium buildup from leaflets may improve valve closure.

Repairing your own valve instead of replacing it may produce better, longer-lasting results and minimize complications such as blood clotting. But repair may not be possible if valves are badly damaged or are degenerated from calcification. If a person had rheumatic fever, the disease can continue even after repair. Some mitral regurgitation caused by coronary artery disease is particularly difficult to treat successfully without replacing the valve.

Valve Replacement

If valve repair or valvuloplasty is not feasible or successful, a surgeon can remove your heart valve and replace it with either a mechanical or a biological substitute (prosthesis). A mechanical valve is made of metal and plastic; a biological valve (bioprosthesis) is made from animal or human tissue. Each type has some advantages and disadvantages that you and your doctor need to consider.

Mechanical valves offer the practical advantage of durability: even if they are placed in a young person, they are likely to last a lifetime. Many models are available; your surgeon may prefer one model over another because of the procedure required to place it, but from your point of view, there is little if any difference between these products. However, there is a tendency for blood to clot around any mechanical valve. A blood clot could clog the valve, or break off and travel elsewhere in the body (including the brain, which could cause stroke). As a result, anyone with a mechanical valve must take warfarin, an anticoagulant medication (see page 172), for life.

A biological valve, unlike a transplanted heart, is not living tissue and usually does not cause rejection problems. The natural tissue is sterilized and treated with preservatives. Several options are available: an animal tissue valve (xenograft or heterograft), usually the aortic valve of a pig; a human valve (allograft), retrieved from someone who has died; or more rarely, the person's own valve (autograft)—for example, the pulmonary valve is moved from the right side of the heart to replace the aortic valve on the left—in what is known as the Ross procedure. (The pulmonary valve is then replaced with a prosthesis.)

The main advantage of a biological valve is that it is much less likely to cause clotting than a mechanical valve. You may need to take anticoagulants for several weeks or months after the procedure, but not permanently. However, the tissue is not as strong as a mechanical valve and more likely to calcify over time. An animal valve might need to be replaced in 10 to 15 years (or even sooner in a child or young adult). A human valve might last longer, but may not be readily available.

Generally, a mechanical valve is a practical choice for a person under 70 years of age who can safely take anticoagulants. A biological valve may be a good choice for an older person, particularly if he or she cannot tolerate anticoagulants, or for a woman who plans to become pregnant (because taking anticoagulants during pregnancy is not safe).

The risks of valve replacement surgery depend on your age, the overall condition of your heart, and other medical conditions. After successful surgery, you will probably be able to return to a normal level of exercise. Any artificial heart valve is subject to infective endocarditis, so you will need to take antibiotics before dental or surgical procedures (see page 194).

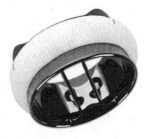

Mechanical heart valve

A mechanical heart valve opens in response to pressure building up behind it, then closes as the pressure diminishes, just as your own valve does. Both the materials and the contours of the valve are designed so the blood flows smoothly through the valve, to minimize the risk of forming blood clots. However, a person with a mechanical valve must take anti-coagulant medications for life.

What to Expect

If you and your doctor decide that repair or replacement of a heart valve is the best option for you, you will probably be able to schedule the operation at a time that is best for you (rather than having an emergency procedure). As for any surgical procedure, do not hesitate to discuss any questions or concerns with your cardiologist and your surgeon. Make sure that they know about all medications you are taking, including over-the-counter drugs such as aspirin. If you smoke, your doctor will recommend that you quit at least 2 weeks (but preferably 6 weeks) before surgery, because smoking can lead to problems with blood clotting and breathing.

Minimally Invasive Valve Surgery

At some specialized medical centers, surgeons perform minimally invasive heart valve surgery, using smaller incisions. The large arteries of the lower body may be used to attach the person to the heart-lung machine in this surgery. The patient stays in the hospital for less time and recovery is shorter and less uncomfortable. These techniques, which are still developing, are not possible in a person with severe valve damage, with more than one valve that requires surgery, or with atherosclerosis, or in a person who is obese.

You will probably be admitted to the hospital the day before surgery or the morning of the procedure. Because general anesthesia is safest on an empty stomach, you will be told not to eat anything after midnight. (If you do, be sure to tell a doctor about it.) You will probably have a chest X-ray, blood tests, urine tests, and an electrocardiogram before the procedure, and you will be given a mild sedative to relax you before you go into the operating room. Your chest will be washed, treated with antiseptic, and shaved if necessary.

You will be given a local anesthetic to numb your arm, and an intravenous line will be inserted to give you anesthesia. After you are completely anesthetized, a tube will be placed down your trachea (windpipe) to connect you to a respirator, and another tube will be threaded through your nose and down your esophagus into your stomach to remove air and fluids from your stomach. A catheter (thin tube) will be inserted in your urethra and up into your bladder to collect urine during the operation and recovery.

Your breastbone will be divided to expose your heart. A heart-lung machine (see page 183) will take over the function of your heart during surgery, so that your heart is immobile while the surgeon works. You will be given anticoagulant medications to prevent your blood from clotting.

Depending on the extent of surgery, the operation will take from 2 to 4 hours. When the valve repair or replacement is complete, your heart will be started again and the heart-lung machine will be disconnected. Most people spend 1 to 3 days in the intensive care unit and about a week in the hospital.

Your recovery from valve surgery may take several months, as your breastbone mends and your heart adjusts. Your doctor will advise you about physical activity, and he or she may recommend a cardiac rehabilitation program (see page 185). You may be able to go back to work in 1 to 4 months, depending on the physical demands of your job. You may need to take anticoagulant medications, either temporarily or permanently, if you have had a mechanical valve replacement (see page 207).

Some people who have mechanical valves can occasionally hear a clicking sound in their chest—the sound of the new valve at work. This is a perfectly normal, and even reassuring, sign that the valve is working properly.

Valve repair or replacement is usually successful. Failure of a new valve is rare, but if you experience signs of valve failure (basically, the symptoms of valve problems, described earlier), tell your doctor immediately. You will also need to be on the alert for signs of infection, such as fever, weakness, chest pain, and shortness of breath. Endocarditis can affect artificial valves as well as natural ones.

13

Stroke and Other Diseases of the Blood Vessels

Astroke is an injury to the brain that occurs when the blood supply to the brain is blocked or when there is bleeding into the brain tissue. A stroke is characterized by the rapid onset of neurological symptoms that last at least 24 hours. Like any other organ in your body, your brain relies on a constant supply of blood, loaded with oxygen and nutrients, to fuel its billions of nerve cells. Deprived of oxygen, these cells quickly begin to die and permanent damage can occur within hours or even minutes.

Your brain cells are highly organized to control every activity in your body, from breathing and movement to your senses; your speech; and thought, emotion, awareness, and memory. The impact of a stroke depends on what part of your brain is damaged, how quickly blood flow is restored, and how quickly other areas of your brain can compensate for the injury.

Stroke is the leading cause of disability in the United States, and the third-leading cause of death after heart disease and cancer. A stroke is the result of cerebrovascular disease, usually atherosclerosis of the blood vessels supplying the brain. Just as with cardiovascular disease, which may build up for decades before a "sudden" event like a heart attack, the conditions that cause a person to have a stroke (a "brain attack") have probably been developing for years. Today medical professionals know much more about how to recognize the symptoms of a stroke early, how to treat it rapidly, and how to rehabilitate someone who has had a stroke to return as much healthy function as possible. Just as importantly, a solid body of knowledge exists about what factors put a person at risk, so you can take steps to prevent a stroke.

Preventing Stroke

Research shows that stroke is more likely in certain groups of people, and there are some risk factors you cannot change. Your age is one such factor: although you can have a stroke at any age, your risk increases as you get older. Generally, more men than women have strokes. However, women are slightly more likely to die if they have a stroke. Your genetic background also plays a role: your stroke risk is higher if one of your parents, grandparents, or siblings has had a stroke. Almost twice as many black Americans die from stroke than white Americans, partly because they are also at greater risk of high blood pressure, diabetes, and obesity.

But many factors contributing to stroke can be controlled or treated. Your overall medical profile is of critical importance. If you have already had a stroke, including a warning or transient ischemic attack (TIA)—in which symptoms reverse in less than 24 hours—you are more likely to have another one. If you have heart disease— including coronary artery disease, irregular heart rhythm, and heart failure—you are at higher risk for stroke. So lifestyle changes and medical treatment for heart disease may prevent stroke.

You can do a lot to lower your risk of stroke by taking these steps:

- Have your blood pressure checked at least once a year. If it is high (more than 120/80 mm Hg), talk to your doctor about how to lower it.

- If you smoke, get help to quit immediately. Cigarette smoking contributes to high blood pressure, damages the lining of blood vessels, and increases the risk of blood clots that can clog arteries.

- Get your cholesterol checked. Talk to your doctor about treatment if your total cholesterol is 200 mg/dL or higher; your LDL (harmful cholesterol) is 130 mg/dL (but 100 dL if you already have heart disease) or higher; your triglycerides are 150 mg/dL or higher; or your HDL (good cholesterol) is 40 mg/dL or lower.

- Ask if you should have your level of C-reactive protein (CRP) checked (see page 132). A high level (3 mg/L) may be a strong indication of cardiovascular risk, including stroke, even if your cholesterol is low. But it is not yet clear what role this test plays in heart disease prevention.

- If you know you have coronary artery disease, an irregular heart rhythm such as atrial fibrillation, congestive heart failure, or a ventricular aneurysm, follow through with your doctor's recommendations for managing the condition.

- If you experience pain in your legs when you walk, talk to your doctor about being tested for vascular (blood vessel) disease (see page 120). Don't just assume that the pain is a back problem or arthritis.

- If you have coronary disease or atherosclerosis anywhere in your body, ask your doctor to check your carotid arteries (in your neck). He or she may listen with a stethoscope over the arteries in the neck for bruits, a type of whooshing sound that may signify blockage.

- If you have diabetes, work with your doctor to keep it under control (see page 105).

- Talk to your doctor about taking aspirin regularly to lower your risk of clot-related strokes (see page 109), particularly if you have already had such a stroke, a TIA, a heart attack, or unstable angina.

- Cut back on saturated fats and sodium (see pages 90–93). Whether you have high blood pressure or not, a low-fat, low-sodium diet may reduce the incidence of stroke.

- Drink alcoholic beverages moderately (one drink a day for women; two drinks a day for men), if at all. Heavy drinking increases blood pressure and raises triglycerides in the blood.

- Be physically active (see pages 75–82). Inactivity, overweight, or both increase your risk of stroke and other related conditions.

Recognizing the Warning Signs

The effects of any type of stroke may be mild or severe, and they may be temporary or permanent. Immediate medical attention to restore blood flow in certain types of stroke can minimize the damage and improve chances of regaining function in the areas affected by the stroke. The first 3 hours after a stroke occurs are the most critical, so you must respond very quickly to symptoms. Most delays in treatment occur because people wait too long to seek treatment. Don't wait.

Transient Ischemic Attacks

A transient ischemic attack (TIA), is often called a ministroke or a warning stroke. It most likely occurs when a blood clot temporarily blocks blood flow to the brain, then is dislodged before permanent

---

Warning Signs of Stroke

If you notice one or more of these signs in yourself or another person, do not delay. Call 911 or the emergency medical service number in your area immediately and get to a hospital:

- Sudden numbness or weakness of the face, arm, or leg, especially on one side of the body only
- Sudden confusion, or trouble speaking or understanding speech
- Sudden trouble seeing, in one or both eyes
- Sudden trouble walking, dizziness, loss of balance, loss of hearing, or loss of coordination
- Sudden, severe, unusual headache with no known cause, or a change in the pattern of headaches, including migraines if you have them

Be prepared to take action:

- Don't ignore any of these signs, even if they go away. Remember that not all the signs occur in every stroke, and early signs may not seem severe.
- Check the time if possible. Medical personnel will want to know when the first warning sign or symptom started.
- If you are with someone who may be having symptoms of a stroke, call 911 or emergency services right away. Expect the person to protest or to deny the symptoms. Insist on taking quick action.

Be prepared for an emergency:

- Keep a list of emergency service numbers next to the telephone or in your wallet or purse.
- Find out which hospitals in your area have stroke centers and 24-hour emergency stroke care and write them down with the list of numbers. Know which hospital or medical facility is closest to you.

---

damage is done. A TIA may last a few minutes or up to 24 hours, but then the symptoms resolve and do not cause permanent damage. A TIA causes strokelike symptoms but does not cause permanent impairment. However, a TIA is an extremely important predictor of another, more serious stroke: about one out of three people who have had one or more TIAs will have a stroke at a later time. But the TIA does not give any information about how soon another potentially disabling or fatal stroke might occur; it could be a matter of days or a year or more.

The only differences between a TIA and a stroke are the short duration of the symptoms, and the fact that no permanent damage is done. But it is essential to get medical attention immediately. A doctor should determine if you have had a TIA or a stroke, or if you have another medical problem with similar symptoms (such as a seizure, fainting, a migraine headache, or another heart condition).

Warning Signs of a TIA

Call 911 or emergency medical services and get to a hospital immediately if you or someone else has one or more of these symptoms of a transient ischemic attack (TIA), no matter how vague they may seem or how briefly they may last:

- Sudden numbness, weakness, or clumsiness in an arm or leg, especially on one side of the body
- Sudden numbness, weakness, or droop in the face, possibly on one side of the body only
- Sudden confusion, trouble speaking, or trouble understanding speech
- Sudden trouble seeing in one or both eyes; might include blurry, blocked, or grayed vision
- Sudden trouble walking, dizziness, loss of balance, or loss of coordination
- Sudden, severe headache without a known cause

Types of Stroke

There are two broad categories of strokes. Most strokes—about three out of four in the United States—are ischemic strokes, meaning that they are caused by a blockage (usually a blood clot) in an artery supplying part of the brain. A TIA (transient ischemic attack) often precedes a larger, disabling ischemic stroke. A hemorrhagic stroke—far less common but more often fatal—results from bleeding within the brain. In either case, the blood flow to part of the brain is disrupted and brain tissue is damaged.

A person who has an ischemic stroke may become disabled by it, because part of the brain dies for lack of blood and the brain cannot replace the lost cells. However, some people eventually recover with few or no lasting impairments. A person who has a hemorrhagic stroke

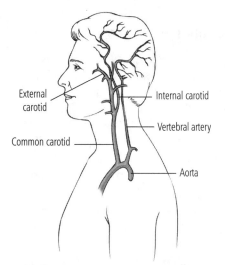

Carotid and vertebral arteries

The common carotid artery arises from your aorta, then branches into the external carotid artery (which supplies blood to your face and scalp) and the internal carotid artery (which supplies the front part of your brain). The vertebral arteries also arise from your aorta, run along your spinal cord, and then branch into the back portion of your brain.

External carotid

Common carotid

Internal carotid

Vertebral artery

Aorta

may die quickly from the pressure the bleeding exerts on the brain. But if he or she survives, the brain may recover at least part or even most of its function.

Ischemic Stroke

An ischemic stroke—by far the most common type—most often occurs when a blood clot develops in one of the carotid arteries (in your neck) and then travels to block one of the arteries supplying blood to the brain. Blood clots are much more likely to form or lodge in carotid arteries already narrowed by atherosclerosis, a condition called carotid artery disease or carotid stenosis (see page 218). A blood clot in the vertebral arteries or on the heart can cause a stroke. Doctors need to know where the clot has formed because it helps indicate the underlying condition that led to the stroke and how to direct treatment.

If a blood clot forms in an artery at the site of the blockage, it is called a thrombus. A thrombus is far more likely to form in an artery with carotid stenosis. Usually this type is referred to as a thromboembolic stroke; that is, the thrombus forms and a small piece of it travels until it lodges in a small artery.

When a blood clot forms somewhere else in the body and travels, it is called an embolus. If the embolus floats into an artery supplying the brain and blocks it, the resulting stroke is called an artery to artery embolus. Again, an artery affected by carotid stenosis is far more likely to cause a traveling clot. Sometimes, an embolus develops in the heart and moves through the bloodstream until it lodges at a point in the branching arterial system where it can go no further. Emboli that come from the heart are often caused by a rhythm disorder called atrial fibrillation (see page 263), which causes a quivering heartbeat within the atrium (the upper chamber of the heart). Because of the abnormal heartbeat, blood pools in the atrium and forms clots that can then move through the heart and into the bloodstream. Emboli from the heart usually cause a sudden onset of symptoms that may improve over time.

Hemorrhagic Stroke

A hemorrhagic stroke occurs when an artery in or on the surface of the brain bursts or leaks, flooding brain tissue with blood. Because a vessel has burst, part of the brain tissue loses its blood supply, and the bleeding also may cause pressure and swelling in or on the brain. In addition, the blood disturbs the function of nearby blood vessels, which become compressed when the first vessel bursts. The severity of the stroke depends on the amount of bleeding. There are two kinds of hemorrhagic stroke, cerebral and subarachnoid, characterized by where the bleeding occurs.

Cerebral hemorrhage is bleeding in and into the brain. It usually happens as a result of a cerebral aneurysm, which is a weak spot in an artery in the brain that balloons out and fills with blood. Chronic high blood pressure (see page 37) is the most common disorder linked with the weakening of blood vessels. If the aneurysm bursts, sometimes strained by high blood pressure, a hemorrhagic stroke occurs. A cerebral hemorrhage can also be caused by a head injury, as in a car accident.

A subarachnoid hemorrhage occurs when a blood vessel on the surface of the brain bursts and the blood spills into the space between the brain and the skull (the subarachnoid space). The blood may remain in the cerebrospinal fluid that fills the space, or it may break through the pia mater (the inner membrane covering the surface of the brain) and seep over brain tissue, but it does not penetrate the brain. The bleeding may be the result of a ruptured aneurysm, or possibly a head injury. The most typical symptom of subarachnoid hemorrhage is a sudden, severe headache.

How Blood Reaches Your Brain

Your brain—which requires about 20 percent of your body's blood supply to function—receives oxygen-enriched blood from your heart through just two sets of arteries. One set, the carotid arteries, run up through your neck; they are the prominent ones you can feel pulsating just under your jaw. The external carotid artery supplies blood to your face, and the internal carotid artery goes into your skull and branches off to supply the front two-thirds of your brain. Many strokes occur as the result of blockage of the carotid arteries.

The other set, the vertebral arteries, parallel your spinal column and join at the base of your skull. This system branches into the brain stem and supplies the back third of your brain. Emboli may also travel through these arteries to the brain, causing a stroke. The jugular veins, running down through your neck, carry blood out of the brain and back to the heart.

Other Vascular Diseases

Strokes and TIAs are perhaps the best known forms of vascular disease, but they may be caused by or related to other forms of peripheral vascular disease including carotid stenosis, peripheral artery disease,

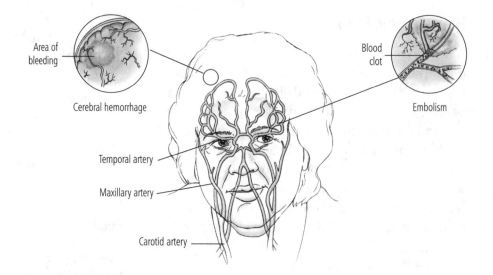

Area of bleeding

Cerebral hemorrhage

Blood clot

Embolism

Temporal artery

Maxillary artery

Carotid artery

Ischemic and hemorrhagic strokes

A stroke occurs when blood supply to part of the brain is disrupted by either a hemorrhage or a blood clot. Most strokes result from an embolism (traveling blood clot) that lodges in an artery supplying brain tissue. Less commonly, a stroke is caused by hemorrhage (bleeding) in or on brain tissue.

aneurysms, and arteriovenous malformations. Each of these vascular diseases may cause symptoms on its own and may, if untreated, lead to stroke.

Carotid Stenosis

If your carotid arteries are affected by atherosclerosis, blood flow to the brain can be reduced by plaque buildup that narrows the artery. Stenosis is the medical term for the narrowing, and doctors may discuss your disease in terms of the percentage of narrowing: 60 percent stenosis means that your artery is 60 percent blocked. The shape and severity of the narrowing contribute to the risk from a clot.

If you have carotid artery disease, you probably have coronary artery disease as well—the process of atherosclerosis is not usually limited to a single part of the vascular system. The same factors—high levels of LDL and triglycerides, high blood pressure, smoking, diabetes, family history, obesity, physical inactivity—contribute to the disease and usually result in a general involvement of the body's vascular system.

Carotid artery disease itself does not have specific symptoms, but the warning signs of a stroke, including TIAs, are indications that blood flow to your brain is getting blocked. However, some people can have serious stenosis without experiencing these symptoms.

Your doctor may suspect that you have carotid artery stenosis during a regular physical examination by listening to the arteries with a stethoscope. A partially blocked artery sometimes causes a characteristic sound (called a carotid bruit) as the turbulence caused by the blood moves past the blockage and makes a soft noise audible with a stethoscope. If your doctor hears a carotid bruit, this means atherosclerosis is present but does not indicate how severe it is. Further tests such as a Doppler ultrasound MRI arteriogram are needed to assess how severe the disease is.

Your doctor may order other diagnostic tests to determine the presence or the extent of the disease: carotid ultrasound to observe blood flow and measure the thickness of your carotid arteries; magnetic resonance imaging (MRI) to get a clear picture of the arteries supplying your brain; ocular tests to measure the pulses in the arteries behind your eye, which may indirectly indicate a blockage in the carotid arteries; or digital angiography and digital subtraction angiography (DSA), which involve injecting a dye into your bloodstream and then taking X-ray images of your arteries. (For more information about these tests pertaining to stroke, see pages 223–225.)

Your doctor will recommend that you make lifestyle changes to slow the development of carotid artery disease and perhaps prevent a stroke (see pages 83–98). If your carotid arteries are less than 50 percent blocked, your doctor may prescribe anticoagulant medications (see page 172), such as heparin or warfarin, or antiplatelet drugs (see page 171), such as aspirin or clopidogrel, to reduce the likelihood of blood clots. You may have to take an antiplatelet agent or warfarin for the rest of your life.

If you have more than 50 percent stenosis in one or more carotid arteries, along with symptoms of decreased blood flow to the brain, your doctor may recommend a carotid endarterectomy (see page 228) or carotid angioplasty (see page 175) to reduce the narrowing more aggressively and help prevent a stroke.

Aneurysms

An aneurysm is an outward bulge or ballooning caused by the pressure of blood pushing against a weakened place in the wall of an artery. Not

Peripheral Artery Disease

Peripheral artery disease (PAD) affects the arteries outside your heart, such as those supplying your arm and leg muscles and the organs in or below your abdomen. These vessels can be damaged or blocked by atherosclerosis (page 152) or blood clots, just like the coronary arteries or the carotid arteries. A person who has PAD is likely to have some degree of coronary artery disease (which can lead to heart attack) or carotid artery disease (which can lead to stroke), or both. The risk factors that contribute to peripheral artery disease are the same as those for coronary artery disease: smoking, diabetes, high blood pressure, and high cholesterol.

PAD can lead to a blood clot in affected limbs, an aortic aneurysm (see page 222), rarer conditions such as Buerger's disease (related to smoking) or Raynaud's phenomenon (which causes numbness, discoloration, or pain in the fingers and hands). If you have PAD, you may experience pain and cramps in your calves, thighs, or buttocks—in the muscles, not the joints. These pains may occur when you walk or exercise and then go away when you rest, a symptom called intermittent claudication. Some people describe the pain in terms that they feel the calves of their legs are being grabbed. Generally, if your pain is severe, or if very little activity triggers the pain, that means your disease is severe. If the disease is advanced, you may have bluish toes or cold feet.

Your doctor may check for PAD with a simple screening test called the ankle-brachial index, which compares the blood pressure in your arms and legs to indicate how well blood is flowing. In a healthy person, the ankle pressure is at least 90 percent of the arm pressure. But if arteries are narrowed, it can be 70 percent or less. Your doctor may confirm a diagnosis of PAD with ultrasound (using sound waves to form an image of your blood vessels) or computed tomographic (CT) or magnetic resonance (MR) angiography.

To treat PAD, your doctor may recommend lifestyle changes such as losing weight, quitting smoking, and getting more exercise. Surgical options include angioplasty (using a balloon-tipped catheter to open the artery), putting in a stent (a supporting device to hold the artery open), or a bypass graft (using an artificial vessel or one of your own veins to create a route around the blockage).

all aneurysms burst; they may remain small and harmless. But if the ballooning area is stretched too far, perhaps aggravated by atherosclerosis, high blood pressure, or the effects of smoking, the aneurysm can rupture.

Aneurysms can occur in any artery, and they typically form where an artery branches. A cerebral (or brain) aneurysm is in an artery supplying the brain. If it bursts, it causes a hemorrhagic stroke (see page 217). Other types of aneurysm include an abdominal aortic aneurysm, located in the aorta (which carries blood from the heart to the rest of the body) below the stomach (see the box on page 222); a thoracic aneurysm, in the part of the aorta that is in the chest; and a ventricular aneurysm, in the left ventricle of the heart. In these locations, if the aneurysm bursts, the person may bleed to death very quickly.

A cerebral aneurysm may be small and not cause any symptoms at all. But if it presses on surrounding nerves or tissues, it may cause headaches, blurred vision, or double vision. Doctors usually detect a brain aneurysm with angiography (see page 146), magnetic resonance imaging (MRI, page 141), or computed tomography (CT, page 139). Treatment will depend on the size and location of the aneurysm, and your overall health. If it is small and you do not have symptoms, your doctor or neurologist may just check it regularly to see if it is enlarging. The risk of stroke increases with the size of the aneurysm.

An aneurysm that ruptures into the subarachnoid space (an area between two of the three membranes surrounding the brain) is a common cause of subarachnoid hemorrhage. The subarachnoid space is filled with cerebrospinal fluid, and the bleeding may remain in the fluid or break through the inner membrane (pia mater) into brain tissue. A major subarachnoid hemorrhage (one that causes you to lose consciousness) can cause permanent damage or death. The most common symptom of a subarachnoid hemorrhage is a sudden, severe headache. A person may also have a stiff neck or be extremely sensitive to light.

The most common treatment is a surgical procedure to place a metal clip at the base of the bulge (see page 229). Another less invasive form of treatment is an endovascular (through the vessel) procedure to place a coiled stent (page 229) in the artery to support the walls.

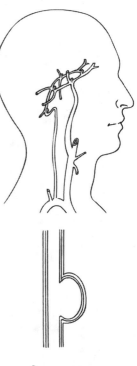

Berry aneurysm

Typical sites of berry aneurysms

A common type of aneurysm is the berry or sacculated aneurysm (see closeup), which is a bulging weak spot on one side of the artery. Cerebral (brain) aneurysms are most likely to occur at certain typical sites in the brain, usually where arteries branch. The cerebral artery system is designed to maximize blood flow to brain tissue, even if small interruptions in flow are present.

Arteriovenous Malformations

A stroke can also be caused by a congenital (present since birth) abnormality in the brain called an arteriovenous malformation. The cause of this abnormality is unknown. An arteriovenous malformation is a tangled mass of vessels, often with abnormal connections between arteries and veins, that can be located anywhere in the brain or spinal cord. Pressure can build up in these vessels and cause a rupture, with subsequent hemorrhage into or onto the brain.

Often, an arteriovenous malformation does not cause symptoms for years. An affected person may experience recurring headaches or seizures if blood starts to leak into the brain or spinal cord. If you have

Screening for Aortic Aneurysm

An abdominal aortic aneurysm (a weakened, bulging spot in the aorta below the stomach) is potentially fatal: if it bursts, you are likely to die very quickly. About 15,000 people a year die from this condition, and doctors think the figure may be much higher because the deaths are often attributed to heart attack or stroke.

Men over the age of 65 who are smokers or ex-smokers are at the highest risk of aortic aneurysm. If a family member has had an aneurysm, the risk is higher. High blood pressure and high cholesterol are also contributing risk factors. The condition is about four times more common in men than in women.

Most aortic aneurysms develop without causing symptoms. Many are detected incidentally, during testing for some other reason. If an aortic aneurysm begins to expand, it may cause pain in the stomach, sides, or back. Sometimes, during a physical examination, a doctor can feel an aortic aneurysm as a soft, pulsating mass in the abdomen.

Some medical experts advise that all men over the age of 65 who have ever smoked (100 cigarettes or more, about five packs) in their lifetime should have an ultrasound to determine if they have an abdominal aortic aneurysm. If one is detected, it can be surgically repaired while it is still small. The effectiveness of the scan is controversial and it may not be covered by insurance, but it could be life-saving. If you are a man over 65 who has smoked, or if you are a woman with several risk factors, talk to your doctor about being tested for aortic aneurysm.

such symptoms, your doctor may recommend that you have an MRI or angiography to detect the malformed vessels.

A treatment plan for an arteriovenous malformation often involves a combination of techniques to remove all or part of the mass or cut off its blood supply before it enlarges and ruptures. Some malformations can be removed surgically. Stereotactic radiosurgery is another technique using radiation to close off abnormal vessels. It can be done only on small masses, and it may take 2 years of treatments to get rid of the entire mass. A third technique, embolization, uses tiny catheters to deliver a liquid glue into the vessels that feed the malformation. Embolization can make surgical removal safer or reduce the size of the mass so that radiosurgery is possible.

If an arteriovenous malformation ruptures before diagnosis and treatment, the person may die suddenly. If the person lives and does not have serious neurological deficiencies from the rupture, emergency surgery may be performed.

Testing for Strokes

If you have had TIAs or other symptoms of stroke, or if you have had a stroke, doctors can perform tests to visualize your brain and its blood supply to determine what part of your brain is affected and define the problems a stroke has caused. Your doctor will consider your personal medical history to decide which tests are necessary. These tests are generally safe and painless and can be done on an outpatient basis (you will not have to stay overnight at the hospital).

Imaging of the Brain

Some tests use imaging technologies to study brain tissue:

- **CT (computed tomography) scanning** uses the X-ray technique to create cross-sectional, "slicelike" pictures of your brain to determine if a stroke has occurred and what kind (ischemic or hemorrhagic). The scan takes about 20 minutes.

- **MRI (magnetic resonance imaging)** involves placing you in a magnetic field and then exposing your head to bursts of energy at a certain frequency. The brain responds with signals that can be used to create a highly accurate image. Doctors can identify the presence, location, and size of aneurysms or arteriovenous malformations that may have caused a stroke. An MRI usually takes about 30 minutes to complete. A new technique called ultrafast MRI, available at some medical centers, takes only 15 minutes or less. Diagnosing and imaging a stroke more quickly in the hospital speeds the delivery of clot-busting drugs (see page 171) that may prevent damage.

- **Angiography** produces an X-ray image (angiogram) of your blood vessels. When it is done to image blood vessels in your brain, it enables doctors to detect stroke and brain aneurysms or hemorrhaging, or to plan surgical procedures. Because it is a more invasive procedure, it is usually done only when other tests have not provided the necessary information. To perform an angiogram on your brain, a catheter (thin tube) will be inserted into an artery, usually in your groin, then guided all the way into the carotid arteries in your neck. A contrast medium (dye) will be injected through the catheter and X-rays will be taken so that your doctor can study the blood flow through your brain. (For complete information about the procedure, see "Cardiac Catheterization," page 142, and "Angiography," page 146.)

Testing the Brain's Electrical Activity

Some tests study the brain's electrical activity:

- **EEG (electroencephalography)** records the electrical activity of your brain. Electrodes placed on your scalp transmit electrical impulses from your brain in a form that can be recorded on paper. The intensity, duration, frequency, and location of the impulses provide information about your brain's function.

- **Evoked response tests** are procedures to measure your brain's ability to process and respond to stimuli in your environment. Electrodes on your scalp will transmit your brain's response. To evoke a visual response, a doctor will flash a light or checkerboard pattern in front of you. For an auditory response, a sound will be introduced into your ear. For a bodily response, a nerve in your arm or leg will be stimulated electrically. The responses will indicate abnormal areas in your brain.

Testing Blood Flow in the Brain

Some tests study vascular function, or how well blood is flowing to your brain:

- **Doppler ultrasound (or carotid ultrasound)** uses high-frequency sound waves to detect blockages in your carotid arteries (in your neck). An instrument called a Doppler probe or transducer is placed on your neck. Ultrasound waves pass into your arteries and are reflected off the moving blood cells. The sound waves return through the transducer at a different frequency that relates to the speed at which the blood cells are moving. This information can detect narrowing or blockages.

- **Digital subtraction angiography (DSA)** is an X-ray procedure in which a contrast dye is injected through a catheter that has been guided into the major blood vessels supplying your brain (see the box on page 217). As the dye circulates, an X-ray machine records its movement so that a doctor can identify and locate the origin of a stroke; the technology "subtracts" the background of bone and tissue to highlight the vessels. DSA uses smaller amounts of the contrast dye than traditional angiography, so it is especially useful for a person for whom the contrast medium presents the risk of kidney disease.

Effects of Stroke

The impact of a stroke can range from relatively subtle to seriously disabling, depending on the type of stroke, the area of the brain affected, and the severity of the brain injury. With rehabilitation, many of these problems can improve. In some people, they will disappear completely as the brain makes new connections to restore lost function. A stroke may affect a person in any of these broad areas:

- **Paralysis, weakness, motor control.** Paralysis or weakness is one of the most common disabilities resulting from stroke. It usually occurs on one side of the body, opposite from the affected side of the brain. It may affect the face, an arm or leg, or the whole side of the body. Everyday activities such as dressing, walking, or picking up objects may be difficult. Some people have difficulty swallowing (dysphasia). Damage to the lower part of the brain may cause coordination problems that affect posture, walking, or balance.

- **Awareness.** Loss of feeling or movement may cause a person to neglect the affected side of their body or ignore objects on that side. They may dress only one side of their bodies or bump into furniture on one side.

- **Sensory disturbances, including pain.** A person may lose the ability to feel touch, pain, temperature, or position. Sensory damage can also cause problems with recognition of common objects or even parts of the body. Some people have pain, numbness, or tingling sensations in affected limbs. A paralyzed limb may "freeze" from lack of movement, causing discomfort. Damage to

Screening for Artery Disease

Some medical experts recommend that anyone over the age of 60—especially people with risk factors for stroke—should be tested for carotid artery disease or peripheral artery disease to help prevent stroke. Two diagnostic tests, carotid ultrasound (see page 224) and the ankle-brachial index (which compares the blood pressure in your arms and legs), can be done to detect artery disease early so that it can be treated with lifestyle changes and medications. These tests are generally done in a hospital. If you are over 60 and have one or more risk factors for stroke (family history, tobacco use, overweight, high blood pressure, diabetes or prediabetes), talk to your doctor about these tests, and find out whether your insurance covers them.

the nervous system can also cause chronic pain, either in affected limbs or elsewhere in the body.

- **Language impairment.** About one out of four stroke patients experiences some difficulty with speech, speech comprehension, reading, or writing. Although stroke does not usually cause hearing loss, damage to a language center may harm the person's ability to understand or respond to the spoken or written word, a condition called aphasia. A person with expressive aphasia has trouble conveying his or her thoughts in words. A person with receptive aphasia has difficulty understanding and processing language, and often speaks incoherently. If the muscles used in speech are affected, the person may have slow, slurred, or inarticulate speech, called dysarthria.

- **Memory and learning.** Some people may have a shortened attention span, poor short-term memory, or difficulty learning a new task. Their ability to connect thought and action may be impaired, so that they have a hard time thinking ahead, organizing tasks, doing things in sequence, or following instructions.

- **Emotions.** Physical damage to emotional centers in the brain may cause mood swings or irrational emotional reactions, called emotional lability, or personality changes. The person may cry or even laugh uncontrollably. Depression after a stroke is common, as a reaction to the disabilities (see page 232).

Treatment for Stroke

Although there is no "cure" for stroke, medications, surgical procedures, hospital care and support during recovery, and rehabilitation are all useful parts of treatment. Because the disease processes that lead to either ischemic or hemorrhagic stroke are different, immediate treatments differ depending on which type of stroke has occurred. For an ischemic stroke—and most strokes are ischemic—early treatment centers on removing the blockage (such as a clot) in the blood vessels and restoring blood flow to the brain. For a hemorrhagic stroke, treatment is either surgery to stop the bleeding, or a procedure to support an aneurysm to prevent rupture. For either type of stroke, treatment of the underlying condition—often some type of vascular disease—may involve medication, surgery, or an angioplasty procedure.

If you arrive at a hospital and doctors determine that you have had a ischemic stroke, you will probably be given antiplatelet drugs (such as aspirin or clopidogrel) and anticoagulant drugs (such as warfarin) to prevent clotting. Your blood pressure may rise as your body tries to compensate for the lack of blood to your brain, so even if your blood pressure is high, your doctors may not want to lower your blood pressure right away.

Tissue Plasminogen Activator (tPA)

The most promising treatment for ischemic stroke is the thrombolytic medication or "clot-buster" called tPA (tissue plasminogen activator), the only drug currently approved for strokes. About 80 percent of all strokes are caused by a blood clot, and tPA dissolves the clot and restores blood flow to the brain. In order to have maximum benefit (that is, restore blood flow to the brain to prevent as much damage as possible), the drug must be given within 3 hours of the onset of the stroke symptoms. Within that time frame, the person must have responded quickly to symptoms and gotten to a hospital, and doctors must have determined what type of stroke has occurred. Currently only about 3 to 5 percent of people who have strokes get to the hospital quickly enough to be considered for tPA.

In most people who have an ischemic stroke, the blood flow to the brain is not completely shut off. Reduced blood supply causes a core area of tissue to stop functioning, and you start to experience symptoms. But a much larger area of cells (called the ischemic penumbra) surrounding the core go into an idling mode, impaired but not yet destroyed. They can survive for several hours in this state. Administering tPA restores the blood supply to these cells.

The use of tPA is not appropriate for every stroke victim, especially not someone having a hemorrhagic stroke. Also, tPA presents some risk of causing bleeding in the brain in some people. Doctors are currently investigating ways to identify such people with blood tests in order to make use of tPA safer. Generally, a person with bleeding ulcers or very high blood pressure is not a good candidate. But the potential benefits of tPA treatment far outweigh the risks in most people. The availability of tPA underscores the importance of responding quickly to stroke symptoms and getting to a hospital with stroke treatment capabilities as early as possible.

Carotid Endarterectomy

Carotid endarterectomy is a surgical procedure to remove plaque that is narrowing a carotid artery. Done to prevent stroke, the procedure is most typically done for a person who has had a stroke or someone who has had symptoms of stroke and has a blockage of more than 50 percent in a carotid artery. Even without symptoms, a person with severe blockage (80 percent or more) may benefit from the procedure.

If you are having a carotid endarterectomy, you will receive a general anesthetic. The surgeon will make an incision in your neck to expose the carotid artery, and will either briefly clamp the artery above and below the blocked area or put in a temporary bypass tube to route blood around the blockage during surgery. The surgeon will open the artery and cut out the plaque and the lining, then close the artery and sometimes patch it with a synthetic or natural material for strength. In some cases, a graft of new vessel is attached to replace the damaged area.

You will probably stay in the hospital for 1 or 2 days, lying flat and turning your head as little as possible. After you leave the hospital, you may experience pain in your neck for 2 weeks or so. There is some risk of stroke or heart attack during the procedure. As with any surgery, it is important to thoroughly discuss the risks and the reasons why your doctor recommends the procedure for you.

Carotid Stents

The Food and Drug Administration has approved one stent device to open blocked carotid arteries. The stent—a wire mesh tube inserted in an artery like scaffolding to hold it open—offers an option to a person with a severely blocked carotid artery (80 percent or more) who is not a good candidate for carotid endarterectomy. Although the procedure, called cerebral angioplasty, is not available in all medical centers, it is a promising development. It is a less invasive procedure and may cause fewer complications than carotid endarterectomy.

Like angioplasty in the coronary arteries (see page 176), placement of a carotid stent involves making an incision in an artery in the groin and then threading a catheter up into the carotid artery. A balloon-tipped catheter opens the artery by pressing the plaque against the walls, and then the stent is positioned in the artery to support it. The stent has a built-in filter to catch debris so it cannot float up into the brain during surgery.

Surgical Clipping of an Aneurysm

If a person has a brain aneurysm (see page 219), either ruptured or unruptured, a neurosurgeon can clip the aneurysm at its base to prevent blood from pushing against the weakened area. The clip either prevents the aneurysm from bursting or, if the aneurysm has broken open, closes it off to stop bleeding in a person who has already had a hemorrhagic stroke.

To perform this operation, the neurosurgeon must open the skull and expose the brain (a procedure called a craniotomy). He or she locates the blood vessel with the aneurysm and carefully separates it from surrounding brain tissue, then applies a spring-loaded metal clip to the base of the bulge. Many types of clips are available to accommodate aneurysms of different sizes or in different locations.

Endovascular Coiling

Endovascular coiling is a technique to repair an aneurysm by inserting a coiled device into the blood vessel. For this procedure, a neurosurgeon makes an incision in an artery in the person's arm or leg and threads a catheter up into the brain to the site of the aneurysm. He or she then guides a soft wire spiral, or coil, into the aneurysm. The coil alters the blood flow and a thrombus (blood clot) forms that cushions the aneurysm and prevents it from bursting. This procedure is desirable because it does not involve opening the skull, but how long this treatment lasts is not yet certain. That is why periodic monitoring—usually with MRI scans (see page 141)—is needed to determine whether weakness in the wall of a blood vessel may progress over time. Not all aneurysms are suitable for coiling.

Both clipping and coiling present the risk that the aneurysm will rupture during the procedure, causing a hemorrhagic stroke. There is also a risk of blood clots causing a stroke during either procedure. Before having either clipping or coiling of an aneurysm, you and your doctor must thoroughly discuss the risks and benefits of these procedures for you.

Rehabilitation after a Stroke

In the first month or so after a stroke, a person may spontaneously regain many lost abilities. But the effects of a stroke often require that you change, relearn, or rethink aspects of how you live. Getting some

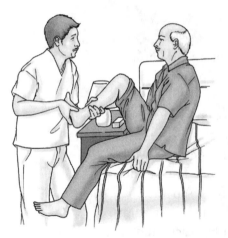

Benefits of physical therapy

If a stroke has impaired physical abilities such as walking, physical therapy is usually begun immediately, in the hospital, to maximize your recovery. You may continue to improve and benefit from physical therapy for weeks or months following discharge from the hospital, especially if you are involved in a rehabilitation program that is structured to increase in intensity and complexity as you recover.

help with rehabilitation is invaluable as part of the process of returning to an active, satisfying life. Although rehabilitation does not reverse the effects of stroke, the goal is to help you be as independent and active as possible. You may find that even a seemingly slight improvement in function can make a big difference in your quality of life and independence. A positive, receptive attitude on your part and the support of family and friends can contribute enormously to a successful recovery.

Rehabilitation can begin as soon as your medical condition is stable. While you are still recovering in the hospital, medical staff will work to improve your physical condition and prevent problems (such as bed sores, stiff joints, falls, and pneumonia) that might result from spending time in bed. With your family members, talk to your doctor or other medical staff about where you can get post-stroke rehabilitation services in your area. Your doctor may recommend that you spend some time in an acute-care or rehabilitation facility that can offer some of the same services

Physical Therapy and Occupational Therapy

To help you recover from stroke, other diseases, or injuries, physical therapists evaluate your condition and design a treatment plan to ensure that you recover to the fullest extent possible. Physical therapy exercises are designed to help you, if necessary, regain balance, walk more normally, use your arms or legs without pain, increase strength and flexibility, and generally improve your everyday functioning. If you need a cane or other walking aid, the physical therapist fits that for you and trains you to use it.

Occupational therapy is targeted to help you regain the ability to do your daily activities, whether you are working or retired. For example, an occupational therapist may help a stroke

patient learn to feed himself or herself and to get in and out of a bathtub or shower. Occupational therapists also work with people to help them walk up and down stairs again and to get in and out of an automobile. If you need any devices to regain your health—for example, a large spoon with a looped handle if you have difficulty holding an ordinary fork or spoon—the occupational therapist will provide those for you and train you to use them.

Physical therapists and occupational therapists complete a professional course of study to do this work and are licensed by each state. Therapy generally takes place in a gym that may be in a hospital, nursing home, or separate office suite.

as a hospital, but in a more comfortable, affordable setting. A long-term-care facility may be necessary if your stroke has caused more extensive disability. Assistance from home health agencies may enable you to return home earlier in your recovery. Other types of therapies may be available as outpatient services at hospitals or clinics.

Your doctor can put together a team of specialists to help you with the specific types of rehabilitation you need. Building up your strength and capabilities may involve work in areas you never thought about before:

Going Home after a Stroke

As you look forward to going home after a stroke, you and your family may need to rethink the home environment with your independence, convenience, and safety in mind. The changes you need to make will depend on the nature of your post-stroke capabilities, but here are some general tips to consider:

- Before you are discharged, arrange for a rehabilitation specialist or occupational therapist to visit your home and do a room-by-room assessment with your partner or family member. Talk about the daily tasks you will be doing and make lists of changes that need to be made before you arrive home or soon after that. You may even arrange to make a trial visit before you go home permanently, because some problems may not be apparent until you get there.

- Your safety is the top priority. Make a safety checklist that includes considerations like fire extinguishers you can reach and a plan for regular smoke detector checks.

- Make sure emergency phone numbers are posted throughout the house.

- Establish easy-to-use communication links. Be sure that you can reach and hold onto the telephone. Install an emergency alarm system that you can activate 24 hours a day.

- Remove clutter throughout the house. If mobility or balance are problems, or if you need a walking aid such as a walker or wheelchair, you may need to get rid of excess or fragile furniture, throw rugs, extension cords on the floor, and other potential hazards.

- Consider brighter lighting throughout the house.

- Talk to a rehabilitation specialist about where to get devices that make tasks easier: dressing and grooming aids, specially designed kitchen implements and eating utensils, laundry baskets on wheels. Hundreds of ingenious products are available.

- Some more major home modifications may be necessary: installing grab bars and railings in the bathrooms and on staircases; widening doorways and lowering counters to accommodate a wheelchair; adjusting or marking water controls to make them easier to use, even for a person with difficulty sensing temperature; getting a stove with front controls; installing organization systems in closets.

- Be ready to experiment. It will take time and experience to find all the resources you need.

- Self-care skills such as feeding, dressing, and bathing
- Mobility skills such as using a walker or wheelchair
- Speech and language skills
- Memory or problem-solving techniques
- Social skills for interacting with caregivers and other people

You may need the services of nurses specializing in stroke rehabilitation, physical therapists, occupational therapists, speech and language pathologists, audiologists, recreational therapists, or nutritionists. Psychologists or psychiatrists, social workers, vocational counselors, or family counselors can help you and your family make the personal and emotional adjustments necessary in your work and home life.

Your partner and family members can play a key role in your rehabilitation program. Your family will need to understand what you have been through and how disabilities may change your life. You and they will be able to handle the situation best if you go through the rehabilitation process together. Gathering information, knowing what to expect, and knowing where to get help and support will be essential for both you and your family. Your doctor or nurse can recommend stroke support groups where you can be with other people who are dealing with the same types of changes and feelings.

Depression after a Stroke

Stroke specialists say that some degree of depression is almost universal—and understandable—among stroke survivors. Even minor or temporary impairment can sap your spirit and confidence. A slow recovery, problems with mobility, or problems communicating can leave you feeling isolated and frustrated. Symptoms of depression may include sleeplessness, withdrawal, irritability, or reluctance to follow through with therapy or medications. Some of these symptoms can slow down your recovery or dampen the enthusiasm of friends or family who care about you. For most people, these feelings can be relieved by talking to friends and family, going to a support group, or perhaps getting counseling from a psychologist or psychiatrist. If the depression persists, your doctor may recommend antidepressant medications.

14

Congestive Heart Failure

Congestive heart failure (CHF) is a serious condition in which the heart is not pumping efficiently so fluid builds up in the lungs and other organs such as the liver. Many people with congestive heart failure are in very stable condition and can live for years with proper treatment. Congestive heart failure may be due either to the heart's inability to fill properly or to a weakening of the pumping action that delivers blood throughout your body. The decreased or inefficient pumping activity causes a backup of fluid—congestion—in your lungs and other body tissues. The condition may develop slowly, often occurring with minor or no symptoms for years, because your heart compensates for its own gradual weakening.

Anything that damages the heart can contribute to heart failure. Today people are living longer and surviving medical problems that over time cause stress on the heart. The exact cause may be hard to determine, but if you have been diagnosed with heart failure, you probably have had one or more of these conditions:

- Coronary artery disease
- Heart attack (myocardial infarction)
- High blood pressure
- Arrhythmia
- Heart valve disease

- Diabetes
- Cardiomyopathy (disease of the heart muscle; see page 249)
- Congenital or genetic heart disease
- Abuse of alcohol and other drugs

Congestive heart failure is both a common disease and a serious disease, so doctors have performed a great many research studies on how to treat it. As a result, doctors' understanding of how to manage the condition is improving all the time. Although there is usually not a cure for heart failure, most people can live a satisfying life for many years with a combination of lifestyle changes, medications, and possibly surgery.

Recognizing Heart Failure

Your heart has more strength than you generally use every day, and if it is damaged it can compensate for some decrease in its pumping strength by enlarging, developing more muscle mass, and beating faster. The body also tries to compensate for a weakening heart by increasing blood pressure and diverting blood away from some less vital organs and tissues in order to maintain blood flow to the heart and brain. These compensating mechanisms may limit the onset of the symptoms of heart failure for a long time. But as the burden on the heart becomes greater, eventually symptoms develop that are the first clues to the presence of heart failure.

By the time you are diagnosed, your heart function may have been declining for some time, although it may seem to you as though heart failure occurred suddenly. Many heart failure symptoms are similar to other conditions, so the symptoms do not necessarily indicate heart failure.

Your doctor will most likely consider the possibility of heart failure if you have a history of heart problems or if you are experiencing shortness of breath, unusual fatigue, and swelling. Using a stethoscope, your doctor can assess you for possible heart failure by listening to your chest for the rales, or crackling

Symptoms of Heart Failure

If you experience any of these symptoms, report them to your doctor:

- Shortness of breath, especially when lying down or with daily activities
- Waking from sleep short of breath
- Unusual fatigue or lethargy
- Coughing, either with exercise or when you lie down
- Coughing up pink-tinged phlegm
- Swelling in your feet, ankles, or legs
- Loss of appetite or a feeling of indigestion
- Abdominal swelling
- Sudden bloating; fluid weight gain
- Palpitations or rapid heartbeat

sounds that indicate fluid in the lungs, the characteristic sound of a heart murmur, or a very rapid irregular heartbeat. Tapping on your chest is another means of detecting fluid in the lungs. He or she will look closely at your neck veins for signs of fluid overload and press on your legs or ankles to detect swelling, which is a sign of excess fluid under the skin. He or she can do several tests to confirm the diagnosis:

- A chest X-ray may reveal an enlarged heart and the buildup of fluids in the lungs.

- An electrocardiogram (ECG; see page 122) can detect changes in the heart rhythm, the thickness of the heart wall, or prior signs of heart damage.

- An echocardiogram (see page 122) will measure the size of the heart and the motion of the heart wall during contraction and relaxation. It can also measure overall function of your heart muscle and detect abnormal heart valve function.

- Exercise stress testing (see page 125) may help determine the cause of your symptoms.

- Nuclear imaging may be needed to assess the overall function of your heart muscle.

- Magnetic resonance imaging (MRI; see page 141) may help identify the cause and assess the heart's overall ability to function.

- Although cardiac catheterization techniques (see page 142) or nuclear imaging (see page 135) are typically not needed to diagnose heart failure, they may provide information about how damaged your heart is, or enable doctors to look for causes of heart failure that can be corrected.

A new blood test measures the concentrations of BNP, a hormone produced in the heart, or NT-proBNP, which measures a key portion of BNP; both are markers of cardiac distress. A high level of these substances suggests the presence of heart failure and how severe it is.

Understanding Heart Failure

It is easier living with heart failure and following through with treatment if you understand what goes on in your body as a result of the condition and how the treatment is going to improve your heart functions.

Heart failure can be caused by dysfunction of either the right side or the left side of your heart, or both. But it usually begins on the left side—the more powerful side that pumps blood out to your body (see pages 6–8). Your left atrium receives blood from the lungs and sends it into your left ventricle, which pumps it out into circulation. If the left ventricle weakens, it cannot keep up with the amount of incoming blood, and fluids start to back up in lung tissue.

When the left ventricle cannot contract sufficiently, this is called systolic failure, and the heart cannot pump enough blood forward and out to the body with each heartbeat. When the muscular walls of the ventricle have become rigid and cannot relax enough, this is called diastolic failure, meaning the heart is stiff and cannot fill with enough blood between contractions. In either case, blood entering the left side of the heart from the lungs starts to back up in lung tissue. When fluid buildup in the lungs' small vessels (capillaries) reaches a critical point, fluid leaks into the air sacs (alveoli) themselves, causing congestion. This fluid accumulation, called pulmonary edema, makes breathing difficult.

You may experience symptoms from this congestion in the lungs in different ways. You may feel breathless only with activity, or you may have difficulty breathing when you lie down, as fluid "pools" in the lungs. Breathing difficulties may awaken you from a sound sleep. You may require additional pillows to breathe more comfortably through the night. Wheezing or coughing, particularly if the cough produces pinkish phlegm, is another sign of fluid buildup in your lungs.

Heart failure can also affect the right side of your heart, due to lung disease or as a result of left-sided failure. The right side of the heart, which receives blood returning from the body and pumps it into the lungs to be enriched with oxygen, is affected by back pressure from a failing left ventricle. As the right side of the heart becomes less able to pump, fluids back up in the veins and engorge tissues and organs throughout the body. This form of edema (swelling) is likely to be most evident in your legs, ankles, and feet. Veins in your neck also may swell. Your abdominal organs—particularly your liver and the abdominal cavity, which includes the intestines—may also be enlarged and tender, causing you to feel nauseous or full.

Also, as the heart's pumping ability declines, general circulation may slow down. Some people experience symptoms related to inadequate blood supply to other organs. If your kidneys are not getting enough blood, they react by retaining fluids, meaning that they are not disposing of water and sodium properly. Normal kidney functions include controlling your acid-base balance and potassium balance in the bloodstream; impaired kidney function also affects your acid-base and potassium levels. This effect contributes to the fluid retention throughout the body.

If your muscles don't get adequate blood, you may feel weaker and more tired than usual, especially when you exert yourself. If your brain is not getting enough blood and oxygen, you may feel light-headed, confused, disoriented, or forgetful.

Medications can strengthen your heart's pumping efficiency in several different ways, and other drugs can relieve fluid retention. Once you have been diagnosed with heart failure, it is important that you are aware of these possible symptoms so that you can notice changes and report them to your doctor. The nature of your symptoms can tell your doctor a great deal about where the heart's pumping action is weakened, what effect medications are having, and how to proceed with treatment so that you can enjoy normal activities.

What Is the "Ejection Fraction?"

Even in healthy people, not all the blood is pumped out of the heart with each heartbeat. During a good strong contraction, the ventricles pump out about 50 to 70 percent of the total volume of blood the ventricles hold when filled. Doctors call this percentage the ejection fraction, and it is one indicator of how efficiently the heart is working as a pump. When a healthy person exercises and the muscles demand more blood, his or her ejection fraction may increase by about 5 percent or more.

In a person with heart failure, the ejection fraction may drop to as little as 20 to 30 percent, which means the heart is pumping out a much smaller fraction of its blood volume. One way the heart tries to make up for its diminished pumping strength is by enlarging, resulting in ventricles that can expand to hold a larger volume of blood. Even if the ejection fraction is only 20 or 30 percent, the extra volume of blood in an enlarged ventricle means that the heart may still pump an adequate amount of blood to supply the body. The heart may also beat more quickly in order to keep enough blood flowing. But these compensatory mechanisms can only work up to a point, often leaving you with no cardiac reserve if the heart is stressed.

Living with Heart Failure

Because a number of medical conditions can cause heart failure, and because the symptoms can be so diverse, treatment for heart failure is highly individualized. Occasionally, heart failure can be resolved by correcting an underlying cause. For example, in some cases doctors can repair a faulty valve, restore blood flow through a blocked coronary artery, or correct an arrhythmia to alleviate heart failure. But certain forms of heart failure probably cannot be reversed. Instead, successful treatment involves adapting your lifestyle to alleviate your symptoms and to slow the progression of the disease; taking medications to strengthen the heart's pumping action and reduce its workload; and, in some cases, having surgery or even a heart transplant. Living with heart failure will certainly mean that you will need to see your physician regularly, and promptly report any changes in your condition.

For most people with mild to moderate heart failure, lifestyle changes, in combination with drug treatment, can enable them to live an active life. Your doctor will advise you to quit smoking if you smoke; lose excess weight if you are overweight; eat a low-fat, low-sodium diet; limit your consumption of alcohol; limit your intake of caffeine; and avoid stress. Most people with heart failure also benefit from an exercise program tailored to the severity of their heart failure and general health; ask your doctor what's appropriate for you.

Monitoring Your Sodium Intake

Because fluid retention is one of the primary symptoms of heart failure, and large amounts of sodium in the diet tend to increase fluid retention, your doctor will probably counsel you to limit your salt intake to 1 to 2 grams, or 1,000 to 2,000 milligrams, per day (see page 91), which is less than 1 teaspoon of salt. Restricting salt helps lower your blood pressure and maximize the effect of some of your medications, such as diuretics. If you have advanced heart failure, you may also be advised to limit your intake of fluids (to no more than about 2 quarts per day).

Because processed foods often contain high amounts of sodium, and it can be difficult to control the amounts of sodium in restaurant food, cooking at home may be the most reliable option. Do not add salt in cooking or at the table; instead, try various spices, herbs, and peppers to season your food. Be careful about salt substitutes, some of which are high in potassium; check with your doctor's office before using any salt substitute. If you do not cook, try to learn to prepare healthful versions of favorite dishes you enjoy. If someone cooks for you, ask him or her to learn to cook the foods you can eat. Bring that person with you to the doctor's or nutritionist's office to get involved.

In many locales, some companies offer heart-healthy meals you can pick up or have delivered. Also, many restaurants now offer menus that help you choose healthier options when you dine out. If the meal is being freshly prepared, you can and should request that the chef refrain from adding any salt.

Monitoring Your Weight and Swelling

It's important to monitor your weight closely to watch for the sudden weight gain indicating that fluids are building up in your body. You can gain water weight before noticeable swelling occurs. To keep accurate track of your weight, try this method:

- Ask your doctor to weigh you and tell you your dry weight—that is, your body weight in the doctor's office without retained fluid—and write it down.
- Weigh yourself every day, preferably in the morning after you urinate. Your weight may vary by as much as 2 pounds, depending on your diet and activity level.
- Write each day's weight down immediately, and compare it to your dry weight (see above or ask your doctor), not yesterday's weight.

Unusual swelling (edema) is another sign of fluid retention. To monitor swelling, watch for visible swelling in your ankles, legs, or hands; your shoes feeling tight; your rings feeling tight; or your clothes feeling tight around the waistline.

If you gain more than 2 pounds in 1 day, or 4 pounds in 1 week, or if you have more swelling than usual, your doctor may adjust your medication or recommend the following:

- Cut the sodium in your diet by 500 milligrams (about ¼ teaspoon) or more each day.
- Decrease the amount of liquid you drink by 1 or 2 cups per day.

Exercise

Moderate exercise can be a good way to deal with the fatigue that you may experience with heart failure, but check with your doctor first. Exercise is also beneficial for your whole body and sense of well-being, and a moderate level of activity will keep you fit. If you have not been physically active, work with your physician to start a safe walking program (see page 80).

If you lead a physically active life, describe your typical activities to your doctor and work out safe and sensible limits. Your doctor may recommend that you avoid strenuous activity, such as heavy lifting, that increases your blood pressure and makes you short of breath. If you have already had an exercise stress test, your doctor may be able to give you exercise recommendations based on the test results.

If you experience severe difficulties breathing while you are exercising, you definitely need to curtail physical activity. During these times, it is important to get more bed rest to reduce your heart's workload and allow fluids in your body to redistribute. When you are feeling stronger, and with your doctor's advice, you can gradually return to a more active routine.

Getting Rest and Sleep

Many people with heart failure experience fatigue that interferes with their usual activities. Fatigue can also be a symptom of worsening heart failure. You can avoid overtaxing your heart and lessen the impact of fatigue in several ways:

- Plan a nap or rest period in your daily routine. Don't wait until you are exhausted to rest. Plan a regular bedtime at night and stick to it.
- Space more strenuous activities throughout the day, with rest periods in between. Plan activities you enjoy for the times of day that you feel the best.
- Take things easy; don't rush. Avoid quick spurts of activity.
- Save your energy in small ways: sit down while you shower and get ready in the morning; sit down during meal preparation; group your activities so you are not going up and down stairs several times a day.

- Avoid vigorous exercise when it's especially hot or cold, or right after a meal.
- Don't hesitate to ask for help from family or friends. Many people will be glad to help you get strenuous tasks done.
- Call your doctor if you or your family observe that your feeling of fatigue is getting worse.

You may have difficulty sleeping comfortably because of breathing problems. To get a better night's sleep, prop your head and shoulders up on pillows, or even try sleeping sitting up. If your medications cause you to get up to go to the bathroom often during the night, talk to your doctor about adjusting the dose or changing the time of day at which you take them.

Treating Heart Failure with Medications

Most people with heart failure will require a combination of medications to achieve the best results. In order to minimize side effects, your doctor may prescribe a drug at a low dose at first, and then gradually increase the dose to an optimum level over the long term. It is always important to take your medications at the prescribed dose, even if you are feeling better. You should plan to refill your medications at least three days in advance so that you do not run the risk of running out of medication and missing any doses. If you are taking your medications and you begin to feel worse or experience a change in symptoms, tell your doctor immediately. You may be able to adjust the dose, take a different drug, or manage the symptoms in another way.

Diuretics: Reducing Fluids and Sodium

You will almost certainly start taking diuretics, often referred to as water pills, to help you urinate more often to get rid of the excess fluids and sodium that are characteristic of heart failure. Reducing fluids in your lungs will help you breathe more easily, and reducing fluids in other parts of the body will minimize swelling and discomfort. There are several different types of diuretics that each act on your body slightly differently. Your doctor will work with you to find a diuretic agent that works at a level that is best for you.

Some diuretics cause your body to lose potassium or magnesium, which can affect your heart rhythms and the effectiveness of other medications. Your doctor may recommend that you eat foods that are rich in potassium: bananas, cantaloupe, grapefruit, apricots, orange juice, potatoes (especially sweet potatoes), prunes, and prune juice. Some people with low potassium may develop symptoms such as leg cramps or fatigue. If your potassium level is low, your doctor may prescribe potassium supplements, but don't take them on your own.

Many people don't like taking diuretics because the intended effect—making you urinate more—is inconvenient. Most diuretics are short-acting, so the greatest effect on urination comes within the first 2 to 3 hours of taking the drug, as with furosemide. However, chlorthalidone, another commonly prescribed diuretic, has longer-lasting effects of about 6 hours. You may find that you can plan your day better if you take your diuretic first thing in the morning, and then again in the late afternoon, so that the medication does not interfere with your day's activities or your night's sleep. Learning how a diuretic seems to affect you is helpful, since it will probably work the same way each time you take it and you can learn to plan accordingly.

Often people who are risk for heart failure are also at risk for bladder problems such as incontinence. Diuretics can cause this problem or

Commonly Prescribed Diuretics

Generic Name	Possible Side Effects
Hydrochlorothiazide, Chlorthiazide	Potassium loss, increases in blood sugar, gout
Hydrochlorothiazide with spironolactone	Dizziness, dehydration
Chlorthalidone	Dizziness, dry mouth, headache, potassium loss
Spironolactone	Dizziness, dehydration, elevated potassium, gynecomastia
Furosemide	Potassium loss, magnesium loss
Bumetanide	Dizziness, headache, potassium loss
Metolazone	Dizziness, headache, nausea, high blood sugar, potassium loss

can make it worse. People are often reluctant to talk to their doctors about personal problems such as incontinence. If your doctor does not ask the appropriate question, ask him or her for advice. The market has responded with a variety of products for men and for women.

Digitalis: Strengthening Heart Contractions

Digitalis (also called digoxin or digitoxin) strengthens your heart's contractions and slows the heart rate, which in turn leads to better circulation and helps reduce swelling in body tissues. See also "Medications for Valve Disease," page 203.

Possible side effects of digitalis, particularly in large doses, may include dizziness, anxiety, confusion, blurry or double vision, nausea, or loss of appetite. However, most of these symptoms are not specific to heart failure or to usage of digitalis. For example, if you are taking a large dose of a diuretic, dizziness can be a sign of dehydration, or it could be a sign of some other illness. As always, report any side effects to your doctor immediately. Your doctor will periodically order a blood test to monitor the levels of digoxin in your bloodstream.

Medications That Ease the Workload

Medications that help your heart include ACE inhibitors and angiotensin receptor blockers (ARBs).

ACE Inhibitors

First prescribed for high blood pressure, ACE inhibitors (angiotensin-converting enzyme inhibitors; see pages 61 and 169), are now widely prescribed for heart failure as well. By blocking the production of angiotensin 2, a hormone that constricts

Coenzyme Q10

Coenzyme Q10, also known as CoQ10 or ubiquinone, is a vitamin-like substance that occurs naturally in every cell in your body. It is involved in biochemical reactions that produce cellular energy. It is an antioxidant, meaning that it protects cells from free radicals, the harmful by-products of cellular activity. It is marketed as a nutritional supplement and is also found in foods such as organ meats, beef, sardines, soybean oil, and peanuts.

Some research has suggested that some people with congestive heart failure have low levels of CoQ10 and can benefit from taking it in the form of supplements. People in these studies received CoQ10 in addition to conventional drugs, so it is difficult to say which treatment was effective. However, one small well-designed study did not show any benefit for heart failure patients from taking CoQ10. Presently, the American Heart Association and the American College of Cardiology say that without more data, CoQ10 cannot be recommended as an effective treatment for congestive heart failure.

No harmful side effects have been reported as a result of taking CoQ10. But it can interfere with the anticlotting drug warfarin, so if you are taking warfarin, make sure you consult your doctor before taking CoQ10.

blood vessels and is found in high levels in people with heart failure, ACE inhibitors have the beneficial effect of enlarging (dilating) the vessels and reducing the work required for the heart to pump blood into the arteries. In a person with heart failure, ACE inhibitors not only reduce symptoms but also lengthen life expectancy. Common side effects include dizziness, low blood pressure, cough, allergic reaction, dangerous increases in potassium levels, and kidney problems.

ARBs

ARBs (angiotensin receptor blockers) are a newer group of drugs most frequently prescribed for high blood pressure but also prescribed for people with heart failure who cannot take ACE inhibitors. Like ACE inhibitors, ARBs work by inhibiting the effects of the hormone angiotensin 2, keeping blood vessels open and lowering blood pressure.

Tips for Taking Medications

If you have heart problems, you may be taking several medications at once. It's not easy to keep track of prescriptions, pills, and schedules, but it's very important to take these powerful drugs exactly as your doctor has prescribed. Here are some ideas to help you and your family members get organized so that your medications become part of a regular, manageable routine.

- Buy a pill organizer, available at any drugstore. This is a set of pillboxes marked with the days of the week and the times of day that you take your medications. At the beginning of each week, fill the pillbox carefully, or have someone do it for you, so that the medications are ready for you when you need to take them. Always keep the pillbox in the same handy place—for instance, on the table where you eat.

- With the help of a doctor or nurse, make a medication chart (see page 299) that lists all the drugs you take, the dosages, the times of day that you take them, and the days of the week that you take them. Put the chart in a prominent place—such as the

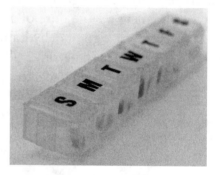

Simplifying your medications

If you have congestive heart failure, you may be taking several medications several times a day. A pill organizer is an inexpensive, simple means of following a complicated drug regimen. The organizers, available at any pharmacy, come in many sizes and configurations to help you sort and schedule your medications.

back of the medicine cabinet door—and make another copy that you can use to fill your pill organizer every week. If you are

Unlike ACE inhibitors, ARBs work not by slowing down the production of angiotensin but by blocking its effects. Common side effects of ARBs include dizziness and headache; be sure to tell your doctor if you experience unpleasant side effects.

ACE inhibitors and ARBs can also increase your potassium levels and affect your kidney function, so your doctor will probably want to do blood tests regularly. You may be advised to avoid some foods or products such as salt substitutes that are high in potassium.

Beta-blockers: Reducing Stress on the Heart

Beta-blockers (beta-adrenergic blocking agents; see also page 167) are another group of drugs prescribed for many heart conditions, including heart failure. A person with congestive heart failure often has

having difficulty, enlist a friend or family member to help you assemble the list and keep it updated anytime there is a change in your medications. Bring that list with you to all doctors' appointments.

- Ask your doctor or pharmacist for written information sheets about the drugs you are taking. Keep them in a file where you and family members can refer to them.

- Don't hesitate to ask your doctor questions about why you are taking a medication or what it does to help your condition. If you don't understand the answers, get a family member or friend to talk to the doctor.

- Develop a routine for taking your medicines every day. But don't hesitate to talk to your doctor about changing the routine if you have a problem. (For instance, you may want to adjust the time when you take diuretics to fit with your sleep patterns or daily schedule of activities.)

- If you miss a dose of medicine, do not take two doses to make up for it. However, if you are not due to take another dose for several hours or until the next day, take the missed dose as soon as you remember it. If you are scheduled to take the next dose in 2 hours or less, just skip the forgotten dose and take the next dose on schedule. Ask your doctor about the correct procedure for handling missed doses.

- If you start to have unpleasant side effects, do not stop taking the drug. Contact your doctor immediately and ask if changes can be made in the drug or the dosage. Some side effects diminish after you have been taking the drug for a while.

- Always be sure to tell your doctor about any other medications, including dietary supplements and over-the-counter remedies, that you are taking. Many drugs can interact with each other.

- If you are having trouble paying for your drugs, talk to your doctor about how to get financial help. Many pharmaceutical companies offer major discounts to those who qualify for help due to financial need.

high levels of catecholamines (hormones that the body produces to withstand stress and exercise) in the bloodstream. By blocking the action of these hormones, beta-blockers slow the heart rate, reduce blood pressure, and reduce the heart's need for oxygen. As a result, the drugs reduce symptoms and help avoid the heart enlargement and decline in heart function that is characteristic of heart failure.

These drugs may also suppress arrhythmias. Beta-blockers commonly prescribed for arrhythmias include carvedilol and metoprolol.

In some people, beta-blockers can cause wheezing or fluid to build up in the body. They may also lower a person's blood pressure. Management of fluids in the body is an important part of your care, so be sure to tell your doctor immediately if you notice signs of swelling, bloating, or rapid weight gain from fluid retention. Excess salt intake is one reason people retain fluids, so restrict salt intake if you notice these signs. You may also need to take a diuretic with the beta-blocker.

Other Heart Failure Medications

Your doctor may prescribe other types of drugs to treat heart failure. These may include aspirin or anticoagulants (see page 109) to prevent blood clots; aldosterone antagonists (diuretics), which block the effects of a stress hormone (aldosterone) that may aggravate heart failure; and hydralazine with isosorbide dinitrate, which reduces the heart's workload, especially in people who cannot tolerate an ACE inhibitor or an ARB. Each of these drugs or drug groups has specific instructions for use and possible side effects. Always ask your doctor or pharmacist for written instructions about a drug you are taking.

Certain calcium channel blockers—such as amlodipine—can be prescribed in some people with heart failure if needed to control blood pressure. Influsions of calcium channel blockers may help improve symptoms of heart failure in some people, but they have not been shown to prolong life.

Treating Heart Failure with Surgical Procedures

For some patients who have severe heart failure or for whom medications are not sufficient, surgical procedures may be recommended to stop further damage to the heart and to improve its pumping ability. Some operations, such as coronary artery bypass surgery or valve surgery, may be used to correct an underlying problem that may be causing or contributing to another heart problem such as an inadequate blood supply.

Other procedures are more specific to the treatment of heart failure. For example, if you have had a heart attack that has damaged the left ventricle (the main pumping chamber), an aneurysm can form (a thin area of tissue that bulges with each heartbeat). An aneurysm in this critical area can rupture, or may contribute to heart failure, aggravating other heart damage you may have. A cardiac surgeon can perform reconstructive surgery on the left ventricle to remove the scar tissue and reshape the left ventricle. The goal of surgery is to reduce your symptoms of heart failure and restore some of the pumping strength of the left ventricle.

Ventricular Assist Device

Another surgical option for some patients is the implantation of a left ventricular assist device (LVAD or VAD). This device is a mechanical pump that supplements the pumping action of a weakened left ventricle. It does not replace the chamber or the heart, but it increases the amount of blood pumped throughout the body. A VAD will partially relieve symptoms of heart failure and may improve the quality of life for a person with severe heart failure. VADs were first developed to "buy time" for someone awaiting a heart transplant and were often referred to as a bridge to transplant. Today, some VADs are implanted for long-term use (which doctors sometimes call destination therapy), eliminating the need for a transplant.

A VAD consists of a pump, a control mechanism, and an energy supply. Some devices are air-driven and others are powered by battery. Both the energy supply and the controls are worn outside your body and attached by wires to the pump. The pump is usually implanted in the body and attached to the heart. Most often, the device is connected to the left ventricle; blood flows from the left ventricle into the pump and is delivered to the aorta (which carries the blood to the rest of the body). If the VAD is implanted on the right ventricle, blood is brought through the pump and into the pulmonary artery to be delivered into the lungs.

VADs are used only in severe cases, either before a transplant or if a transplant is not possible. A very small or thin person might not have enough body surface area to support the device, and people with kidney failure, liver disease, blood-clotting disorders, lung disease, or persistent infections may not be good candidates. The surgery carries definite risks, including bleeding, blood clotting, respiratory failure, kidney failure, infection, stroke, or failure of the device itself. Research continues to try to develop safer VADs for a wider group of patients.

Cardiac Resynchronization

Cardiac resynchronization (also sometimes called biventricular pacing) is a relatively recent development in the treatment of heart failure patients. Heart failure is often caused by a condition called cardiomyopathy (weakened or enlarged heart muscle; see the box on page 249). Many people who have cardiomyopathy and heart failure—as many as 40 percent—also have an abnormality in the heart's electrical system that causes uncoordinated contractions of the heart muscle. This irregular contraction still further reduces the heart's ability to pump effectively. Cardiac resynchronization involves installing a specific type of pacemaker to restore coordinated pumping action in the ventricles.

In a person with a healthy heart, the electrical impulse that triggers a heartbeat originates in the right atrium, then travels along nerve routes, called the left and right bundle branches, that fan out into the left and right ventricles (see pages 10–12). These routes enable the electrical signal to stimulate the left and right ventricles simultaneously.

In some people with heart failure and cardiomyopathy, there is a delay (usually in the left bundle branch) that causes the right ventricle to contract a split second before the left ventricle. A cardiologist can see this abnormality on an electrocardiogram (ECG).

A unique type of pacemaker—a cardiac resynchronization therapy device, or CRT pacemaker—corrects this problem. In addition to the two leads in a conventional pacemaker (in the right atrium and right ventricle; see page 272), a CRT device has a third lead implanted into a vein on the surface of the left ventricle. Through these leads, the CRT device can stimulate both ventricles simultaneously and restore coordinated contractions.

You may be a good candidate for cardiac resynchronization therapy if you have moderate to severe symptoms of heart failure, you have cardiomyopathy, and you have the characteristic electrical delay in the ventricles. If you are also at risk of rapid heartbeat (fibrillation; see page 265), you may benefit from a still more specialized device that defibrillates as well. This device combines a CRT device with a standard implantable cardiac defibrillator (ICD; see page 275). The combined device is called a cardiac resynchronization therapy defibrillator (CRDT). (For more information about what to expect during the implantation of a pacemaker device, see page 273.)

Most people who have had CRT devices implanted experience fewer symptoms of heart failure, are able to tolerate exercise better, and have a better quality of life. Some people may experience these benefits immediately after the procedure, while for others it may take several weeks or months before they see an improvement in their condition. However, even though cardiologists are careful to select only those

What Is Cardiomyopathy?

Cardiomyopathy literally means disease of the heart muscle, which can alter the structure of the heart. The condition can significantly diminish the heart's pumping ability, resulting in heart failure. It is a leading reason for heart transplant. Unlike many types of heart disease, it frequently affects younger people. It occurs in both sexes and in different racial groups.

Often, doctors do not know the cause of cardiomyopathy. Some forms, particularly hypertrophic, are most often inherited, so it helps to know if it has occurred before in your family. Some cases may be caused by viral infection, severe high blood pressure over a long period, prior heart attacks, or alcohol abuse. More research is needed to better understand the causes and treatment for this complex disease.

Cardiomyopathy can be difficult to recognize, and therefore may go untreated. Different forms of the disease result in different types of damage. A dilated cardiomyopathy occurs because the walls of the heart chambers weaken and cannot contract sufficiently. By contrast, the heart wall thickens in hypertrophic cardiomyopathy. Restrictive cardiomyopathy causes loss of elasticity in the walls that restricts the ability of the heart to fill with blood. Ischemic cardiomyopathy is the result of scarring from heart attacks.

The symptoms of cardiomyopathy include unexplained symptoms of heart failure: shortness of breath, bloating, fainting, fatigue, and chest pains. If you have such symptoms, see your doctor immediately. Tests including angiography, echocardiography, electrocardiography, and MRI may help confirm a diagnosis. Each case of cardiomyopathy requires an individualized strategy for treatment, which may include medications, implantation of a pacemaker, or other surgical procedures.

patients they believe will benefit from a CRT device, some people do not improve after the device is implanted. You and your cardiologist need to discuss in detail whether this operation is desirable for you.

Heart Transplantation

In a person whose heart is irreparably damaged, for whom medication, surgical procedures, and mechanical devices are no longer effective, replacement of the diseased heart with a healthy one is the only option. Today, most people who receive heart transplants have either advanced coronary artery disease or cardiomyopathy that is likely to be fatal in less than 3 years. Transplant recipients who have the best results are generally under the age of 65, do not have serious medical problems other than their heart problem, do not have conditions that will interfere with the medications needed after transplantation surgery, and are willing to follow a strict regimen of medication and lifestyle.

If your cardiologist recommends a heart transplant and you are willing to undertake the procedure, he or she will contact a transplantation center. The transplant center team will discuss your case and thoroughly evaluate the severity of your condition. They will also do an in-depth analysis to exclude the possibility of other diseases. The team will talk to you at length about the medication routine you need to follow after the surgery, along with extensive follow-up doctor visits and testing. Heart transplantation is a costly procedure, so if you do not have insurance or other resources to pay for the surgery, you may be able to work with hospital social workers or financial officers to find other sources of funding.

Matching Heart Donors and Recipients

Once you are found eligible, your name will be added to a national list of people waiting for a donor heart to be transplanted. The wait may be long, because the demand for donor hearts is much greater than the supply. An organization called the United Network for Organ Sharing maintains the computerized waiting list. Your position on the list depends in large part on the stability of your medical condition while you wait, your need for medications or mechanical assistance while you wait, and how long you can be expected to live without a transplant.

Your position on the list may change if your condition changes. People whose condition deteriorates may move up in priority on the list, while those whose health improves may move down on the list.

You also have to wait to be matched with a suitable donor heart. The heart must be approximately the right size for your body, and its blood type and tissue type must be compatible with yours. In the event of a transplant, your body's immune system will identify the donor heart tissue as a foreign substance and attempt to reject it. Tissue typing involves matching characteristics of your immune system with that of the donor heart to minimize the danger of tissue rejection—one of the chief risks of any kind of transplant surgery.

Of course, the wait for a donor heart is a difficult, uncertain time. You will need to prepare yourself for the imminent possibility of surgery by quitting smoking, if necessary; refraining from the use of alcohol or any drugs other than prescribed medications; exercising to build your strength and stamina; and controlling conditions such as high blood pressure or diabetes. You will almost certainly be on constant, powerful medications (such as digitalis), and your heart may need mechanical assistance, such as a ventricular assist device (VAD; see page 247). Your cardiologist will monitor your condition very closely during this period to ensure that you are ready for surgery on extremely short notice.

As a transplant candidate, you must carry a pager at all times, and keep a suitcase packed so that you can go to the hospital immediately if a donor heart is found for you. In the event that a transplant is performed, you can expect to stay at the hospital for approximately 2 weeks.

Transplantation Surgery

Once you have arrived at the hospital, a final evaluation and laboratory tests will be done. You will be prepared for surgery and given a general anesthetic. For experienced surgeons, the transplantation surgery itself is straightforward. To perform the operation, surgeons will open your chest by cutting through the sternum (breastbone) and exposing your heart. You will be connected to a heart-lung machine (see page 183), which will assume the functions of your heart and lungs during the operation. Surgeons will disconnect your diseased heart from the major blood vessels and remove it. They will position the donor heart in your chest and attach the major blood vessels to it. Then they will transfer function from the heart-lung machine back to your body. Often the warmth of blood passing through the donor heart starts it beating. If it does not start shortly, doctors will administer an electrical shock to get it started. They will close the chest incision and the surgery is complete.

In relatively rare cases, the body will not accept the donor heart. This "graft rejection" is immediately apparent, and doctors will need to remove the heart and look for another match for a second transplant. A VAD or artificial heart may be inserted temporarily.

After a successful transplant, your recovery will include several days in an intensive care unit. Your condition will be constantly monitored, including regular heart biopsies. A heart biopsy requires taking a tissue sample from the transplanted heart through a tube inserted in your neck or groin. It is the only way doctors can ensure that your body is accepting the new organ. Medications will be given to alter the immune response—that is, to prevent your body's immune system from attacking the heart. You will probably be able to get out of bed in 3 or 4 days, and you may be able to go home in 10 days to 3 weeks after surgery.

For approximately 3 months after the transplant, you will have to return to the hospital regularly for checkups, including continued heart biopsies to look for early signs of rejection. You will be assigned to a transplant coordinator, who will be able to answer your questions and help you get any kind of medical assistance you need. Over time you will have periodic evaluations to make sure that you do not have significant blockages developing in your coronary arteries, because even if blockages are occurring, you may experience fewer symptoms of angina with your new heart, due to severing of nerve fibers during the transplant surgery.

After Transplant Surgery

The most dangerous immediate risk of heart transplantation is not the surgery itself but rejection of the heart tissue. You will need to take immunosuppressive drugs (such as cyclosporine and corticosteroids) that counteract the immune response. These drugs make your body more vulnerable to infection, especially in the first 3 months or so after surgery. Even after your recovery is complete, you will need to take extra precautions against infection, such as avoiding public places

Donor Hearts

A donor heart comes from a person who has given consent for organ donation after his or her death and who has died of an illness or accident that has left the heart undamaged. Approximately 2,300 hearts become available each year for transplant, far fewer than are needed for waiting transplant recipients. After a person dies and has been identified as a donor, the process of readying the heart for transplant must move very quickly, because a heart can live for only about 4 to 6 hours outside the body. The heart must be checked for normal function and for blood type, tested for evidence of infection, and then removed. Through the coordinated efforts of the United Network for Organ Sharing and heart transplant programs across the country, the donor heart is matched with a suitable recipient and transported to the appropriate transplant team.

Because of the critical need for donor organs, many states and medical organizations have made education about organ donation a priority. In the event of a death, a single donor may be able to benefit several lives by providing healthy organs (heart, lungs, liver, kidneys, pancreas, corneas). If you have any questions about how you or someone you know can become an organ donor, contact your local hospital or the secretary of state's office in your state.

during flu season, being careful about handling animals, and getting immediate medical treatment for even minor signs of infection.

You will need to take immunosuppressive medication for the rest of your life, and you may experience side effects. These include trembling of the hands, elevated cholesterol levels, and high blood pressure, which in turn may require additional medication. These medications may be adjusted often, depending on the side effects and the presence or absence of rejection. Over the long term, the immunosuppressive drugs increase the risk of skin and lymphatic cancer, so you must take careful precautions to avoid sun exposure.

Outcomes of Transplantation

Most recipients of donated hearts live significantly longer than they would have without the transplants. Many enjoy reasonably active lives, including moderate exercise and a return to work. Of course, a heart-healthy lifestyle and regular monitoring are essential.

Heart-Lung Transplantation

If a person has severe lung disease that has also affected the heart, most often pulmonary hypertension (high blood pressure in the vessels in the lungs), a heart-lung transplant can be performed. This procedure is undertaken only when all other medical and surgical options have failed. The chances of success are greatest if the recipient is under age 45.

To accomplish a heart-lung transplant, surgeons remove the donor's heart and lungs by severing the trachea, aorta, and the connection between the heart and the venae cavae (the two major veins that carry blood into the right side of the heart). The blood vessels between the heart and lungs are left intact. The recipient's heart and lungs are removed. Then the donor lungs are reattached to the recipient's trachea first, the heart is attached to the aorta, and finally the blood vessels are connected.

Availability of donor organs for a heart-lung transplant is a serious problem, because lungs begin to deteriorate very shortly after death. The recipient of such a transplant must take immunosuppressive drugs for life.

15

Arrhythmias

Every second or so, an electrical impulse originating in the right atrium of your heart travels through the heart and triggers a single heartbeat, or contraction of the heart. A group of specialized cells in the muscle tissue, called the sinoatrial (SA) node, initiates the signal, acting as your heart's natural pacemaker. The impulse travels through the four chambers of your heart in a carefully timed sequence to stimulate the rhythmic contractions that pump blood through your body (see pages 9–10).

Any change or interruption in the electrical signal that throws off this rhythm is called an arrhythmia. The heart may beat too fast, too slow, or in an irregular pattern. Arrhythmias can occur in people with normal hearts or those with underlying disease. Throughout the course of your lifetime, your heart will occasionally skip a beat or palpitate slightly, and these brief variations are completely harmless. Some people have minor arrhythmias that never cause a problem. However, in some arrhythmias, the pumping action of the heart can be seriously affected, or it can cause symptoms of palpitation (awareness of the abnormal heartbeat), light-headedness, or fainting. If you have another heart condition, such as heart failure, an arrhythmia is more likely to cause a problem for you.

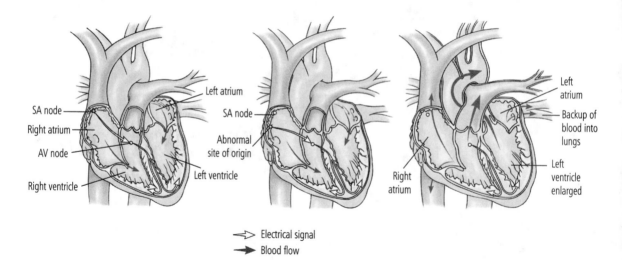

Left atrium

SA node

Right atrium

AV node

Right ventricle

Left ventricle

SA node

Abnormal site of origin

Right atrium

Left atrium

Backup of blood into lungs

Left ventricle enlarged

⇨ Electrical signal

→ Blood flow

Healthy heartbeat

In a normal heartbeat, the sinoatrial (SA) node is the pacemaker that initiates an electrical impulse and paces the normal sequence through the electrical pathways in the structures of the heart.

Abnormal origin of impulse

In some forms of arrhythmia, the electrical impulse originates somewhere other than the sinoatrial node, and the heartbeat starts early or quickens. As a result, less blood is moved through the heart with each contraction.

Backup of blood

Some arrhythmias, in which the impulse originates outside the SA node, cause the heartbeat to be irregular and ineffective. The ventricles may enlarge in an effort to keep blood moving. Blood may back up into the lungs, causing congestive heart failure.

Some people are born with an irregular heartbeat. Other cardiovascular conditions, such as high blood pressure, valvular disease, heart failure, or coronary artery disease can be factors; diabetes can also contribute (see page 105). Substances such as caffeine, tobacco, alcohol, cocaine and prescribed medication, some over-the-counter cough and cold medications, diet pills, and some herbal remedies can affect the pattern of your heartbeat (see page 267). Stress can also cause arrhythmias in some people, as the body releases adrenaline, the stress hormone. Low levels of or an imbalance of electrolytes such as low potassium levels may cause or worsen an arrhythmia. Your doctor may order a blood test to check your electrolytes, to make sure there is no correctable problem causing your arrhythmia.

Treatment, therefore, may include lifestyle changes and control of other conditions, taking an antiarrhythmia medication, avoiding some medications, nonsurgical procedures, or surgery (for instance, implantation of a pacemaker) to restore a normal heartbeat. Your doctor may refer you to a heart rhythm specialist, called an electrophysiologist.

Types of Arrhythmia

Irregularities in your heart rhythms can be described by the effect they have on the speed of your heartbeat (acceleration or deceleration) and where they occur in your heart (in the atria or in the ventricles). Another type of arrhythmia, called heart block, is a partial or complete interruption in the transmission of the electrical impulses between the upper and lower chambers of your heart.

Bradycardia and Tachycardia

An irregular heartbeat can be either too slow (bradycardia) or too fast (tachycardia). A healthy person generally has a resting heart rate of 60 to 100 beats per minute.

Bradycardia, a heart rate of less than 60 beats per minute, may not be a medical problem. A physically active person whose heart pumps very efficiently may have a lower heart rate that is not at all abnormal. But a very slow heart rate can become a problem if the brain does not receive enough blood, causing symptoms such as light-headedness or fainting.

Bradycardia most commonly affects older people because with age-related damage of the heart's electrical system, all the impulses from the atrium may not get to the ventricle. It may be caused by damage to the sinoatrial node (where the electrical pulse begins) or to the biological "wires" that connect the upper chambers (atria) to the lower chambers (ventricles). This damage may be brought on by heart disease, aging, a genetic defect, or some drugs or medications. Medications or a temporary pacemaker can speed up the heart's contractions temporarily. A pacemaker is also a long-term treatment.

Tachycardia, a very rapid heart rate of more than 100 beats per minute, can take many forms, depending on where in the heart it occurs. Fibrillation, perhaps the most serious form of tachycardia, causes the heart muscle to quiver instead of contracting rhythmically. (For symptoms, see page 258.) The heartbeat is not only too fast but uncoordinated as well. Both tachycardia and fibrillation, in various forms, can be treated with medications, surgery, or mechanical devices.

> ### Symptoms of Bradycardia
>
> Call your doctor if you have prolonged or recurring episodes of these symptoms:
> - Fatigue
> - Shortness of breath (with minimal activities)
> - Pulse less than 50
> - Light-headedness
> - Fainting or near-fainting

Heart Block

Heart block is a condition in which the sinoatrial node sends a normal electrical impulse, but the signal does not travel through the atrioventricular node and into the ventricles as it should. Therefore, there may be inefficient contraction of the ventricles. It usually occurs as a result of aging, or because the heart is scarred from chronic heart disease such as coronary artery disease or from valvular heart disease (which a person may be born with). Prior heart surgery may also cause scarring. Certain medications that slow the electrical conduction through the heart—for example, digitalis, beta-blockers, or some calcium blockers—can worsen heart block.

Heart block is classified into three groups, according to how severe it is. In first-degree heart block, the electrical impulse moves too slowly through the atrioventricular node. Your doctor may refer to the PR interval, which is a part of an ECG recording that measures the amount of time it takes for an impulse to get from the atria into the ventricles (see page 265). If your PR interval is longer than 0.2 seconds, you have first-degree heart block. If your heart rate and rhythm are normal, there may be nothing wrong with your heart. In fact, some highly conditioned athletes also have first-degree heart block. Usually, you will not require treatment for a first-degree heart block. If you are taking medications such as digitalis (see page 243) or beta-blockers (see page 167), the drug may be causing the condition.

If you have second-degree heart block, some signals from your sinoatrial node do not reach your ventricles. In most people with second-degree block, impulses are progressively delayed in the atrioventricular node with each heartbeat until a full beat is skipped. This is called a Mobitz type of block. You may have no symptoms, or you may experience some dizziness, but the condition is not serious. On an ECG, the skipped beat will show up as a P wave that is not followed by a QRS wave—a tracing of a contraction in the atria that did not activate the ventricles (see page 265). In a Mobitz type II heart block, the interval between the P wave and the QRS wave remains constant, but the atrioventricular node intermittently blocks the electrical impulses. A Mobitz type I block may pass on its own, but a Mobitz type II block is generally more serious and requires that you have a pacemaker implanted (see page 272).

In a person who develops third-degree or complete heart block, no signals at all are passing from the atria into the ventricles. To compensate, the ventricles use their own secondary pacemaker to contract and keep blood moving. But the heartbeats generated this way are slow and cannot maintain full heart function. On an ECG, the relationship between the P wave and the QRS wave is completely abnormal (see page 266). A person with third-degree heart block may lose consciousness, may develop heart failure, and is at risk of cardiac arrest. A mechanical pacemaker must be implanted on an emergency basis. If it is not possible to put one in right away, a temporary pacemaker device can be used to keep the person alive until surgery can be done.

For all types of heart block, the decision of whether to implant a pacemaker is based on the severity of the bradycardia symptoms. In some cases, the deciding factor is how slow your heart rate has become.

Ventricular Arrhythmias

Generally, an arrhythmia in the ventricles is a more serious condition than one in the atria, because the ventricles perform the heart's essential pumping functions. Most serious ventricular arrhythmias occur in association with other forms of heart disease, rather than as an isolated problem. A healthy person may have numerous isolated extra heartbeats originating in the ventricle, and a person with normal heart function usually does not require treatment. Ventricular tachycardia is made up of several of these irregular heartbeats in a row.

Premature Ventricular Contraction

Premature ventricular contractions occur when your ventricles contract too soon and interrupt the normal heartbeat. They may happen without warning, and often occur after you have consumed caffeine or taken over-the-counter medications that contain ephedra or ephedrine. By themselves, premature contractions may be harmless and often do not require treatment. But if you have another heart condition such as cardiomyopathy or heart failure, premature ventricular contractions can be a warning of more serious or prolonged rhythm disturbances such as ventricular tachycardia or ventricular fibrillation.

Ventricular Tachycardia

In a person with ventricular tachycardia, a series of ventricular contractions originates from a spot within the ventricles, and the heartbeat quickens—from 100 to 250 beats per minute. The initial concern with this form of tachycardia is that the arrhythmia may interfere with the ability to pump blood, and the person may become dizzy or faint. But ventricular tachycardia may deteriorate without warning into ventricular fibrillation, which is life-threatening.

Therefore, ventricular tachycardia is considered a medical emergency. The goal of treatment is to stop the rapid heartbeat, with electrical shock (defibrillation) if necessary, and then to prevent it from recurring. If the heart cannot return to a normal rhythm, it may go into ventricular fibrillation, which can be fatal in minutes.

Ventricular Fibrillation

Ventricular fibrillation is the most dangerous form of arrhythmia, requiring immediate emergency attention. In this form of extreme tachycardia, several impulses may be firing from different locations in the heart, and the heart contractions are in chaos. Although the heart rate may be as high as 300 beats per minute, the heartbeats are completely ineffective and very little blood leaves the heart. Since the brain is the organ most sensitive to the loss of oxygenated blood, ventricular fibrillation causes unconsciousness. Someone should call 911 or emergency medical services immediately and begin cardiopulmonary resuscitation (CPR) immediately if you are not breathing properly. Electric shock (defibrillation) is usually essential to restore heart rhythm, to prevent severe damage to the brain and other organs. Cardioversion (see page 271) may be used to deliver the necessary shocks. As many as 250,000 people die suddenly each year from ventricular fibrillation.

A defibrillator (sometimes called an automated external defibrillator, or AED) is an electronic device that emergency medical services personnel or other trained "first responders" use to deliver shock to someone whose heart is fibrillating. These defibrillators are now available in many public places such as health clubs and airports.

Long Q-T Syndrome

Long Q-T syndrome is a rare disorder of the heart's electrical system, in which the time between the electrical activation and relaxation of the ventricles (the Q-T interval as represented on an ECG; see page 266) is delayed. As a result, the process of recharging the heart at the end of each heartbeat is interrupted. Serious ventricular arrhythmia may occur. The syndrome is usually an inherited disease, although it can be caused by some medications, stroke, or a neurological disorder. It most often affects children or young adults who may be otherwise very healthy.

The main symptom of long Q-T syndrome is blacking out, or fainting. A person with the disorder does not necessarily have the characteristic abnormal beat all the time. It may occur during physical exercise, intense emotion (such as fright, anger, or pain), or at the sound of a startling noise. The syndrome can be difficult to diagnose because the abnormal beat may not occur during a routine ECG, and because a healthy child does not usually have ECG tests, there is no opportunity to diagnose the syndrome.

A person with long Q-T syndrome may be vulnerable to an abnormally rapid heartbeat, which may lead to a form of ventricular tachycardia (called torsade des pointes) that causes the heart to pump ineffectively. If the brain does not get enough oxygen as a result, the person may faint. If the heart cannot return to a normal rhythm, it may go into ventricular fibrillation (see page 260), which can be fatal in minutes.

Treatment for long Q-T syndrome most often involves taking beta-blocker drugs, which prevent or reduce the symptoms. For some people, an implantable cardioverter defibrillator (ICD; see page 275) may be necessary to stop ventricular fibrillation.

If you or someone in your family has the syndrome, talk to your doctor about the safety of strenuous activities, such as participation in recreational sports. Once treatment is effective, you may be able to participate in moderate activity, or make sure that you exercise with a family member or friend who knows how to get help if you faint. Families with members who have long Q-T syndrome may benefit from having access to automated external defibrillators (AED; see page 155).

Supraventricular Arrhythmias

An arrhythmia that occurs in either of the two atria of your heart, located above your ventricles, is considered a supraventricular (or atrial) arrhythmia.

Supraventricular Tachycardia

Supraventricular (or atrial) tachycardia is a regular but very rapid heartbeat (more than 100 beats per minute) involving the upper chambers of the heart. It can occur in several different forms, when regions of the atria other than the sinoatrial node (the natural pacemaker) develop the ability to fire electrical impulses repetitively. The path that these "extra" impulses take determines what type of tachycardia you have.

Home Defibrillators

You can now purchase a device called an automated external defibrillator (AED), without a prescription, that you can use at home on someone who is experiencing cardiac arrest. The device delivers a shock to the person's heart to restore normal heart rhythm. The Food and Drug Administration (FDA) has reviewed this product and has ruled that it is safe and effective for use by people with no training beyond the written instructions and video that come with the device.

To use the defibrillator, the person must set up the device and place the pads on the victim. The device "diagnoses" whether the person needs a shock, and then issues voice and visual commands to the user to deliver the shocks. The device is intended for use only on someone who is not breathing normally and does not respond when shaken. Special considerations as to pad placement must be made for people who already have implanted pacemakers or implantable defibrillator (ICD) units.

By FDA regulation, the manufacturer of the defibrillator must systematically track purchasers so that they can be notified in the event of a recall.

If you choose to purchase a do-it-yourself defibrillator, it is important to remember that your first steps, before you initiate the defibrillator, should be:

- Call 911 or the emergency medical services in your area.
- Apply CPR, to get oxygen to the person's vital organs quickly.

The American Heart Association says that there has not yet been enough study done to recommend either for or against use of a home heart defibrillator.

In one type (atrioventricular nodal reentrant tachycardia), electrical impulses travel in an abnormal circular path around the atrioventricular node between the atria and the ventricles, causing the heart to beat with each circle. Another form, called Wolff-Parkinson-White syndrome, occurs when there is an extra electrical pathway between the atria and ventricles that causes electrical impulses to arrive at the ventricles too soon, resulting in a rapid heart rate. Some are caused by short circuits or extra electrically active tissue in the heart. It turns out that these "reentry circuits" are the most common mechanism.

If you have supraventricular tachycardia, you may experience palpitations or a sense that the heart is fluttering or racing. Often these symptoms occur abruptly with little or no warning. Some people have shortness of breath, chest pressure or pain, or light-headedness. These sensations may last for a few seconds or several hours. The symptoms can be alarming, but usually supraventricular tachycardia is not life-threatening. Of course, if you have these symptoms, you should have your doctor diagnose and treat your condition. Treatment with drugs (see page 268) can relieve symptoms, or a cardiac ablation procedure (see page 269) can cure the condition.

If you have severe symptoms and go to the emergency room, doctors may give medications that can stop the supraventricular tachycardia and thus relieve your symptoms rapidly. Also, if the type of tachycardia you have has not yet been diagnosed, an ECG performed while you are experiencing the symptoms is very helpful in determining the best long-term treatment.

Atrial Fibrillation

Atrial fibrillation (AF) is the most common type of arrhythmia in the United States, occurring in 5 to 10 percent of all people over 65. People over the age of 80 are especially vulnerable, too, although it can occur in some people who are 40 or younger. In a person with AF, the electrical impulse from the sinoatrial node accelerates as it spreads across the atria, causing these upper chambers of the heart to quiver, contracting rapidly and irregularly—at rates of 400 to 600 beats per minute. A specialized structure between the atria and the ventricles, the atrioventricular node, acts as a safeguard, stopping one or two of every three signals from the atria before they reach the ventricles. But the ventricles still beat too rapidly and irregularly.

AF may occur without any associated heart disease. However, it is commonly linked with hypertension (high blood pressure), coronary artery disease, mitral valve disease, pericardial disease, lung disease, cardiomyopathy, or thyroid disease. When AF occurs, it is important to slow the ventricular rate and then look for the cause and treat that.

Several different forms of AF can occur, and the symptoms can vary widely. Some people experience AF only occasionally, with symptoms such as palpitations that last from a few seconds to a few days before subsiding spontaneously; this form is called paroxysmal atrial

The Valsalva Maneuver

If you have been diagnosed with supraventricular tachycardia, your doctor may mention a technique called the Valsalva maneuver to help you control minor palpitations yourself. The technique works like this: Lie down, then take a deep breath and hold it while you bear down as you if you are having a bowel movement. Coughing may produce a similar effect. Unfortunately, this maneuver does not always work.

But if you have more severe symptoms—such as light-headedness, shortness of breath, or chest pain—or if these symptoms persist after you try the maneuver, don't delay getting to a hospital. Lie down and have someone call 911 or your emergency services number immediately.

fibrillation. In a person with persistent AF, episodes do not stop by themselves, and drugs or other treatments—such as ablation (see page 269) or cardioversion (see page 271)—are required to restore normal heart rhythm. Permanent AF is constant and does not respond to treatment. In these situations treatment focuses on heart rate control and prevention of blood clots. AF can cause symptoms of fatigue or shortness of breath and lead to fluid buildup. Over time the heart rate may slow to the point of causing bradycardia (see page 257).

For many people, the experience of AF is unpleasant—causing a sensation of palpitation and unwellness—but not necessarily harmful. Treatment can relieve the symptoms, and AF is generally unlikely to advance to a more serious condition. But having palpitations can be frightening and worrisome. If you experience palpitations for the first time, you should always get medical attention to diagnose the problem.

AF can cause blood to pool in the atria, which can lead to blood clots. If a clot travels from the heart into a smaller artery in the brain, it can cause a stroke. About 15 percent of strokes occur in people with AF, and among those with AF, the rate of strokes is about 5 percent per year. Once AF is diagnosed, your doctor may prescribe warfarin, a blood thinner, which prevents blood clots from forming and reduces the risk of stroke by two thirds. Risk factors for blood clots associated with AF include advanced age, diabetes, high blood pressure, previous heart damage, and a history of stroke.

Left untreated, AF can cause a chronic increase in heart rate, which can weaken the ventricles over time and cause heart failure. But most people seek treatment before this occurs.

Atrial Flutter

Atrial flutter is another common form of arrhythmia in which the atria beats rapidly but relatively regularly. It usually occurs when electrical impulses are trapped in an endless loop, typically in the lower right atrium. Although the atria may be contracting as quickly as 300 times per minute, the atrioventricular node allows only some of those beats to pass into the ventricles. Still, the ventricles are contracting too quickly and the heart is not pumping as efficiently as it needs to. Atrial flutter or atrial fibrillation often occurs as a consequence of a heart attack or surgery on the heart or lungs.

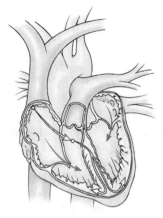

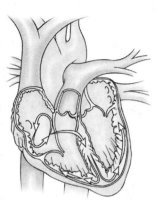

Normal heartbeat   Circling signals in atrial flutter

Atrial flutter

Atrial flutter occurs when impulses from an abnormal site cause an extremely rapid but regular heartbeat. Only a fraction of the beats are allowed past the AV node and into the ventricles, but the ventricles still contract too quickly and the heartbeat is inefficient.

An episode of atrial flutter may last from a few seconds to several hours, causing palpitations, some chest pain, shortness of breath, or light-headedness. Treatment may involve medications (see page 268) or cardioversion (see page 271).

For other people the atrial flutter can persist until treated, or it may get worse and deteriorate into atrial fibrillation. If atrial flutter persists, medications tend to be less effective, and cardiac ablation (see page 269) may be required.

Recording Your Heartbeat

Your electrocardiogram (ECG) is a measurement and graphic representation of the electrical impulses that generate your heartbeats. On an ECG, the sequence of electrical impulses as they occur with each heartbeat is labeled with letters of the alphabet from P through T. The P wave represents the impulse as it moves through your atria. The PR segment is the period during which the impulse goes through the atrioventricular node (between the upper and lower chambers of your heart). The QRS complex is created as the impulse moves through the ventricular node. The T wave is the recovery period during which your heart muscle relaxes and prepares for the next beat.

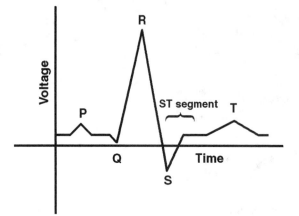

Tracing an electrical impulse

A healthy heartbeat—a single electrical impulse traveling through your heart in less than a second—forms a characteristic set of waves that are recorded on an ECG reading. An injured or malfunctioning heart cannot conduct the impulse normally. Alterations in different parts of the waves provide clues about the location, extent, and nature of injury or malfunction.

Diagnosing Arrhythmias

Once your doctor diagnoses an arrhythmia through your symptoms or an examination, he or she will need to determine where it originates and whether it requires treatment; that is, whether it is causing symptoms or putting you at risk for more serious problems in the future.

The electrocardiogram (ECG; see page 122) is a very important tool that your doctor uses to diagnose and study your arrhythmia. The ECG records and measures the path and timing of your heart's electrical impulses from their origin in the sinoatrial node, through the atria, through the atrioventricular node, and into and through the ventricles. However, the standard ECG can only record the electrical activity that takes place during the short time that the machine is hooked up to you.

Ambulatory ECG methods enable your doctor to study longer periods of the heart's activity while you go about your normal routine. Ambulatory ECGs are available in the form of a Holter monitor (see page 124), which you wear for 24 to 48 hours and which provides a continuous readout. Your doctor compares the ECG recordings with your account of your activities and symptoms to see if an arrhythmia is occurring, how often it occurs, and how it relates to the daily log of your activities. Also, the effectiveness of any antiarrhythmic medications you may be taking can be monitored. However, if your arrhythmia is very infrequent, 48 hours of Holter monitoring may not capture it.

An event monitor (see page 124) is another ambulatory ECG, one that allows for longer recording—as long as 30 days. You activate the device yourself if you sense symptoms. The monitor's recording system is "looped" to continuously record and erase, so that when you activate it, it can retrieve data from 1 to 4 minutes prior to that time.

Your doctor may want to order exercise stress testing (see page 125) to see if an arrhythmia is brought on by exercise. If you have had fainting spells, you may be asked to have a tilt-table study (see page 147) to observe how your heart responds to a change in position. This information helps your doctor determine how to prevent fainting episodes. Echocardiography (see page 132) may also be used to determine if there is structural heart disease that may be causing arrhythmias.

Electrophysiologic studies (see page 147) are done in a hospital setting to more specifically study an arrhythmia, test the effect of medications, and perform some treatments such as catheter ablation. Electrophysiologic studies are generally done by threading catheters through the veins

Substances That Can Affect Heart Rhythm

Thousands of substances have the potential to affect the electrical signals that stimulate your heartbeat. The impact of any one of them on you can range from harmless to severe. If you are diagnosed with a heart arrhythmia, be aware of your own exposure to some of these substances, and talk to your doctor about how they might be affecting your symptoms, the effects of your medications, or your overall heart health.

- Caffeine in coffee, soft drinks, tea, or chocolate
- Alcohol
- Tobacco, including secondhand smoke
- Diet pills
- Some over-the-counter cough and cold remedies (especially those with pseudoephedrine)
- Some herbal remedies (such as ephedra or ephedrine)
- Prescription drugs (such as antianxiety, antipsychotic, or antiarrhythmic medications)
- Bronchodilators, whether prescription or over-the-counter
- Automobile emissions
- Industrial pollution
- Paint thinners
- Propane gas
- Hazardous substances in the workplace (such as carbon monoxide)

into your heart in order to record electrical signals and stimulate the heart to induce an arrhythmia, to provide more precise information about your heart rhythms. Because the test requires that catheters are placed in your veins, it is described as an invasive study. However, with proper preparation, electrophysiology studies can be performed with little or no discomfort and are among the safest of all invasive tests. Also, importantly, if possible, some arrhythmias are treated or cured at the same sitting during your electrophysiologic studies, with only a small risk to you.

Electrophysiology studies require taking periodic X-rays via fluoroscopy during the procedure to determine where the catheter is within the heart. In some cases, transesophageal echocardiography (TEE; see page 134) may be used.

Treatment with Medications

Antiarrhythmic medications slow down rapid heartbeats and regulate irregular or premature heartbeats. Generally, these drugs work by blocking chemical reactions that promote electrical conduction. They act to either suppress abnormal electrical impulses or slow down transmission of impulses as they are conducted through heart tissue. As a result, your heart beats more rhythmically and you experience fewer symptoms.

You may be given these medications intravenously during an emergency situation, or they may be prescribed for you to take orally for an indefinite period. Certain antiarrhythmics, such as amiodarone, cause side effects such as increased sensitivity to sunlight. This drug may also affect your vision, the thyroid, or the lungs. Many people are surprised to learn that an antiarrhythmic drug can in fact cause an arrhythmia or make an existing one more frequent or more severe.

You and your doctor will need to carefully consider the balance of benefits and risks of medication. Your doctor will also do thorough testing and monitoring, either with Holter monitoring, electrophysiologic studies, or both, to determine what drug works best for you. The electrophysiologic testing indicates how well a medication is controlling your symptoms, exactly how it alters your heart's rhythm, and how well it protects your heart from an arrhythmia induced during the study.

Apart from these antiarrhythmics, medications such as calcium channel blockers (see page 168) or beta-blockers (see page 167) may be prescribed.

If you have atrial fibrillation, which can make you more susceptible to blood clots, you will probably also take an anticoagulant (see page 172) or an antiplatelet medication (see page 171). As with all medications, drug interactions with antiarrhythmics are always a concern; be sure to let your doctor know about other medications you are taking, including over-the-counter drugs and herbal remedies.

Nonsurgical Treatments for Arrhythmias

Great advances have been made in nonsurgical treatments for certain types of arrhythmias. These techniques, including ablation and electrical cardioversion, may restore normal heart rhythms, reduce or eliminate symptoms, and reduce or eliminate the need for medications or surgical procedures (such as implantation of a pacemaker or an internal cardioverter-defibrillator).

Catheter Ablation

Catheter ablation is now widely used to treat many types of tachycardia (rapid heartbeat), including atrial fibrillation, atrial flutter, and atrial tachycardia, as well as some ventricular tachycardias. To perform catheter ablation, a doctor specializing in the treatment of arrhythmias (an electrophysiologist) threads one or more electrode-tipped catheters into the heart chambers and uses some form of energy—usually radiofrequency—to destroy (ablate) abnormal tissue that is generating extra impulses. The area of tissue that is eliminated is very small (about one-fifth of an inch across) and is not significant to overall heart function. A small, harmless scar forms at the site, and normal heart rhythm resumes.

The procedure has a high success rate and a low risk of complications, and requires only mild sedation and local anesthetic. It causes little or no discomfort, and most people can return to their daily activities in a few days. Many people are cured of their tachycardia, so they no longer need to take antiarrhythmic medication.

How Ablation Is Done

If you have ablation done, your doctor will probably tell you to stop taking any antiarrhythmic medications for several days before the procedure. At the hospital, you will be given a mild sedative and a local anesthetic. The doctor will make one or more small punctures in your groin and in one side of your neck, your elbow, or just under your collarbone. He or she will thread catheters through your veins or arteries and into the heart. The procedure is done with X-ray guidance via fluoroscopy in real time, so the doctor can see the progress of the catheter.

Then the doctor often needs to start an episode of tachycardia in order to determine exactly where the arrhythmia is coming from. Using recordings of electrical activity from inside the heart, he or she "maps" the tissue to locate the problem area. Once the site is identified and the ablation catheter is positioned, the radiofrequency energy is turned on and the abnormal tissue is destroyed. To ensure that all abnormal tissue has been eliminated, the doctor may test you with medications or electrical stimulation to see if the tachycardia can be induced again. If it can be, he or she repeats the ablation procedure. When the tachycardia can no longer be initiated, the catheters are removed. The entire procedure lasts from 2 to 4 hours.

You will stay in the hospital for at least a few hours, while doctors watch for recurring symptoms, rhythm disturbances, or bleeding from the catheterization sites. You may be able to go home after this observation period, or you may need to stay overnight.

You can probably be moderately active, walking and climbing stairs, almost immediately. Many people go back to work or school in a few days. Your doctor may recommend that you take aspirin for 2 to 4 weeks to thin your blood so that clots do not form at the ablation sites in your heart. You will probably return for a follow-up visit to the electrophysiologist in a few weeks.

Complications from ablation are rare but can be serious. Depending on the type of arrhythmia treated, and where in your heart the ablation is done, you could develop heart block (requiring a pacemaker) or experience bleeding around the heart. However, the chance of heart attack, stroke, or death from ablation is quite rare.

In people with supraventricular arrhythmia and no other heart disease, a complete cure of tachycardia is achieved by ablation more than 95 percent of the time. In people with ventricular arrhythmia, the cure rate is also high.

In people with other heart problems, such as a previous heart attack resulting in heart muscle damage or in heart muscle problems, an internal defibrillator is almost always implanted as well (see page 275).

Rather than curing the tachycardia entirely, catheter ablation helps reduce the number of times the defibrillator is activated. Sometimes to achieve a cure, though, more than one session of ablation is needed.

Cardioversion

Cardioversion is the medical term for restoration of your heart's normal rhythm. Cardioversion can be done either chemically (with drugs) or electrically (with shock). Atrial fibrillation, ventricular tachycardia, and ventricular fibrillation are the types of arrhythmia most commonly treated with cardioversion. Ventricular fibrillation, the most serious type of arrhythmia, can only be treated with electrical shock.

IV line for sedation

Oxygen tubes

Pad for delivery of shock

Pulse oximeter to measure oxygen levels

Restoring normal rhythms

A cardioversion procedure delivers a carefully timed and measured shock across your heart, through pads placed on your chest and back. The shock stops your abnormal heart rhythm and the heart resumes a normal rhythm. The level of shock is generally less than that of a defibrillator.

If your doctor chooses to treat your atrial fibrillation with antiarrhythmic drugs, he or she may give you the medications to take at home. But first you take blood thinners for several weeks. Or the doctor may admit you to the hospital to give you the antiarrhythmia drugs either intravenously or by mouth, where hospital staff can check to see how you respond to treatment, and equipment can be used to monitor your heart rate and rhythm. Your symptoms, the medication your doctor is giving you, and the presence of other heart conditions (if any) will be factors in this decision.

If your doctor recommends electrical cardioversion (sometimes called direct-current or DC cardioversion), the procedure will be done in a hospital. It involves delivering a synchronized electrical current through paddles that touch your chest wall and allow the current to travel to your heart. The shock causes all of your heart cells to contract simultaneously, which stops the abnormal electrical signals without damage to the heart. Then the heart returns to a normal heartbeat.

How Electrical Cardioversion Is Done

Before you have a cardioversion done, your doctor will probably prescribe blood thinners such as warfarin for 3 to 4 weeks to reduce your risk of blood clots. If you take other medications, you should take them as usual unless you are told otherwise. On the day of the procedure, do not eat after midnight. Also, do not use any skin lotions on your back and chest, because they could interfere with the cardioversion apparatus.

In the hospital, you will be given an intravenous sedative, possibly by an anesthesiologist. The doctor will place cardioversion pads (or paddles) on your chest and back, on either side of your heart. The pads are connected to an external defibrillator so that your heart rhythms can be monitored and regulated. Once you are asleep, the doctor will deliver the shock so that the current flows across your heart. If the first shock does not restore your normal heart rhythm, the doctor can deliver gradually increased levels of current.

After the procedure, you will probably awaken quickly without any memory of the experience. You may have some minor chest discomfort or skin irritation where the pads were placed. You will probably be able to go home within an hour after the procedure. Have someone else drive you home, and do not drive or try to make any important decisions for the rest of the day, until the effects of the sedative are entirely gone. You will need to continue taking warfarin until your physician tells you to stop; periodic blood tests will check your clotting time.

Electrical cardioversion restores normal heart rhythms about 90 percent of the time. About half of the people who have the procedure relapse within a year; if so, the procedure can be repeated.

Surgical Treatments for Arrhythmias

In addition to drugs and nonsurgical procedures, several types of surgery can restore your heart's rhythm. Implantation of a pacemaker can treat bradycardia (slow heartbeat); an internal cardioverter-defibrillator can correct more serious arrhythmias; or a procedure called maze surgery can be performed on some people with atrial fibrillation.

Pacemakers

A pacemaker is a battery-powered unit that regulates your heart's rhythm. Most pacemakers are implanted in people whose sinoatrial node is firing too slowly as a result of age, heart disease, or heart medications; the pacemaker takes over for the sinoatrial node if it fails to start. In a person with heart block, the device replaces a blocked pathway. Today pacemakers not only "pace" your heart's rhythm but also have a "demand" sensor that can speed up or slow down your heart rate in response to your activity level, just as your heart would naturally.

The device itself, which is about the size of a man's watch, contains a battery and an electronic pulse generator, with either one or two leads that are threaded into your heart. The device is programmed to read whether your heart rate is within an acceptable range for you. If it is not, the pacemaker generates an electrical impulse to stimulate a heart beat at an appropriate rate. A single-chamber pacemaker has one lead that is positioned in one heart chamber, the right atrium or ventricle; a dual-chamber unit has two leads that are threaded into both the right atrium and the right ventricle. The pacemaker can remain in place for several years before the batteries require replacement.

For people with heart failure or with certain physical characteristics, a third lead may be placed in the back of the heart through a side vein. This is called biventricular pacing. While more complicated to perform than the usual insertion of a pacemaker, this procedure can make some people with heart failure feel much better by coordinating the heart's contractions.

How a Pacemaker Is Implanted

To have a pacemaker implanted, you will need only a mild sedative and a local anesthetic in the area of your upper chest. First the doctor makes a small incision in the skin under the collarbone. The thin, coated leads are threaded through a blood vessel under your collarbone and positioned in your heart under X-ray. Then they connect the leads to the pacemaker unit and slip it under your skin, also just under your collarbone. You will notice only a small bump at the site. The procedure will be over in 1 to 2 hours, and complications are rare. Serious or life-threatening complications occur in less than 1 percent of cases. Infection of the pacemaker is rare but generally requires that the pacemaker be removed. Sometimes less serious complications can occur such as bleeding, collapse of a lung, or the pacemaker's leads may need repositioning.

You will probably be able to return to your routine activities in a few days. Your doctor may tell you to avoid heavy lifting or vigorous movement of your arm on the side of the pacemaker.

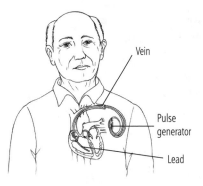

Vein

Pulse generator

Lead

An implantable pacemaker

A pacemaker is comprised of a pulse generator and one or two leads (wires). After the leads are threaded through a blood vessel, they are connected to the generator, and the generator is tucked under the skin near your collarbone. The leads carry signals from your heart to the generator, which reads the signals and sends impulses as needed to pace your heart.

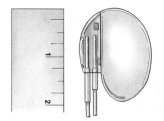

A compact device

The body of a pacemaker, which holds the pulse generator and batteries, is only about 2 inches long. You may be able to see and feel it under your skin, but it is very unobtrusive.

Living with Your Pacemaker

You will need to have regular checkups. The checkups are more frequent until the pacemaker site heals completely; then they occur about every 3 to 6 months, for monitoring. Your doctor will evaluate your pacemaker by moving an electronic programmer over the device. The programmer relays information about pacemaker function and the life of the battery, and it can also change the programming (pacing instructions) of the device if necessary. In addition to the office checkups, your doctor may also give you instructions for how to have some monthly evaluations done by telephone.

When the battery begins to wear down, your pacemaker will slow down somewhat, but it won't stop suddenly. Your doctor will be able to detect the first warnings that the battery is running down before you have any sensation of it. When the battery needs replacing, you will need surgery to implant a new device. This procedure requires local anesthetic, but because the leads usually do not need replacement, the procedure is somewhat simpler than the original implantation.

Your doctor will also give you an identification card that provides specific information about the device you have. It is important to show this card to health-care professionals and to airport security staff (see the box on page 276).

Once your pacemaker is in place and the implant site has healed, you most likely can participate in all of your usual activities. You and your doctor can review any possible restrictions—such as full-contact sports—that might apply to you. Always feel free to ask your doctor about any questions you have about appliances, medical procedures, or other considerations that you think might affect your pacemaker (again see the box on page 276). In general, it's a good idea to be aware of your surroundings and alert for any circumstances that might interfere with the electronic circuitry in your pacemaker.

Although your pacemaker is not likely to restrict your life in significant ways, it is important to remember that there are many things your pacemaker cannot do. It cannot protect you, for instance, from a heart attack caused by blocked arteries. It also cannot necessarily replace your need for medications, including heart-related drugs for conditions such as high blood pressure, angina, or even other forms of arrhythmia.

Implantable Cardioverter-Defibrillators

The internal cardioverter-defibrillator (ICD) is a battery-operated unit, only slightly larger than a pacemaker, that is implanted under your skin to monitor and correct your heart's rhythm. All current ICDs also function as pacemakers. An ICD is usually placed in a person with a damaged heart (as from a heart attack) who has had or is at high risk of having life-threatening heart rhythms, such as ventricular tachycardia or ventricular fibrillation. It may also be used for some people with severe atrial fibrillation.

An ICD can deliver the same sort of low-energy, imperceptible pulses that a pacemaker does. Furthermore, the ICD monitors the heart using the same technology. Defibrillators are different from pacemakers in that they also monitor for very fast heart rates as well as for bradycardia. The ICD can also deliver higher-energy pulses (shocks) to the heart when it detects more serious or sustained rapid arrhythmias. These stronger impulses are called defibrillation shocks, and they are often life-saving.

A person with an ICD can feel these stronger impulses—usually a single shock, but sometimes a series of them—and they are often described as feeling like a quick thump or kick in the chest. Depending on the level of consciousness you have at the time of the shock, it may be painful (if you are not sedated) or may not be painful (if you have received sedatives).

Like a pacemaker, an ICD has two parts: a pulse generator, including a battery and electronic circuitry, and a system of coated leads tipped with electrodes. Newer devices are as small as a pager. They are also designed to provide a controlled burst of impulses, called overdrive pacing, at the first sign of ventricular tachycardia. If that does not restore normal heart rhythms, the device delivers defibrillation shock.

The devices make decisions on what type of therapy to give based on how fast the heart rate is. The devices are also equipped to regulate bradycardia (slow heartbeat) if that occurs. They also have a memory to record arrhythmic episodes and do some internal electrophysiologic testing.

In a person who has experienced prolonged ventricular arrhythmia, the ICD is more effective than antiarrhythmic drugs at preventing sudden death. The device may also similarly prevent cardiac arrest in a person who is considered at high risk of developing such arrhythmias. Before you are considered as a candidate for an ICD, your doctor must rule out other causes of the arrhythmia, such as a heart attack, myocardial ischemia (inadequate blood flow to the heart; see page 161), or chemical imbalance and drug reactions, which can be treated in other ways.

Safety and Your Implantable Device

Both pacemakers and ICDs monitor your heart electrically. Therefore, very large electrical fields or magnetic fields can potentially influence the devices. The larger or closer the magnetic field or electrical field is to you, the more likely your pacemaker or ICD will be affected. These are general guidelines about equipment or technology in your environment and its potential for affecting your pacemaker or implantable cardioverter-defibrillator (ICD; see page 275). Always consult your doctor in detail about any questions or concerns you have.

Little or No Risk

• *Home appliances* such as electric drills, remote controls for a TV, microwave ovens, heating pads, and CB or ham radios. (Some of these appliances have remote potential to interfere with a single heartbeat, but most people can continue to use these items. However, it's a good idea not to stand next to a microwave oven while it's on.)

• *Dental equipment.* (Some people report they can feel an increased heart rate during drilling.)

• *Diagnostic radiation*, such as X-rays.

• *Electroconvulsive (shock) therapy* for certain mental disorders.

Some Caution or Risk

• *Most cellular telephones* do not affect pacemakers or ICDs, but as technology changes, some newer phones using newer frequencies might affect you. Ask your doctor about any new developments, and watch for news reports about relevant studies. As a safeguard, use the ear opposite your device when you use a cell phone.

• *Radiofrequency ablation*, a technique to treat some arrhythmias (see page 269), can affect your device. Your doctor will need to carefully evaluate your pacemaker during and after treatment.

• *Short-wave or microwave diathermy*, a medical

How an ICD Is Implanted

The procedure for placing an ICD is very similar to that for a pacemaker (see page 273). At the hospital, you will be given a sedative and then a local anesthetic. The cardiologist or surgeon will make an incision in the skin and then tunnel the leads through blood vessels into your heart, or onto its surface. Then he or she will tuck the ICD into a pouch of skin under the collarbone or somewhere above the waistline. The leads will be attached to the pulse generator. Electrophysiologic testing will be done to check out the device. The entire procedure takes about 2 hours.

You will probably stay in the hospital overnight. You may be prescribed some antiarrhythmic medications, too. These drugs may lessen the need for high-energy shocks from your ICD. The recovery time, the pain after the procedure, and risks of the procedure are very similar to those of a pacemaker.

technique used in some types of physical therapy for arthritis and some surgical procedures, can cause damage to pacemaker devices.

- *Radiation therapy (used for treating cancer)* can damage a pacemaker or ICD, and the risk increases with the dose of radiation given. Your device should be shielded and carefully monitored during therapy.

- *Transcutaneous electrical nerve stimulation (TENS)*, a therapy for acute or chronic pain, may briefly inhibit some pacemakers. This affect can be managed by reprogramming the pacemaker.

- *Extracorporeal shock wave lithotripsy (ESWL)* is a noninvasive treatment that delivers a series of shocks to the kidneys to break up kidney stones, so that they can be excreted in your urine. Your pacemaker will need to be adjusted for the ESWL procedure and again afterward.

Serious Risk: Avoid These Situations

- *MRIs* People with pacemakers or ICDs are not allowed to have magnetic resonance imaging because of the strong magnetic fields used.

- *Antitheft systems, metal detectors,* and *airport security* do not cause symptoms in most people, and you can go through them. But you should be aware that many businesses have hidden antitheft systems near their doorways. You should not stand near an antitheft device or metal detector longer than is necessary, and do not lean against such a system. If you need to be scanned with a handheld metal detector (at an airport, for example), warn security personnel about your implanted device and ask them to be brief or to use an alternate search system if possible.

- *Arc-welding equipment, power-generating equipment, outdoor power lines,* and *powerful magnets (such as in medical devices, heavy equipment, or some motors)* can inhibit pacemakers. If you work with or near such equipment, discuss your exposure with your doctor.

Source: Adapted from the American Heart Association.

After Implantation

After your ICD is installed, you will need to return to the doctor's office for monitoring every 1 to 3 months. Your doctor can evaluate the ICD function electronically by moving a programming wand over your chest. By this means, he or she can determine what kinds of impulses have been delivered, whether they worked, whether they need modification, and how much energy is left in the battery. When the energy level in the battery is down to a predetermined level, you will be scheduled for replacement surgery. The battery usually lasts from 3 to 5 years, depending on how many shocks it delivers. Usually, replacement surgery is somewhat simpler than the original implantation because the leads do not need to be replaced. Some ICDs can also be checked periodically by telephone.

Many people feel some apprehension about the possibility of receiving unexpected defibrillation shocks. You may need to continue to take antiarrhythmia medications to reduce the risk of needing a shock from the implanted device. Some shocks are small, and some people don't notice them. When you do receive a stronger shock, it may feel like a jolt, thump, or blow to the chest. Some people black out during periods of fibrillation, so they don't feel the shock; see "Living with an ICD," next section, on driving if you have an implanted ICD. If someone is touching you during the shock, he or she may feel a tremor, but will not be harmed by it in any way.

You and your doctor can discuss what to do if your ICD delivers a shock. Your doctor may tell you to call him or her if you feel a shock, or if you feel ill after the shock.

Apart from the discomfort of a sudden defibrillation shock, possible side effects of ICD placement include some sensitivity at the site of the implant, especially in very slender people; very rare problems with infection; and some cosmetic issues (the device is visible under the skin). If you feel apprehension about the shocks or concern about your need for an ICD, ask your doctor about a support group, where you can talk with other ICD "users" and medical staff.

You will also be given an identification card that provides specific information about your ICD. Carry it with you at all times, and show it to health-care professionals and airport security.

Living with an ICD

As with a pacemaker, your ICD can interact with some devices in your environment with electromagnetic or radiofrequency fields. Review the interactions with implantable devices (see page 276), and talk to your doctor in detail about how devices in your environment, medical procedures, or your activities might affect your ICD.

Driving is a major consideration for a person with an ICD. Your ICD may take an interval of 5 to 15 seconds or longer to detect arrhythmias and deliver treatments, during which you might feel dizzy or even faint. Therefore, you are usually advised to avoid driving, and other activities, such as piloting or scuba diving, that would put you and others at risk if you were to lose consciousness. In some states, these restrictions are law. Review this issue with your doctor carefully. Some people who go for long periods without shock or symptoms are allowed to return to driving, but only with the advice of a doctor.

Maze Surgery

In some people with chronic atrial fibrillation, an operation called the maze procedure involves making a series of incision lines within the heart to create a maze that blocks electrical pathways through the heart muscle. This surgery is done in a person for whom medications, a pacemaker, or other treatments have not been effective. A likely candidate might be a person with uncontrolled atrial fibrillation, for whom the chief danger is that blood will pool in the upper chambers of the heart (the atria); this pooling increases the tendency of the blood to clot, which could lead to a stroke. The surgery may be performed with certain other types of heart surgery to prevent atrial fibrillation after the operation.

The procedure is major surgery, done with the patient under general anesthesia. The surgeon must split the breastbone to expose the heart and transfer the functions of the heart and lungs to a heart-lung machine (see page 183) during the procedure.

The surgeon makes a number of small incisions in both the left and right atria. These incisions form a pattern that will direct the heart's electrical impulses into the ventricles and block extra impulses. As the incisions heal, scar tissue forms that cannot conduct electrical impulses, so the new pathways are permanently established. The surgery takes about 3 hours. Sometimes a pacemaker is implanted, too.

Recovery from maze surgery requires about 1 week in the hospital. You may need diuretics to prevent fluid accumulation, and antiplatelet medication such as aspirin to prevent blood clots. You may experience pain from the chest incision, and fatigue for 2 to 3 months after surgery. Most people can go back to normal activities, including work, in about 3 months.

The maze procedure has been adapted to a less invasive technique, similar to a catheter-based ablation technique for atrial fibrillation. The technique allows the radiofrequency to be directed to the outside of the heart. This technique is complementary to less-invasive catheter-based ways to perform ablation of atrial fibrillation through the veins.

16

Women and Heart Disease

During the latter half of the twentieth century, many breakthroughs in medicine advanced understanding of the risk factors that put someone at risk for coronary artery disease, how to control those factors to prevent disease and improve quality of life, and early interventions during heart attacks. Most of the groundbreaking studies were conducted on men, and doctors and the public alike thought heart disease was largely a threat to middle-aged or older men.

However, in 1991 a major study focused on the inadequacies in medical care for women with chest pain. Since that time, doctors and hospitals have paid increasing attention to diagnosing, treating, and preventing heart problems in women. While the death rate for men with heart disease has dropped impressively in the last 25 years, the death rate for women with heart disease has just kept going up.

As studies emerge that acknowledge and explore the disparities—in symptoms, preventive advice, and treatment—between women and men with coronary artery disease, one stark fact stands out. Today, cardiovascular disease is the number one killer of women in the United States. Heart disease claims more than 10 times as many women's lives each year as breast cancer. Both women and their doctors have a lot of work to do to bring those frightening numbers down. The best strategy is first to identify a woman's risk factors for coronary heart disease and then address her risk factors to prevent heart disease altogether or to improve her survival and quality of life.

Differences between Men and Women with Heart Disease

Some of the differences between men and women have to do with how coronary artery disease develops and presents itself. Current clinical studies done on women may help explain some of these differences more fully:

- Premenopausal women who neither smoke nor have diabetes rarely have coronary artery disease. In menstruating women, natural estrogen from the ovaries has effects that prevent the formation of plaque in the arteries and lowers cholesterol. However, when menopause starts and their bodies make much less estrogen, women become at greater risk of heart attacks.

- Women tend to have heart attacks later in life than men do—about 10 years later. A woman's risk of heart attack is relatively low before menopause. By the time a woman has a heart attack, she is older and may have other diseases as well that complicate recovery.

- Heart attacks are more severe in women than in men. In the first year after a heart attack, women are nearly twice as likely to die as men are. In the first 6 years after a heart attack, women are almost twice as likely as men to have a second one.

- Women have different symptoms of heart attack than men. Both sexes report the classic chest pain that spreads across the upper body, but women are more likely to have other atypical chest pains and more generalized symptoms (see page 286)—for example, indigestion, fatigue, back pain, or shortness of breath—that are harder to identify as indicators of a heart attack.

- Results of some routine diagnostic tests are less accurate in women than in men. For example, an exercise stress test is more likely to give a false positive diagnosis in younger women.

- Women with diabetes—an increasingly common disease, and more common in women than in men—are much more likely to die of coronary artery disease than are men with diabetes. These women often do not have symptoms suggestive of coronary artery disease, but they begin to have coronary artery disease even before menopause.

Emerging studies also suggest ways in which, in general, women may be cared for differently than men when they seek medical help for heart problems:

- When women are assessed for their risk of heart attack, they are more likely to be mistakenly assigned to a lower-risk category, so they get less advice about preventive care.

- Women wait longer before going to an emergency department for possible signs of heart attack and may be more likely to be sent home with another diagnosis (for example, indigestion or anxiety), while men are more likely to be diagnosed and treated for a heart attack.

- Cardiovascular imaging methods such as stress echocardiography, which work as well for women as for men, are less frequently ordered for women.

- Treatments such as balloon angioplasty and stenting to open blocked arteries are done less frequently for women.

- Coronary artery bypass surgery was historically of higher risk to women than to men. Generally, women were older than men when they were referred for possible surgery, so they often had more severe disease at the time of surgery.

- Women may have smaller coronary arteries, making surgery technically more challenging.

- Women recuperating from heart surgery may be older and frailer, and they may be single or widowed—having less support and help than their male counterparts having heart surgery.

Each one of these findings represents a complex mix of medical factors and cultural attitudes. Some gaps in treatment are already closing, as national health organizations and hospitals adopt new guidelines to address the unique needs of women. The awareness gap is closing too—more women today understand that cardiovascular disease is an equal-opportunity killer. Whether the differences in care are based on gender differences or gender bias, the message is clear: women and their doctors need to work harder to protect women's heart health.

Prevention: Everyone's Best Bet

A healthy lifestyle is the best means of preventing heart disease in both women and men. Once you know that you too can develop heart disease, you can start to take advantage of all the knowledge about prevention that is now available. The process of analyzing your own personal risk of heart disease, and then eliminating or diminishing as many risk factors as you can, is exactly the same for a woman as for a man.

Risk Factors for Women

What puts a woman at risk for heart disease? You can't control your age, when menopause occurs, your family's medical history, or your genetic predisposition to high cholesterol, high blood pressure, or diabetes. But you can change many aspects of your lifestyle to improve your overall health and your heart health in particular (see chapters 2–7). The first step is to talk to your doctor and ask for the tests you need so that you *know your numbers*:

- **Blood pressure.** This simple examination (see page 40) gives you immediate results.
- **Lipid profile.** This blood test gives you your total cholesterol, LDL and HDL, and triglyceride levels (see page 129). Other blood tests for risks (homocysteine and C-reactive protein) may be useful, too.
- **Fasting plasma glucose.** This test diagnoses diabetes.
- **Weight and body mass index.** Obesity is a particularly important risk factor for women. Studies have shown that a woman's pre-menopausal weight as early as age 18, as well as her weight gain throughout adulthood, impacts her risk of heart disease. Obesity also combines with other risk factors such as diabetes and smoking to cause an even higher risk of coronary artery disease.

With these test results in hand, you and your doctor can discuss your personal risk and what you can do to give your heart a longer, healthier life. You and your doctor can use a risk calculator tailored to women; ask your doctor about which risk score is best. These results will indicate whether you are at low, moderate, or high risk of cardiovascular disease. If you have already had conditions such as a heart attack, stroke, diabetes, or chronic kidney disease, you will automatically be considered high risk. If you have a genetic cholesterol problem, you may also be in the high-risk category.

When you and your doctor have determined your risk level, you can better establish a plan for prevention, and an appropriate level of treatment, if needed. For example, a woman at low risk of heart disease might be fine just fine-tuning her exercise plan and improving her diet. A woman at intermediate risk may be advised to follow these lifestyle patterns with closer attention to controlling blood pressure or high cholesterol, and her doctor may also recommend preventive aspirin therapy. A woman at high risk is the most likely to benefit from preventive lifestyle changes and medications.

How Women Can Prevent Heart Disease

Some of the positive, preventive lifestyle changes your doctor will recommend are especially important for women, but all these changes are fundamentals of heart health:

- Know your family history. Whether you are male or female, your risk is increased if a male or female family member had heart disease at an early age.

- Stop smoking cigarettes (see pages 69–74) and avoid secondhand smoke. Women taking birth control pills who smoke are at increased risk of blood clots and stroke. Ideally, young women who smoke should quit anyway, but especially if they are pill users. Women over 35 who smoke should not take oral contraceptives.

- Get at least 30 minutes of exercise daily (see pages 75–82), or work up to an hour a day if your doctor says that is a good goal for you. You don't have to join an expensive gym; studies have shown that women benefit from walking 30 minutes a day.

Emotional Health and Heart Disease

Although the relationship of psychological factors to heart disease is still unclear, there is some evidence to suggest a relationship between cardiovascular disease on the one hand and stress and depression on the other. Stress may not independently cause heart disease, but stress may lead to risky behaviors such as smoking or overeating. Thus, managing stress makes sense in terms of your overall health, including your heart health.

Stress may also cause symptoms that mimic heart disease. Women may first present in the emergency department with symptoms such as fatigue, shortness of breath, anxiety, palpitations, or indigestion, rather than the classic symptom of chest pain (see pages 286–288). Physicians may interpret these symptoms as stress-related and fail to test for heart disease. You may be advised simply to "take it easy." Even if you agree you are under stress, be persistent about asking questions or inquiring about tests of your heart function, especially if the symptoms are new to you and you are at risk for heart disease.

- Eat a heart-healthy diet (see pages 83–98).
- Maintain a healthy weight (see pages 99–104).
- Work with your doctor to manage high blood pressure and high cholesterol, using medications in addition to lifestyle changes as necessary. Postmenopausal women tend to have higher cholesterol than men of comparable age.
- Pay close attention to your triglyceride levels, because they are more closely linked to heart disease in women then in men. A normal triglyceride level is less than 150 (see page 29).
- Work with your doctor to manage diabetes or prediabetes, which are more strongly linked to heart disease in women than in men. In fact, women with diabetes are at the same high risk for heart disease as are men with diabetes.
- Talk to your doctor about the preventive use of aspirin for you. Some studies suggest that aspirin may not prevent a first heart attack in women under 65, but may be helpful for many women over 65. Aspirin may also help lower the risk of stroke in women.
- Work on stress management (see the box on page 285).

Women's Symptoms

Perhaps one of the most surprising findings to emerge from recent research on women and heart disease is the fact that their symptoms differ significantly from those of men. The classic symptoms of heart disease (see page 156) can occur in either men and women. But women and their doctors need to know that women are less likely to experience the crushing chest discomfort lasting 20 minutes or more that signals a heart attack in many men. Women may have no pain at all, or they may have more transient discomfort. Women are more likely to report:

- Fleeting chest discomfort that comes and goes away in a few minutes, or vaguer chest pains that can easily be mistaken for indigestion (see page 158).
- Shortness of breath
- Weakness or fatigue
- Cold sweats
- Dizziness

- Back pain (in the upper back between your shoulder blades)

When women who have had heart attacks are asked about any new or unusual symptoms in the month before the attack occurred, they may not report any chest discomfort. Although chest pain may be the first sign of a heart attack, women often mention severe fatigue, trouble sleeping, shortness of breath, indigestion, or anxiety. These are more general symptoms that may be easy to dismiss as just the signs of aging or a busy schedule. It's important to be on the lookout for new patterns of symptoms that you can't explain. Many studies have shown that when women have symptoms of a heart attack, many stay home and delay a trip to the hospital because they do not realize they are having a heart attack. It is vital to seek emergency medical attention if you have heart attack symptoms.

Many women—perhaps especially older women—don't want to complain, don't want to cause trouble, or don't want to acknowledge how bad they are feeling. But this reluctance may just delay treatment that could be life-saving.

The bottom line is that you need to be aware of the possible significance of these symptoms, and you need to take them seriously when you notice them:

- If you notice an unusual pattern of symptoms that you can't explain, see your doctor as soon as possible and describe the symptoms. Also, be alert to subtle changes in your ability to perform daily tasks. Say that you are concerned about the possibility of

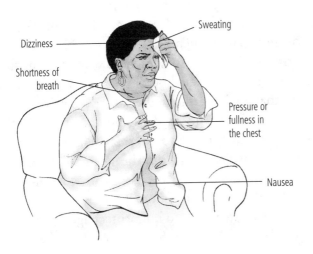

Dizziness

Sweating

Shortness of breath

Pressure or fullness in the chest

Nausea

Women's symptoms

A woman may experience symptoms of a heart attack quite differently than a man does. Although some women report the crushing chest pain that is considered the classic sign of heart attack, many women say they have vaguer symptoms such as fatigue, dizziness, cold sweats, nausea, or trouble sleeping. If you have a pattern of symptoms that you can't explain, talk to your doctor, and ask about the possibility of heart tests.

heart attack. If you don't feel that your complaints are taken seriously, consider talking to another doctor.

- If you notice symptoms of a heart attack that last for more than 5 minutes, call 911 or emergency medical services immediately.

- When you go to the emergency room, describe your symptoms in as much detail as possible and tell the staff you are concerned about the possibility of a heart attack. Don't hesitate to ask for tests—such as an ECG or a cardiac enzyme test—to determine if you are having a heart attack.

Special Issues for Women

At various stages of her life, a woman faces issues that can impact her heart health in unique ways. How do birth control pills, pregnancy, menopause, and hormone replacement therapy affect your cardiovascular system? As cardiovascular research focuses more closely on women, the effect of estrogen on a woman's heart is still being studied.

Estrogen and Heart Disease

A woman's risk of heart disease is much lower than a man's until menopause, largely because of the protective effect of the female hormone estrogen. The effect is not fully understood, but estrogen appears to affect positively both cholesterol levels and the blood vessels themselves in younger women. When estrogen production stops at menopause, this protective effect is lost. A woman's risk of heart disease goes up, and at age 65 it begins to approach that of a man.

For decades, hormone therapy has been a mainstay of treatment to alleviate the symptoms of menopause, such as hot flashes. Numerous studies suggested that hormone therapy also protected women against heart disease and osteoporosis, just as their body's own estrogen does. The consensus opinion was that while hormone therapy poses increased risk of breast cancer and some other cancers, the benefits appeared to far outweigh the risks in most women. However, in the 1990s, when the National Institutes of Health analyzed data from the Women's Health Initiative—large, long-term clinical trials on thousands of women—it authoritatively concluded that the form of hormone therapy used in the study (estrogen and medroxyprogesterone) did not protect against heart disease, and it actually caused a small but significant increase in the risk of heart attacks, strokes, and blood clots in the women in the study. Estrogen alone caused a similar increase in clots but not heart attacks in women in their sixties. However, estrogen alone provided some protection against heart attacks for women in their fifties.

These findings were startling, and today, the American Heart Association offers these recommendations:

- Women who have coronary artery disease should not take hormone therapy for the purpose of preventing cardiovascular disease.
- Hormone therapy should not be prescribed or continued solely to prevent heart disease or stroke.

Does this mean that you should not take any form of hormone therapy during menopause? Not necessarily. It means that you and your doctor will have to weigh your individual risk of disease—including heart disease, osteoporosis, and cancer—against the benefits of different types of hormone therapy for you. The Women's Health Initiative showed that women taking hormone therapy had substantially fewer spine and hip fractures, and fewer cases of colon cancer. Hormone

---

Q&A

Q. I have severe hot flashes and no family history of heart disease, blood clots, or breast cancer. If I take hormone therapy for my hot flashes, how long can I take it?

A. If you use estrogen alone or with progestin for your symptoms of menopause, it's best to use the lowest effective dose for the shortest possible time. Talk to your doctor at least annually to reassess your need for hormones and to discuss any new information that might influence your decision. We still don't know for sure what safe short-term use of hormone therapy might be. The Women's Health Initiative found increases in the number of women with blood clots and stroke within 1 year, and an increase in breast cancer within 4 years for those taking estrogen and progestins. You and your doctor might decide that a slightly elevated risk is acceptable to you. Just be aware of the risks. Smoking and having diabetes also raise the risks.

Most women who experience menopausal hot flashes have them for 4 years or less. Apart from hormone therapy, you may be able to reduce the severity of your symptoms in a number of ways: wear layers of light clothing; lower the thermostat at home; avoid spicy foods, caffeine, and alcohol; and try biofeedback techniques or relaxation exercises. Also, though hormone therapy is the most effective treatment for hot flashes, other prescription drugs such as clonidine may help alleviate symptoms, but to a lesser degree.

replacement therapy is still the most effective treatment for hot flashes, night sweats, and other symptoms of menopause. If you are now taking hormone therapy, or thinking of taking it, you and your doctor should discuss risk factors for coronary artery disease and any needed tests.

If you have been taking estrogen, or estrogen plus progestin, to prevent osteoporosis, talk to your doctor about the pros and cons of nonhormonal treatments.

Pregnancy and Heart Disease

Pregnancy puts additional demands on a woman's heart. When you are pregnant, your blood volume gradually increases by as much as 50 percent. Your heart beats faster and pumps out more blood with each contraction to handle the extra work of supplying blood to the uterus, placenta, and developing fetus. For a woman who has a cardiovascular disease such as congenital heart disease, coronary artery disese, a heart valve disorder, high blood pressure, or diabetes, pregnancy poses some serious concerns for both mother and fetus. Women with elevated pressures in the blood vessels of the lungs (pulmonary hypertension) or weakened heart muscles (cardiomyopathy) are advised to avoid pregnancy.

Today many women with different forms of heart disease, or other high-risk factors, safely deliver healthy babies. But you need to plan your pregnancy very carefully, consulting with both your gynecologist and your cardiologist. Your doctor will want to discuss with you how your heart problems might put you or your fetus at risk. He or she will tell you what symptoms to watch for that might signal a problem. You will also need to discuss your medications, because some drugs—even over-the-counter remedies—may not be safe to take during pregnancy. Your doctor will either prescribe safer drugs or change your dosages. You will also need frequent testing throughout your pregnancy to monitor your health and that of your baby.

Because pregnancy has a profound effect on a woman's cardiovascular function, some women with healthy hearts develop problems while they are pregnant. You may have a heart murmur (an audible sound of blood moving through your heart) that you haven't had before. Usually these heart murmurs are harmless, but your doctor will want to determine the cause to be sure that your heart valves are functioning normally. You may develop an arrhythmia (a fast or slow heartbeat) as a result of your pregnancy, or you may have one that was previously unknown but causes symptoms due to the added stress of pregnancy. Your doctor will probably want to do an ECG or have you wear a heart monitor to investigate the arrhythmia. You probably will not need treatment, but if you do, your doctor will explain the effect on you and your fetus. Rarely, near the end of pregnancy or even right after delivery, women may develop signs of heart failure (see page 234). These symptoms require immediate attention and treatment.

You may develop high blood pressure, especially during the third trimester, which is why your doctor checks your blood pressure frequently during pregnancy. High blood pressure caused by pregnancy usually goes away after childbirth but may occur later in life. But a form of high blood pressure, called preeclampsia, is a serious complication of pregnancy and requires immediate medical attention.

Birth Control Pills

The estrogen in birth control pills raises blood pressure, blood sugar levels, and the risk of blood clots in some women, increasing the overall risk of heart attack and stroke. Using the pill may worsen the effects of other risk factors such as smoking, diabetes, or overweight. These risks tend to increase as a woman gets older, but they lessen as soon as she stops taking the pill. However, the risks of the pill are very small compared to the risks of pregnancy, so for most women—especially those in their twenties and early thirties—the use of birth control pills is safer overall than using a less effective contraceptive, with the resulting risk of unintended pregnancy.

Much of this information derives from studies done on women taking early, high-dose forms of birth control pills. The level of estrogen in the pill is substantially lower now. Generally, you can safely use the pill if you don't smoke and you don't have high blood pressure, diabetes, or other heart disease risk factors—even if you are over 40. But if you are on the pill, *don't* smoke. If you smoke and are over 35, you are strongly advised not to take birth control pills because of the high risk of a serious side effect such as stroke. If you are thinking of going on the pill, be sure to tell your doctor about any risk factors for heart disease in you or your family.

Appendix

Managing Your Health Care

If you or someone in your family develops a heart problem, you may begin a relationship with a cardiologist and other medical specialists you have not encountered before. You may learn a new vocabulary, make significant changes in your lifestyle, take more medications than you have taken previously, and see your doctor more frequently for checkups and tests. You will feel more comfortable and follow through with treatment better if you are satisfied with the decisions you have made and are confident with the medical information and advice you get from your doctor along the way. The following information is designed to help you and your family organize and manage your heart health care.

Finding a Specialist

Your primary-care physician may recommend that you see a cardiologist. If you are in a health insurance plan or you need a doctor who accepts Medicare, your choices may be somewhat limited. Ask your insurance company or your employer's health-care plan administrator for a list of participating doctors. To choose a specialist, you have a number of sources for referrals. Your primary-care physician (family practitioner, internist, or gynecologist), with whom you already have a good relationship and who knows you, may be able to give you some names. You can also consult family or friends who may have been treated by a cardiologist in your area.

If you cannot get a personal referral, or think you need more names of doctors to choose from, you can get names of qualified specialists in several ways:

- Call a medical center near you that specializes in cardiovascular care and ask for names of cardiologists who are accepting new patients.

- Call a state or local medical society for a list of member specialists, call a university hospital or medical school for a list of affiliated specialists, or contact your local office of the American Heart Association.

- Consult Doctor Finder, a physician referral service offered by the American Medical Association. This service can provide names of licensed physicians in your area, organized by specialty, with basic professional information that has been verified for accuracy and authenticated by accrediting agencies, medical schools, residency training programs, and licensing boards. It also offers a list of local and state medical societies, with contact information. To contact Doctor Finder, also called AMA Physician Select, follow the links on the home page of the American Medical Association Web site (www.ama-assn.org).

Understanding Credentials

Before you select a specialist, it's a good idea to find out as much as you can about him or her. You may see these terms among a doctor's credentials:

- **Board certification.** This term means that the doctor has been certified by the American Board of Medical Specialties (ABMS). To become board-certified, a doctor must complete medical school and a residency and pass a comprehensive examination in his or her chosen specialty (such as cardiology). To find out if a doctor is board-certified in cardiology (or another specialty), call ABMS at (866) 275-2267, or visit the ABMS Web site (www.abms.org). Also, if you look up a doctor on Doctor Finder on

the AMA Web site (see above), you will find any board certification listed for each doctor. Many cardiologists have subspecialties such as electrophysiology (treatment of arrhythmias) or interventional cardiology; it is helpful to ask these doctors if they have completed fellowships or earned certificates in their subspecialty.

- **FACC (Fellow of the American College of Cardiologists).** To become a Fellow of the American College of Cardiologists (a medical specialty society), a doctor must be board-certified in cardiology, must have been personally sponsored by another fellow, and his or her credentials must have been reviewed by peers (other cardiologists).

Doctors get better with experience. When choosing a surgeon, ask how many times he or she has performed the procedure you need. Also find out how often the doctor has treated people with diagnoses similar to yours. As you are choosing your cardiologist or other specialist, remember that this relationship is long-term. You need to have a doctor with whom you feel comfortable and in whom you are confident. Look for a doctor with whom you feel you can achieve good two-way rapport—someone who listens to your concerns, clearly answers your questions, and explains your medical situation and choices in terms you can understand.

Getting a Second Opinion

There are a number of circumstances under which you will need or want to get an opinion from more than one doctor. Your health insurance company may require a second opinion for certain procedures or operations. If so, the insurance company may help you find another doctor to consult, and will pay for the cost of the services. Medicare may also pay for a second opinion.

You may wish to get a second opinion for a variety of reasons. If there are several options for treatment for your condition, you may want to explore those options with doctors who specialize in certain procedures or therapies. If the treatment you are considering has significant risk or will seriously affect your lifestyle, work, or family, you may want to gather as much information as you can. If a diagnosis is unclear or if a treatment is not working as well as you hoped, you may want another perspective. Or you may not feel confident about the initial recommendation or the doctor.

Getting more than one opinion is a common medical practice, and you do not need to be concerned about offending your doctor by doing so. Keep in mind that if getting the second opinion is your own choice, you may have to pay for it yourself; check with your health-care plan to be sure. But cost should not be the deciding factor. Your comfort with your ultimate decision is valuable. (To find a qualified specialist for a second opinion, you can use the same resources mentioned on page 293.)

Let your doctor know that you plan to get a second opinion. Ask your doctor's office to forward your medical records to the doctor giving the second opinion, so that there will not be unnecessary

Questions to Ask a New Doctor

When you are choosing a doctor or specialist, you may take into account some personal preferences, such as age or gender. Feel free to ask questions of the doctor to get a better sense of his or her medical experience and credentials, and to get a clear picture of how you will experience working with his or her office. Here are a few questions you may wish to ask:

1. How long have you been in practice? Where did you practice before you came here?

2. What is your specialty or area of particular interest?

3. Are you board-certified, and in what specialty or specialties?

4. How many years of residency training or fellowship did you complete?

5. Do you belong to professional organizations, such as the AMA, the state or local medical society, or a medical subspecialty society?

6. At what hospitals do you practice?

7. Do you accept my insurance coverage, whether Medicare or a private plan?

8. How many patients have you treated with my condition?

9. How many procedures have you performed like the one I am considering?

10. What are your office hours?

11. How long does it take to get an appointment for a routine problem? For an urgent problem?

12. About how long does it take to get on your surgery schedule?

13. If I have an emergency, whom do I call, and can I get an answer from a doctor or nurse the same day?

duplication of tests. If the diagnosis or recommendation from the second doctor is different from the first, it does not necessarily mean that one is right and the other is wrong. There is room for different interpretations of test results, and for different strategies for managing complex problems. Ultimately, the choices are yours to make, and having more than one source of information is often productive. If you receive different opinions from two specialists, ask your primary-care doctor to help evaluate your options.

Preparing for an Appointment

You can make the best use of your time, and your doctor's, by preparing in advance for an appointment. If you are seeing a doctor for the first time, he or she will ask questions about your personal and family health history. You can also anticipate that the doctor will need to know all the medications you are taking, including over-the-counter drugs and alternative remedies.

If you have had cardiac tests done at other hospitals, bring copies of the test results to your appointment. It is also helpful to have information on your cardiac history such as dates of any events such as a heart attack and dates of any surgery. You may find it easiest to write down this information beforehand so that you can refer to it as needed. Answer questions as specifically, briefly, and truthfully as possible. Your doctor will ask about past health issues and personal habits only as they relate to your current health concerns.

The doctor will also ask about your symptoms. Try to explain them as clearly as possible. Think about any pattern you observe about your symptoms. Do they occur at a certain time of day, after a meal, when you exercise, or when you are under stress?

Bring along a memo pad and pen. When you are talking to your doctor, listen carefully to what he or she tells you about your diagnosis or recommendations. Take notes. If you hear any terms you don't understand, or if a diagnosis or instructions are not clear, ask the doctor to clarify the information before going on. If you wish, take along a family member or friend who can step in to hear your doctor's recommendations. Also, ask if the office has handouts on various heart diseases and surgical procedures or if the doctor has a Web page or recommends a Web site.

After you get home, think back over the appointment. If you still have questions or can't remember the next step, call the office and get the answers you need. Read as much as you can about your condition, making sure that the source is reliable. Look for medical information from national health-care organizations such as the American Heart Association or the American Diabetes Association, medical specialty societies, and the government.

Try to follow instructions about medications and lifestyle as closely as possible, to give treatment the best chance of working as intended. If you are having trouble with a specific aspect of your treatment, call the doctor's office and ask how to solve the problem.

Keeping Medical Records

You may find the following charts helpful for collecting information and keeping it up to date. Tell a family member or friend where you keep these records in case they ever need to refer to them. This is especially helpful if you travel or move to another city.

Personal Health History

Fill out the following form:

Name _____

Sex _____   Birth date _____   Age _____

Place of birth _____   Ethnicity _____

Medical History

Current Conditions	Year Diagnosed
_____	_____
_____	_____
_____	_____
_____	_____
_____	_____

Previous Operations	Year	Hospital
_____	_____	_____
_____	_____	_____
_____	_____	_____
_____	_____	_____

Previous Injuries/Medical Conditions	Year
_____	_____
_____	_____
_____	_____

Mental Illnesses	Year Diagnosed
_____	_____
_____	_____

Current Prescription Medications

Medication	Dose	Length of Time You Have Taken the Medication
_____	_____	_____
_____	_____	_____
_____	_____	_____
_____	_____	_____
_____	_____	_____
_____	_____	_____

Current Nonprescription Medications

Medication	Dose	Length of Time You Have Taken the Medication
_____	_____	_____
_____	_____	_____
_____	_____	_____
_____	_____	_____

Drug Allergies

Medication	Reaction
_____	_____
_____	_____

Social History

Marital status: Married, divorced, or single   No. of children _____

Sexual history:

   No. of sex partners in your lifetime _____

   Sex of sex partners: Male, female, or both

   Practice safe sex? Yes or No

Lifestyle

Tobacco
Have you ever used tobacco products? Yes or No
No. of cigarettes smoked per day _____
No. of cigars smoked per day _____
No. of years you smoked _____
Amount of chewing tobacco or snuff used per day _____
No. of years you used chewing tobacco or snuff _____
Have you ever quit? Yes or No

Alcohol
No. of drinks per week _____
Have you ever quit? Yes or No
Have you abused alcohol? Yes or No

Illicit drugs
Have you ever used illicit drugs? Yes or No
Which drug(s) have you used? _____
When was your last use? _____

Exercise
Do you exercise regularly? Yes or No
If yes, what type of exercise? _____
How often do you exercise per week? _____
Length of exercise sessions _____

Vaccinations

Vaccination	Year of Last Vaccination	Vaccination	Year of Last Vaccination
Tetanus/diphtheria	_____	Varicella (chickenpox)	_____
Pneumococcal vaccine	_____	Hepatitis A	_____
Flu vaccine	_____	Hepatitis B	_____
Measles, mumps, rubella	_____	Meningitis	_____
Polio	_____		

Family Health History

Relative	Living (yes/no)	Age at Death	Medical Conditions and/or Cause of Death
Father	_____	_____	_____
Mother	_____	_____	_____
Partner	_____	_____	_____
Brothers	_____	_____	_____
	_____	_____	_____
Sisters	_____	_____	_____
	_____	_____	_____
Grandparents			
Paternal grandfather	_____	_____	_____
Paternal grandmother	_____	_____	_____
Maternal grandfather	_____	_____	_____
Maternal grandmother	_____	_____	_____
Uncles and aunts	_____	_____	_____
	_____	_____	_____

Doctors

Current Doctor(s)—Medical Specialty	Address	Phone No.
Primary doctor		
_____	_____	_____
_____	_____	_____
_____	_____	_____

Past Doctor(s)—Medical Specialty	Address	Phone No.
Primary doctor		
_____	_____	_____
_____	_____	_____
_____	_____	_____

Health Insurance

Health insurance company _____

Your identification no. _____

Phone no. of insurance company _____

Glossary

This glossary defines some terms related to the cardiovascular system, preventive health care, and medical care for heart disorders. For specific diagnostic tests, drugs, and most disorders, please refer to the index. Words in *italics* appear elsewhere in this glossary.

ablation   Removal or destruction of tissue using a surgical scalpel, laser, electrical current, or other method. See also *cardiac ablation*.

aneurysm   An outward bulge in the wall of an artery or the heart, caused by the pressure of blood pushing against a weakened spot. Aneurysms can occur in any artery; they may be abdominal, thoracic, ventricular, or cerebral.

angina pectoris   Chest discomfort or pain as a result of inadequate blood flow to the heart; usually described as a pressure, burning, or squeezing sensation, often associated with physical or emotional stress and relieved by rest. The discomfort may radiate to the arm or neck.

angioplasty   A procedure to open a clogged coronary artery by inserting a balloon-tipped catheter that, when inflated, compresses the blockage against the arterial walls.

antiarrhythmic   A drug that prevents or corrects an abnormal heart rhythm by blocking, firing, or slowing the transmission of abnormal electrical impulses in heart tissue.

anticoagulant   A drug that prevents the formation or enlargement of blood clots by inhibiting one step in the clotting process; these drugs are often called blood thinners, although they do not truly thin the blood. Examples include heparin and warfarin.

antioxidants   Substances that slow or prevent oxidation. Although oxidation is necessary for the human body to function, it may also help cause diseases such as atherosclerosis. Vitamins such as E, C, and beta carotene (a form of vitamin A) are antioxidants and may help protect against cell damage in the arteries caused by oxidation.

antiplatelet agent A drug that prevents formation or enlargement of blood clots by interrupting the process by which platelets (elements within the blood that are involved in clotting) adhere to arterial walls and begin to stick together. Aspirin is an antiplatelet medication.

aorta The major artery that arises from the left ventricle, goes into the chest, and descends into the abdomen, carrying oxygen-rich blood to the body. In the pelvis the aorta divides into arteries that extend into the legs.

aphasia Impairment of a language center in the brain, often the effect of a stroke, that harms the person's ability to understand (receptive aphasia) or respond (expressive aphasia) to the spoken or written word.

apoB Shorthand term for apolipoprotein B, a component of LDL cholesterol that signals the presence of particularly small, dense, dangerous cholesterol particles in the blood.

arteriovenous malformation A mass of abnormal blood vessels, which contains connecting arteries and veins, in the brain, spinal cord, or other organ. This can grow and cause stress on nearby organs and keep them from working properly.

atherosclerosis A disease process that roughens and inflames the interior walls of arteries, causing the accumulation of *plaque* that narrows the channel of the blood vessel. This is commonly known as hardening of the arteries.

atrioventricular node An area of electrical cells in the heart, located between the atria and ventricles, through which electrical impulses travel from the atrium into the ventricles.

atrium Either of the two upper chambers of the heart, in which blood is received and held before passing into the ventricles. The right atrium receives deoxygenated blood from the body; the left atrium receives oxygenated blood from the lungs.

biventricular pacing Electrical pacing in both ventricles. See *cardiac resynchronization therapy*.

blood glucose A type of sugar in the blood, absorbed from foods or produced by the body's metabolizing of starches or other sugars, which circulates in the blood and is the major source of energy for body cells. The blood glucose level is abnormally elevated in people with diabetes.

body mass index A formula for assessing a person's weight relative to height; an indicator used to define overweight, obesity, and morbid obesity.

bradycardia A slow heart rate, usually defined as less than 60 beats per minute.

bypass surgery, coronary artery A surgical procedure to restore adequate blood supply to the heart by using a length of healthy blood vessel to create a detour around a blocked coronary. Also called coronary artery bypass grafting, or *CABG*.

CABG Coronary artery bypass grafting; pronounced "cabbage." Also called CAB (coronary artery bypass).

calcium   A mineral and essential element in the blood, which, if abnormally low or high, may cause problems. Calcium is a major constituent of bone but may accumulate in the plaque that forms in blood vessels, leading to *atherosclerosis*.

cardiac ablation   Removal or destruction of heart tissue for the purpose of treating an arrhythmia. See also *ablation*.

cardiac arrest   Abrupt stoppage of the heart, usually as a result of rhythm problems.

cardiac output   The amount of blood the heart pumps in a minute, calculated by multiplying the *stroke volume* by the number of times the heart beats each minute.

cardiac resynchronization therapy (CRT)   A treatment for congestive heart failure using a pacemaker that stimulates both ventricles simultaneously; also called biventricular pacing.

cardiomyopathy   Disease of the heart muscle tissue, which may be a cause of *congestive heart failure*.

cardiovascular   Pertaining to the heart and blood vessels.

cardioversion   Restoration of the heart's normal rhythm; may be chemical (with drugs) or electrical (with shock).

carotid artery   Either of two major arteries passing through the neck that provide blood to the brain; blockages in these arteries may cause strokes. The flow of blood within this artery is the pulse that you can feel on either side of your neck.

carotid artery disease   *Atherosclerosis* (plaque buildup) in the carotid arteries.

carotid endarterectomy   A surgical procedure to remove plaque from the carotid arteries.

catecholamines   Hormones, including epinephrine and norepinephrine, that the body releases in response to stress; beta-blocker drugs modify the body's response to these hormones.

catheter ablation   A procedure to treat rapid heartbeat by destroying heart tissue where abnormal electrical impulses originate, usually using radiofrequency pulses.

cholesterol, blood   A natural, waxy substance (lipid) that circulates in the bloodstream. Cholesterol is an essential component of cells and an important building block for many hormones. Excess cholesterol places a person at risk of coronary artery disease.

cholesterol, dietary   A fatlike substance (lipid) that is found in many foods such as meats, eggs, and dairy products.

claudication   Pain, discomfort, numbness, or fatigue in the limbs, caused by partly or totally blocked arteries that limit blood flow and as a result impair oxygen delivery to muscles. The symptoms result when there is an imbalance of oxygen supply and oxygen demand.

congenital   Present since birth.

congestive heart failure Decreased or inefficient pumping ability of the heart, causing a backup of fluid into lungs and other body tissues.

coronary artery disease A condition such as *atherosclerosis*, blood clots, or coronary artery spasm that blocks blood flow through the arteries supplying the heart itself.

C-reactive protein (CRP) A chemical by-product of inflammation in the body; found in the bloodstream. An elevated CRP level may be a predictor of heart disease.

CT scanning Computed tomography imaging, used to detect abnormalities in the heart and blood vessels (and other parts of the body).

DASH Dietary Approaches to Stop Hypertension; a low-fat, low-cholesterol diet plan, with a low-sodium component, that lowers blood pressure by promoting the excretion of salt in the urine. The diet is rich in fruit and vegetables.

defibrillation Delivery of an electrical shock to restore normal heart rhythm to heart muscle that is in *fibrillation*, an extremely rapid, quivering form of abnormal heartbeat.

diabetes A disease in which high levels of glucose (a simple sugar) build up in the blood because the hormone *insulin* is in short supply or is not working efficiently. The primary type of diabetes discussed in this book is diabetes mellitus, type 2, which is usually not insulin-dependent.

diastole The phase of the heartbeat during which the heart muscle relaxes, the ventricles expand, and blood flows into them from the atria. It is represented by the lower, or second, number in your blood pressure reading. See *systole*.

echocardiography Ultrasound technology used to image the heart.

edema Accumulation of fluid in body tissues, causing swelling or bloating.

ejection fraction The percentage of the total volume of blood the ventricles hold that is pumped out in one contraction; about 50 to 70 percent in a healthy person.

electrophysiology, cardiac Study of the mechanisms, function, and performance of electrical activities in specific regions of the heart. This helps pinpoint the source of an arrhythmia, to help guide treatment.

embolus A blood clot (or air bubble) that travels from its origin through the bloodstream to a site distant from its origin. An embolus may obstruct a blood vessel.

endocarditis, infective Infection of the lining of the heart chambers (*endocardium*) or the heart valves.

endocardium The membrane lining the cavities of the heart, composed of smooth muscle cells and elastic fibers.

enhanced external counterpulsation A treatment for angina in which pressure cuffs compress blood vessels to increase the return of blood to the heart during the heart's resting (diastolic) phase.

fibrillation An abnormal heart rhythm in which heart muscle contractions are extremely rapid and uncoordinated; the muscle is essentially quivering.

folic acid   A B-complex vitamin that helps reduce the level of *homocysteine*, a body chemical that if elevated may increase the risk of heart disease.

hardening of the arteries   See *atherosclerosis*.

HDL   High-density lipoprotein; the "good" cholesterol carrier that brings cholesterol from cells to the liver to be metabolized.

heart attack   Stoppage of the flow of oxygen-rich blood through one of the coronary arteries that nourish the heart muscle, causing tissue damage or tissue death. Also called a *myocardial infarction*.

heart block   Partial or complete blockage of electrical impulses as they pass through the *atrioventricular node*, between the atria and the ventricles. This may cause symptoms and require a pacemaker.

heart disease   In this book, a general term referring to any disease of the heart and blood vessels.

heart failure, congestive   See *congestive heart failure*.

heart-lung machine   A machine that temporarily assumes the functions of the heart and lungs during heart surgery, oxygenating the blood and pumping it back into the body, so that surgeons can operate on a heart that is not beating.

heart murmur   A characteristic sound that your doctor hears through a stethoscope when blood flows abnormally through the heart.

heart rate   The number of times the heart beats (contracts) per minute.

high blood pressure   A condition in which the force of moving blood against arterial walls is greater than normal; also called hypertension.

high-density lipoprotein   See *HDL*.

Holter monitor   A portable, battery-powered device to record the heart's electrical activity, usually over a period of days.

homocysteine   An amino acid in the blood that, at high levels, may be a risk factor for some cardiovascular diseases, including stroke and peripheral artery disease.

hypertension   See *high blood pressure*.

ICD   Internal cardioverter-defibrillator; a device placed in a person with serious ventricular arrhythmias that functions as a pacemaker and can also deliver an electrical shock to the heart in the event of ventricular *tachycardia* or ventricular *fibrillation*.

implantable cardioverter-defibrillator   See *ICD*.

inotropic agent   A drug that increases the contraction strength of the heart muscle; digitalis is an inotropic medication.

insulin   A hormone produced in the pancreas that is essential to convert sugars in the blood and in food into energy for body cells.

insulin resistance   A condition that includes hypertension, hyperlipidemia, and the type of obesity that results in an apple-shaped torso; in insulin resistance, the body does not efficiently use the *insulin* it makes.

insulin resistance syndrome   A cluster of risk factors that increase the likelihood that a person will develop type 2 diabetes, elevated cholesterol levels, and cardiovascular disease; the underlying causes are overweight, inactivity, and heredity. Also called metabolic syndrome.

ischemia   Insufficient blood and oxygen supply to an organ or tissue; myocardial ischemia refers to lack of blood to the heart muscle.

isolated systolic hypertension   A form of high blood pressure in which only the systolic or pumping pressure is elevated.

LDL   Low-density lipoprotein; the harmful cholesterol carrier that delivers cholesterol to body cells in the blood.

lipid panel   A fasting blood test that measures the cholesterol—including HDL, LDL, and total score—and triglycerides in your bloodstream.

low-density lipoprotein   See *LDL*.

magnesium   A mineral and an element in blood that, if abnormal in amount, may cause arrhythmias (irregular heart rhythms).

maze procedure   A surgical method to create a maze of permanent new electrical pathways through heart muscle to treat chronic atrial *fibrillation*.

metabolic syndrome   See *insulin resistance syndrome*.

MIDCAB   Minimally invasive coronary artery bypass; a procedure that allows surgeons to perform coronary artery bypass while the heart is still beating through small incisions in the chest wall, without use of a heart-lung machine. See also *portCAB*.

MRI   Magnetic resonance imaging, which is used to detect abnormalities in the heart and blood vessels.

myocardial infarction   The medical term for *heart attack*; an event leading to some tissue death (infarction) in the heart muscle (*myocardium*) because of blockage of a coronary artery.

myocardium   The working muscle tissue of the heart.

nuclear medicine   The use of radioactive technology to image the heart or study heart function.

omega-3 fatty acids   A beneficial form of fat, found in foods such as fish, flaxseed, and soybeans, that slows the growth of plaque in the arteries, among other protective cardiovascular effects.

pacemaker   A battery-powered device that is implanted under the skin to regulate or initiate heart rhythm.

palpitation   The abnormal awareness of one's heartbeat. This may be due to an arrhythmia (irregular heartbeat).

pericarditis   Infection or inflammation of the membrane surrounding the heart (*pericardium*); can cause pain that is easily mistaken for a heart attack.

pericardium   The two-layered membrane surrounding the heart; the outer layer anchors the heart in the chest cavity and the inner layer encases the heart muscle itself.

peripheral artery disease (PAD)   Blockages in the arteries that are distant from your heart, caused by plaque buildup in those arteries.

plant sterols, stanols   Plant-based forms of cholesterol that can be substituted for animal-based forms in products such as margarines, to help lower LDL cholesterol.

plaque An accumulation of fatty substances, cholesterol, and debris that can build up on the walls of arteries, narrowing the channel through which blood flows.

plaque, vulnerable (or soft) A type of *plaque* buried within the arterial walls, enclosed in a thin shell; the shell can rupture and can lead to blockage of the arterial channel.

portCAB Port-access coronary artery bypass (also called PACAB); a surgical procedure to perform coronary artery bypass through small incisions (ports) in the chest wall. See also *MIDCAB*.

potassium A mineral and an essential element that helps balance fluid content in body cells. An imbalance in the body's potassium supply may cause arrhythmias (irregular heart rhythms).

prediabetes A condition in which blood glucose levels are higher than normal, but not high enough to be considered diabetes (fasting levels between 100 and 125 mg/Dl). Also called impaired glucose tolerance, or impaired fasting glucose. This may occur with *insulin resistance syndrome*.

prehypertension A condition in which blood pressure is higher than normal (above 120/80 mm Hg but below 140/90 mm Hg), putting a person at higher risk of developing *high blood pressure*.

proarrhythmia Increased occurrence of existing arrhythmias, a serious reaction to antiarrhythmic medications in some people.

prolapse The sagging of an organ or structure (such as the leaflets of the mitral valve).

PTCA Percutaneous transluminal coronary *angioplasty*.

pulmonary Pertaining to the lungs.

regurgitation In heart valve disorders, back flow or back leakage, when blood enters a heart chamber and then leaks backward through a faulty valve.

respiration The exchange of oxygen and carbon dioxide at a cellular level between the red blood cells and air in the lungs; see also *ventilation*.

restenosis After an angioplasty to open a blocked artery or heart valve, the renarrowing or constriction of the same area where the procedure was done.

rheumatic fever An inflammatory systemic disease, often afflicting the heart valves, that develops as a result of untreated strep throat; now rare in the United States, Canada, and Europe because of the widespread use of antibiotics to treat strep.

secondary hypertension High blood pressure as a result of another problem, such as a kidney abnormality, a structural defect in the aorta, or some types of hormonal abnormality.

sinoatrial (SA) node An area of specialized tissue in the right atrium that generates electrical impulses to stimulate and pace heart contractions; the heart's natural pacemaker.

sphygmomanometer The standard instrument used to measure blood pressure, comprised of a cuff, pressure gauge, and bulb for inflation and deflation.

statin Any one of a group of drugs prescribed for high cholesterol that works by blocking the activity of an enzyme (HMG CoA reductase) involved in the body's cholesterol production.

STEMI   ST elevation myocardial infarction; a severe heart attack demonstrated by a rise in one portion (labeled ST) of a wave on an electrocardiogram.

stenosis   The narrowing or obstruction of an opening or channel; in heart disorders, it may refer to the narrowing of an artery or the obstruction of the opening in a heart valve.

stent   A piece of tubing that acts as a scaffold to prop open the walls of an artery and keep plaque compressed behind it. A drug-eluding stent is coated with slow-release medications to prevent the growth of scar tissue. The stent becomes part of the artery wall. See *angioplasty*.

sternum   The breastbone.

stroke   Injury to the brain as a result of lack of blood supply or bleeding in or onto brain tissue; a "brain attack."

stroke volume   The amount of blood the left ventricle pumps out in a single contraction.

sudden cardiac death   Abrupt death from heart disease, as a result of blocked arteries or an arrhythmia (irregular heartbeat).

supraventricular   Above the level of the ventricles, in the upper chambers of the heart; as in supraventricular tachycardia (which is a rapid heartbeat that originates from abnormal electrical impulses in the atria).

syncope   The medical term for fainting.

systole   The phase of the heartbeat during which the heart muscle contracts and the ventricles squeeze blood out of the heart. This is the upper, or first, number of the blood pressure reading. See *diastole*.

tachycardia   A rapid heart rate, more than 100 beats per minute.

thrombolytic agent   A drug that dissolves blood clots, administered intravenously in a hospital; a "clot-buster." See *tPA*.

thrombus   A stationary blood clot on the wall of an artery or within the heart.

TIA   Transient ischemic attack; a temporary blockage of blood to a part of the brain. Often called a ministroke or warning stroke.

tPA   Tissue plasminogen activator; a clot-busting thrombolytic medication used to restore blood flow to the brain in the event of a stroke. It must be given within 3 hours of the onset of symptoms.

trans fat   A type of fat formed in the manufacture of some processed foods that raises harmful LDL, lowers protective HDL, and increases the risk of blood clotting.

transient ischemic attack   See *TIA*.

transmyocardial revascularization   A surgical laser technique to improve blood flow to the heart in a person with *atherosclerosis*, by creating new channels in heart muscle.

triglyceride   A form of fat occurring in the body and in food; excess calories are converted to triglycerides and are stored in the body's fat cells.

Valsalva maneuver   A technique involving bearing down briefly. This may help control minor heart palpitations.

valve, heart   Any one of four structures, constructed of multiple flaps that control the one-way flow of blood through the heart chambers by closing at specific times during the process of the heart's pumping blood to the body. The four heart valves are the tricuspid, pulmonary, mitral, and aortic valves.

valvuloplasty   A procedure to open a stiffened or fused valve using a balloon-tipped catheter.

vasodilator   A medication that widens arteries and reduces resistance to blood flow in order to reduce the workload of the heart and lower blood pressure; an ACE inhibitor is a vasodilator.

vegetation   An accumulation of microorganisms and scar tissue on diseased heart valves; see *endocarditis, infective*.

ventilation   The mechanical movement of air into and out of the lungs; breathing. See *respiration*.

ventricle   Either of the two lower chambers of the heart, which contract rhythmically to pump blood out of the heart. The right ventricle pumps blood into the lungs; the left ventricle pumps blood out to the rest of the body.

ventricular assist device (VAD)   A mechanical pump implanted in the heart that supplements the left ventricle, used to treat heart failure.

waist circumference   A measurement of the natural waistline, used to gauge distribution of body fat.

white-coat hypertension   A temporary increase in blood pressure during a medical checkup. See *high blood pressure*.

Women's Health Initiative   A federally funded, major research study by the National Institutes of Health to investigate hormone replacement therapies. It was started in 1993 and involved more than 161,000 women.

Index

Page numbers in italics refer to illustrations.

heart rate, 18, 113
  measuring of, 120
  resting, 13
  target, 13, 78
  when sleeping, 13
heart transplantation, 163, 250–254
  donor hearts, *253*
heart valve problems, 189–209, 256
  common causes of, 190–195
  fen-phen and, 195
  medications for, 203–204
  one-way flow of blood, 15, 189,
    190
  regurgitation and stenosis, 189
  symptoms of, 190–191
  valve repair, 204–206
  valve replacement, 206–209
  the valves, 8, 189, *190*
  See also specific problems
Helicobacter pylori, 132
hemoglobin, 15
hemorrhagic stroke, 215–216, 217,
  218, 220
heparin, 172–173, 182, 219
herbal remedies, 256, 269
herbs, 92
heredity
  diabetes and, 66, 106
  family medical history, 119, 121,
    218, 285
  heart disease and, 20, 21, 153
  high blood pressure and, 41, 67
heterograft, 206
high blood cholesterol. *See* cholesterol, blood
high blood pressure (hypertension),
  2, 20, 37–68, 97, 99, 185,
  198–199, 218
  aneurysms and, 217
  antihypertensives. *See* antihyper-
    tensives
  arrhythmias and, 256, 263
  categories of blood pressure,
    43–45
  diabetes, type 2, and, 110

diagnostic tests, 40–41
essential or primary, 41, 67
exercise and, 44, 52–53
eye damage and, 2, 40, 43
groups at higher risk, 63–68
guidelines, 2, 43, 44
home monitoring of, 55–59, 58
lifestyle changes and, 44, 46–55
living with, 67
medications. *See* antihypertensives
medications affecting, 42, 63
pregnant women and, 64–65, 290,
  291
prehypertension, 2, 43–44
preventing, 46–55
pulmonary, 201, 202, 254, 290
as risk factor for other illnesses,
  37–68, 111
risk factors, 41–42, 153
secondary, 41, 66
smoking and, 70
statistics, 2, 37
as symptomless, 42, 43
treatment strategies, 45–46
"white-coat," 39, 55
women and, 41, 64–65, 286
Hispanic women, high blood pressure in, 64
HMG CoA reductase inhibitors. *See*
  statins (or HMB CoA reductase
  inhibitors)
Holter monitoring, 124, 266, 267,
  291
homocysteine levels, testing, 131
hormone therapy, 65, 288–290
hot flashes, 289, 290
hydralazine, 62
  with isosorbide dinitrate, 246
hydrochlorothiazide, 60, 242
  with spironolactone, 242
hyperglycemia, 66
hypertension. *See* high blood pressure (hypertension)
hypertrophic cardiomyopathy, 134,
  249

ibuprofen, 164
iliac arteries, 14
immune system, 16
immunosuppressive drugs, 252, 253, 254
implantable cardioverter-defibrillators (ICD), 249, 261, 270, 275–279
  safety issues, 276–277
implantable loop recorder, 125
incontinence, 242–243
indapamide, 60
indigestion, 156, 157, 282, 285, 287
infarction, 153
  cerebral. *See* stroke
  myocardial. *See* heart attack
infective endocarditis, 190, 191, 194, 197, 198, 199, 200, 201, 202, 203, 207, 209
  overview of, *192*, 192–193
inferior vena cava, *6*, 7, 15
inflammation in the arteries, 132, 153–155, 174
innocent heart murmurs, 191
insulin, 105
insulin resistance. *See* type 2 diabetes
insulin resistance syndrome, 63, 107
intermittent claudication, 111
intravenous pyelography, 40–41
iodine-based dye, allergy to, 139, 140, 144, 146
iron, 87, 89, 96
ischemia, 151, 153, 162
  silent, 161
ischemic cardiomyopathy, 162–163
ischemic stroke, 174, 215, 216, *218*
isolated systolic hypertension, 45
isotope stress test (thallium stress test), 136–138
isradipine, 169

JAMA (Journal of the American Medical Association), 76
jaw pain, 156, 157–158

jugular veins, 217
juvenile diabetes. *See* diabetes, type 1

kidney damage, high blood pressure and, 42–43
kidneys, 245
  congestive heart failure (CHF) and, 237
  the heart's interaction with, 18
  high blood pressure and, 2, 40

labels, reading nutrition, 92, 93–95, *94*
laser angiography, 177
LDL (low-density lipoprotein, or "bad" cholesterol), 24, *24*, 26, 99, 130, 200, 218
  exercise and, 75
  guidelines, 27–29, 212
  lowering, measures for, 29–36, 54
left ventricular assist device (LVAD), 247–248, 252
leg pain, 213
legumes, 89
leukocytes. *See* white blood cells (leukocytes)
lifestyle changes, 165, 180, 219, 220
  See also specific changes, e.g., diet; exercise; stress
light-headedness as heart attack symptom, 156, 160–161, 162, 168
lipid profile, 25–26, 34, 129–130, 284
  interpreting the results of, 26–29
lipids, 23
lipoproteins, 24, *24*
  high-density. *See* HDL (high-density lipoprotein, or "good" cholesterol)
  low-density. *See* LDL (low-density lipoprotein, or "bad" cholesterol)
  very low-density (VLDL), *24*, 110
liquids. *See* beverages
lisinopril, 61, 170
liver, 23, *24*

losartan, 61
lovastatin, 34
lungs, 5, 16–17, *17*
    heart-lung machine, 182, *183*, 204, 208, 251, 252, 272
    heart-lung transplantation, 254
lymphocytes, 16

magnesium, 96, 242
magnetic resonance angiography, 141
magnetic resonance imaging (MRI), 41, 141, 178, 219, 221, 222, 223, 235, 249, *277*
    nicotine patches and, 72–73
mammary arteries, 182
margarines, 32, 90
maze surgery, 279–280
meats, 87–88
mechanical heart valve, 206, *207*, 208–209
medical history, 118–119, 121, 148
medical records, keeping, 297–300
medications
    for angina, 165–170
    antibiotics. *See* antibiotics
    anticoagulants. *See* anticoagulants
    antidepressants, 115
    antihypertensives. *See* antihypertensives
    anti-inflammatory, 164, 173
    antiplatelet agents. *See* antiplatelet drugs
    for arrhythmias. *See* antiarrhythmics
    arrhythmias caused by, 256, 258
    birth control pills, 22, 65
    blood clots, to treat. *See* blood clots
    cholesterol-lowering. *See* cholesterol-lowering medications
    for congestive heart failure (CHF), 241–246
    for high blood pressure. *See* antihypertensives
    hormone therapy, 65, 288–290
    immunosuppressive, 252, 253, 254
    medical history, 119
    nicotine replacement, 54, 73, 74
    over-the-counter. *See* over-the-counter drugs
    tips for taking, 244–245
    for valve disease, 203–204
    See also specific drugs and conditions
menopause. *See* postmenopausal women
mercury blood pressure monitors, 58
metabolic syndrome, 63, 107
methyldopa, 62
metolazone, 61, 242
metoprolol, 61, 168, 246
Mexican Americans, 20
MIDCAB, 188
migraine headaches, 167, 169
milk products. *See* dairy products
minerals. *See individual minerals by name*, e.g., potassium
mineral supplements, 95
minimally invasive coronary artery bypass (MIDCAB), 188
minimally invasive valve surgery, 208
ministroke. *See* transient ischemic attack (TIA)
minoxidil, 62
mitral valve, 8, 190, *190*, 196–98, 263
    prolapse, 196
    regurgitation, 197, 206
    stenosis, 197–198
Mobitz II-type heart block, 258–259
Mobitz-type heart block, 258
monounsaturated fats, 30, 31, 90
MRI. *See* magnetic resonance imaging (MRI)
multidetector CT scans, 140
multiunit gated blood pool scan (MUGA), 138–139
murmurs. *See* heart murmurs
myocardial infarction. *See* heart attack
myocardial ischemia, 151, 153, 162
    silent, 161

myocardium, 7
myoglobin, 131

nadolol, 168
National Heart, Lung, and Blood Institute, 47
National Institutes of Health, 47, 100, 179, 288
nervous system, 18
neuropathy, 111
neurotransmitters, 18
New York City Department of Health, 30
niacin, 87
nicardipine, 169
nicotine. *See* smoking
nicotine gum, 73
nicotine inhalers, 73
nicotine lozenges, 74
nicotine nasal sprays, 73
nicotine patches, 72–73
nicotine replacement products, 54, 72–73
nicotinic acid (niacin), 35
nifedipine, 169
911, calling, 155, 157, 174
nisoldipine, 169
nitroglycerin, 156, 166–167, 178
nonsteroidal anti-inflammatory drugs (NSAIDs), 173
norepinephrine, 11, *62*, 113, 167
NT-proBNP, 235
nuclear imaging, 121, 135–139, 235
  nuclear stress test, 41
nuclear magnetic resonance lipid test, 130
nutrition. *See* diet

obesity. *See* overweight and obesity
occupational therapy, 230, 232
oils. *See* fats and oils, dietary
omega-3 polyunsaturated fats, 27, 31, 88, 89
open-heart surgery, 204
ophthalmoscope, 40

oral contraceptives. *See* birth control pills
oral glucose tolerance test (OGTT), 107, 108
osteoporosis, 52, 83, 288
over-the-counter drugs, 207, 290
  arrhythmias and, 256, 259
  blood pressure and, 63
  drug interactions, 203, 269
  nicotine replacement, *73*
  sodium in, 93
overweight and obesity, 3, 97, 99–104, 132, 218, 284, 286
  body mass index (BMI), 99, 100–102
  children and, 1, 68, 100
  factors contributing to, 99–100
  fat distribution, 99, 102, 107, 132
  heart disease and, 21, 99
  peripheral artery disease and, 111
  shortness of breath, 160
  See also weight; weight loss
oxygen transport. *See* circulatory system; respiratory system

pacemaker generator, 183
pacemakers, 164, 248, 272–275, *274*
  CRT, 248, 249, 250
  safety issues, 276-277
pain pumps, 184
palpitations, 255, 263, 285
  See also arrhythmias
pancreas, 105
pancreatitis, 29
paroxysmal atrial fibrillation, 263–264
pedometers, 77, 82
percutaneous transluminal coronary angioplasty (PTCA). *See* angioplasty
perfusion (flow) defect, 136
perfusionist, 183
perfusion scan (thallium stress test), 136–138
pericardiocentesis, 164